CLINICAL REVIEW.COM

CLINICAL REVIEW OF SURGERY

D1108898

ABSITE PREPARATION

SECOND EDITION

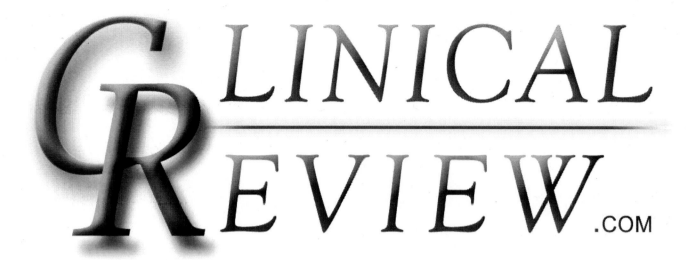

CLINICAL REVIEW OF SURGERY

ABSITE Preparation

SECOND EDITION

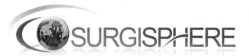

SURGISPHERE CORPORATION

United States of America

2008

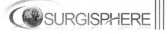

Clinical Review of Surgery
ABSITE Preparation

Inquiries should be addressed to:

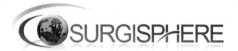

Surgisphere Corporation
3611 Witherspoon Blvd
Suite 111
Durham, North Carolina, USA 27707
www.Surgisphere.com

Second Edition

Cataloging-In-Publication Data

Surgisphere Corporation
Clinical Review of Surgery, ABSITE Preparation
470 p.   cm.
1. Surgery.   2. Medicine
I. Surgisphere Corporation   II. Clinical Review of Surgery
ISBN 9780980210316   C6168
                                  617 SUR   2008901178

Although information herein is based on the author's extensive experience and knowledge, it is not intended to be a substitute for the services of a qualified healthcare professional.

01 / 10 9 8 7 6 5 4 3 2

Second Edition © Surgisphere Corporation 2008. All Rights Reserved.
First published in 2005.

SECTIONS

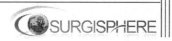

TABLE OF CONTENTS

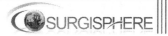

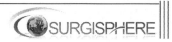

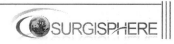

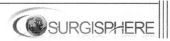

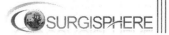

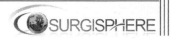

TABLES AND FIGURES

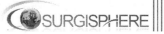

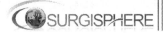

ABBREVIATIONS

5-ASA	5-aminosalicylic acid	ARF	Acute renal failure	CLD	Clear liquid diet
5-FU	5-fluorouracil	AS	Aortic stenosis or Ankylosing spondylitis	CLL	Chronic lymphocytic leukemia
5-HIAA	5-hydroxyindolacetic acid			CML	Chronic myeloid leukemia
5-HIAA	5-hydroxyindolacetic acid	ASA	Aminosalicylic acid, Aspirin	CMV	Cytomegalovirus
5-HT	5-hydroxytryptamine	ASD	Atrial septal defect	CNS	Central nervous system
AAA	Abdominal aortic aneurysm	ASLO	Antistreptolysin-O	CO	Cardiac output
ABC	Airway, breathing, circulation	AST	Aspartate transaminase	COPD	Chronic obstructive pulmonary disease
ABE	Acute bacterial endocarditis	ATC	Anaplastic thyroid cancer		
ABG	Arterial blood gas	ATG	Antithymocyte globulin	CPAP	Continuous positive air pressure
ABO	Blood types	ATIII	Antithrombin III		
ABVD	Adriamycin, bleomycin, vinblastine, decarbazine	ATN	Acute tubular necrosis	CPK	Creatine phosphokinase
		ATP	Adenosine triphosphate	CPM	Central pontine myelinolysis
ACD	Anemia of chronic disease	AVM	Arteriovenous malformation	CPPD	Calcium pyrophosphate deposition disease
ACE	Angiotensin converting factor	AVN	Avascular necrosis		
ACE	Angiotensin-converting enzyme	BAL	Bronchoalveolar lavage or Dimercaprol	CR	Creatinine
				CRAO	Central retinal artery occlusion
AChR	Acetylcholine receptor	BCG	Bacillus Calmette-Guerin	CREST	Calcinosis, Raynaud phenomenon, esophageal dysmotility, sclerodactyly, telangiectasia
ACLS	Advanced cardiac life support	BCx	Blood cultures		
ACTH	Adrenocorticotrophic hormone	BMD	Bone mineral deficiency		
		BMI	Body mass index		
AD	Autosomal dominant or Alzheimer disease	BMR	Basal metabolic rate	CRF	Chronic renal failure or Corticotropin-releasing factor
		BMS	Bone marrow suppression		
ADH	Antidiuretic hormone	BMT	Bone marrow transplant or Behavior modification therapy	CRH	Corticotrophin releasing hormone
AFB	Acid-fast bacilli				
AFP	Alpha fetoprotein	BPH	Benign prostate hypertrophy	CRP	C-reactive protein
AI	Adrenal insufficiency	BPM	Beats per minute	CSA	Cyclosporine A
AIHA	Autoimmune hemolytic anemia	BPPV	Benign paroxysmal positional vertigo	CSF	Cerebrospinal fluid
				CT	Computed tomography
AIN	Allergic interstitial nephritis	BRBPR	Bright red blood per rectum	CTD	Connective tissue disease
ALL	Acute lymphocytic leukemia	BUN	Blood urea nitrogen	CVA	Cerebrovascular accident
ALT	Alanine transaminase	CA	Cancer	CVD	Collagen vascular disease or Cerebrovascular disease
AMA	American Medical Association or Antimitochondrial antibodies	CABG	Coronary artery bypass graft		
		CAD	Coronary artery disease	CXR	Chest x-ray
		CAGE	Cut down, Annoy others, Guilty feelings, Eye-opener in the morning	DBP	Diastolic blood pressure
AMI	Acute myocardial infarction			DCIS	Ductal carcinoma in situ
AML	Acute myelocytic leukemia			DCM	Dilated cardiomyopathy
ANA	Antinuclear antibodies	CAH	Congenital adrenal hyperplasia	DES	Diffuse esophageal spasm
ANCA	Antineutrophil cytoplasmic antibodies			DEXA	Dual-energy x-ray absorptiometry
		C-ANCA	Cytoplasmic ANCA		
ANF	Atrial natriuretic factor	CaDPTA	Calcium trisodium	DI	Diabetes insipidus
Anti-SM	Antibodies to striated muscle	CBC	Complete blood count	DIC	Disseminated intravascular coagulation
Anti-TPO	Antithyroid peroxidase	CCK	Cholecystokinin		
APA	Antiphospholipid antibody	CD	Crohn disease	DIP	Distal interphalangeal joint
APAP	p-aminophenol	CEA	Carcinoembryonic antigen	DKA	Diabetic ketoacidosis
APC	Adenomatosis polyposis coli	CES	Cauda equina syndrome	DLCO	Diffusability of carbon monoxide
APE	Acute pulmonary edema	CHD	Congenital heart disease		
APKD	Adult polycystic kidney disease	CHF	Congestive heart failure	DM	Diabetes mellitus
		CHOP	Cyclophosphamide, hydroxydaunomycin, vincristine, prednisone	DMARD	Disease-modifying antirheumatic drug
APR	Acute phase reactant			DMD	Duchenne muscular dystrophy
AR	Autosomal recessive or Aortic regurgitation			DMSA	Succimer
		CI	Cardiac index	DNA	Deoxyribonucleic acid
ARDS	Adult respiratory distress syndrome	CK	Creatine kinase	DOE	Dyspnea on exertion
		CK-MB	MB fraction of CK		

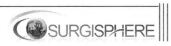

DRE	Digital rectal exam	GCA	Giant cell arteritis	HIPPA	Health information privacy protection act
dsDNA	Double stranded DNA	GCS	Glasgow coma scale		
DSE	Dobutamine stress echocardiogram	GERD	Gastroesophageal reflux disease	HIT	Heparin induced thrombocytopenia
DT	Delirium tremens	GETA	General endotracheal anesthesia	HIV	Human immunodeficiency virus
DTR	Deep tendon reflex				
DUB	Dysfunctional uterine bleeding	GFR	Glomerular filtration rate	HL	Hodgkin lymphoma
DVT	Deep vein thrombosis	GGT	Gamma glutamyl transpeptidase	HLA	Human lymphocyte antigen
EBV	Epstein-Barr virus			HNPCC	Hereditary nonpolyposis colon cancer
ECF	Extracellular fluid	GHB	Gamma-Hydroxybutyrate		
ECG	(EKG); Electrocardiogram	GIP	Gastric inhibitory peptide	HPV	Human papilloma virus
ECM	Extracellular matrix	GM-CSF	Granulocyte-macrophage colony-stimulating factor	HRT	Hormone replacement therapy
ED	Erectile dysfunction				
EDTA	Edetate calcium disodium	GRP	Gastrin releasing peptide	HS	Hereditary spherocytosis
EDV	End diastolic volume	HACEK	*Haemophilus aprophilus, Actinobacillus actinomycetemcomitans, Cardiobacterium hominis, Eikenella corrodens, Kingella kinkae*	HSIL	High-grade squamous intraepithelial lesion
EF	Ejection fraction				
EGD	Esophagogastroduodenoscopy			HSP	Henoch-Schönlein purpura
EHEC	Enterohemorrhagic *E. coli*			HSV	Herpes simplex virus
EIEC	Enteroinvasive *E. coli*			HUS	Hemolytic uremic syndrome
ELISA	Enzyme-linked immunosorbent assay	HAV	Hepatitis A virus	IBD	Inflammatory bowel disease
		HbA	Adult hemoglobin	IBW	Ideal body weight
EMG	Electromyography	HbA1C	Hemoglobin A1C	IC	Inspiratory capacity or Immunocompromised
EOM	Extraocular muscles				
EPO	Erythropoietin	HBcAbIgG	Hepatitis B core antibody immunoglobulin G	ICA	Intracranial aneurysm or Internal carotid artery
ERCP	Endoscopic retrograde cholangiopancreatography				
		HBcAbIgM	Hepatitis B core antibody immunoglobulin M	ICD	Implanted cardioverter and defibrillator
ERV	Expiratory reserve volume				
ESR	Erythrocyte sedimentation rate	HBcAg	Hepatitis B core antigen	ICF	Intracellular fluid
		HbcAgIgM	Hepatitis B core antigen immunoglobulin M	ICP	Intracranial pressure
ESRD	End stage renal disease			IDDM	Insulin-dependent diabetes mellitus
ESV	End systolic volume	HBeAb	Hepatitis B "e" antibody		
ET	Endotracheal tube	HBeAg	Hepatitis B "e" antigen	IgA	Immunoglobulin A
ETEC	Enterotoxic *Escherichia coli*	HBIG	Hepatitis B immunoglobulin	IGF	Insulin-like growth factor
FAP	Familial adenomatous polyposis	HbS	Sickle cell hemoglobin	IgG	Immunoglobulin G
		HBsAb	Hepatitis B surface antibody	IHSS	Idiopathic hypertrophic subaortic stenosis
FEF	Forced expiratory flow	HBsAg	Hepatitis B surface antigen		
FENA	Fractional excretion of sodium	HBV	Hepatitis B virus	IMA	Inferior mesenteric artery
FEV	Forced expiratory volume	HCC	Hepatocellular carcinoma	IML	Intermediolateral column
FFA	Free fatty acid	HCM	Hypertrophic cardiomyopathy	INH	Isoniazid
FFP	Fresh frozen plasma	HCT	Hematocrit	IPF	Idiopathic pulmonary fibrosis
FNAB	Fine needle aspiration biopsy	HCTZ	Hydrochlorothiazide	IRV	Inspiratory reserve volume
FOBT	Fecal occult blood test	HCV	Hepatitis C virus	ITP	Immune thrombocytopenic purpura
FRC	Functional reserve capacity	HCVAb	Hepatitis C virus antibody		
FSH	Follicle stimulating hormone	HD	Hemodialysis	IVC	Inferior vena cava
FTA-ABS	Fluorescent treponemal antibody absorption test	HDV	Hepatitis D virus	IVDA	IV drug abuser
		HEV	Hepatitis E virus	IVF	Intravenous fluids
FTC	Follicular thyroid cancer	HGPRT	Hypoxanthine-guanine phosphoribosyl transferase	IVIG	Intravenous immune globulin
FUO	Fever of unknown origin			IVP	Intravenous pyelogram
FVC	Forced vital capacity	HGV	Hepatitis G virus	JVD	Jugular vein distension
GABA	Gamma amino butyric acid	HHNC	Hyperosmolar hyperglycemic nonketotic coma	JVP	Jugular venous pulse
GAS	Group A streptococcus			LA	Left atrium
GBM	Glomerular basement membrane or Glioblastoma multiforme	HHV	Human herpes virus 8	LAD	Left anterior descending branch of LCA
		HIDA	Hepatobiliary iminodiacetic acid		
				LCA	Left coronary artery
GBS	Guillain-Barré syndrome			LCIS	Lobular cancer in situ

LCX	Left circumflex branch of LCA	MPGN	Membranoproliferative glomerulonephritis	PE	Pulmonary embolism or Plasma exchange
LDH	Lactate dehydrogenase	MPTP	1-methyl-4-phenyl-1, 2, 3, 6-tetrahydropyridine	PEEP	Positive end expiratory pressure
LEEP	Loop electrosurgical excision procedure	MR	Mitral regurgitation	PEG	Polyethylene glycol
LES	Lower esophageal sphincter	MRA	Magnetic resonance angiography	PET	Positron emission tomography
LFT	Liver function test	MRI	Magnetic resonance imaging	PFO	Patent foramen ovale
LGA	Large for gestational age	MS	Multiple sclerosis or Mitral stenosis	PFT	Pulmonary function test
LH	Lutenizing hormone			PGE	Prostaglandin E
LHF	Left-sided CHF	MTC	Medullary thyroid cancer	PHA	Paroxysmal hemolytic anemia
LLSB	Lower left sternal border	MUGA	Multigated acquisition scan	PHP	Pseudohypoparathyroidism
LMWH	Lower molecular weight heparin	NAC	N-acetyl cystine	PICA	Posterior inferior cerebellar artery
LOC	Loss of consciousness	NBTE	Nonbacterial thrombotic endocarditis	PIF	Prolactin inhibiting factor
LP	Lumbar puncture	NC	Nasal cannula	PIGA	Phosphatidylinositol glycan class A gene
LPL	Lipoprotein lipase	NFT	Neurofibrillary tangle		
LSD	Lysergic acid diethylamide	NG	Nasogastric tube	PIP	Proximal interphalangeal joint
LSE	Libman-Sacks endocarditis	NH	Nursing home	PLD	Partial lipid dystrophy
LSES	Low socioeconomic status	NHL	Non-Hodgkin lymphoma	PMI	Point of maximal impulse
LSIL	Low-grade squamous intraepithelial lesion	NIDMM	Non-insulin dependent diabetes mellitus	PML	Progressive multifocal leukoencephalopathy
LUSB	Left upper sternal border	NIH	National Institute of Health	PMN	Polymorphonuclear lymphocyte
LV	Left ventricle	NK	Natural killer cells		
LVF	Left ventricular function	NMDA	N-methyl-D-aspartate	PND	Paroxysmal nocturnal dyspnea
LVH	Left ventricle hypertrophy	NMJ	Neuromuscular junction	PNH	Paroxysmal nocturnal hemoglobinuria
LWN	Lown-Ganong-Levine syndrome	NMS	Nuclear medicine scan		
Mab	Monoclonal antibody	NPH	Normal pressure hydrocephalus	PO	Per os
MAC	*Mycobacterium avium* complex	NPO	Nil per os	PO2	Oxygen pressure
		NS	Normal saline	PP	Pulse pressure
MALT	Mucosa-associated lymphoid tissue	NSAID	Nonsteroidal anti-inflammatory drug	PPD	Purified protein derivative
MAO	Monoamine oxidase			PR	Pulmonary regurgitation
MAP	Mean arterial pressure	NSCLC	Non-small cell lung cancer	PRN	As needed
MCA	Middle cerebral artery	NSR	Normal sinus rhythm	PS	Pulmonary stenosis
MCD	Minimal change disease	OA	Osteoarthritis	PSA	Prostate specific antigen
MCHC	Mean corpuscular hemoglobin concentration	OME	Otitis media with effusion	PSC	Primary sclerosing cholangitis
		OR	Operating room	PSGN	Poststreptococcal glomerulonephritis
MCP	Metacarpophalangeal joint	OSA	Obstructive sleep apnea		
MCV	Mean corpuscular volume	OT	Occupational therapy	PT	Prothrombin time or Physical therapy
MDI	Metered dose inhaler	PAC	Premature atrial contraction or Pulmonary artery catheter		
MDMA	3,4-methylene dioxymethamphetamine			PTC	Percutaneous transhepatic procedure or papillary thyroid cancer
MDS	Myelodysplastic syndrome	PAN	Polyarteritis nodosa		
MEN	Multiple endocrine dysplasia	P-ANCA	Perinuclear ANCA	PTCA	Percutaneous transluminal coronary angioplasty
MG	Myasthenia gravis	PAS	Periodic acid shift		
MGUS	Monoclonal gammopathy of uncertain significance	PAT	Paroxysmal atrial tachycardia	PTH	Parathyroid hormone
		PBC	Primary biliary cirrhosis	PTHrP	Parathyroid hormone related peptide
MI	Myocardial infarction	PCA	Posterior cerebral artery		
MM	Multiple myeloma	PCO2	Carbon dioxide pressure	PTT	Partial thromboplastin time
MMR	Measles, mumps, rubella vaccination	PCP	*Pneumocystis carinii* pneumonia or phencyclidine	PTU	Propylthiouracil
				PUD	Peptic ulcer disease
MMSE	Mini mental status exam	PCR	Polymerase chain reaction	PV	Polycythemia vera
MOPP	Mechlorethamine, vincristine, procarbazine, prednisone	PCWP	Pulmonary capillary wedge pressure	PVC	Premature ventricular contraction
		PD	Parkinson disease	PZ	Peripheral zone
				RA	Rheumatoid arthritis

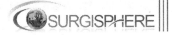

RAA	Renin-angiotensin-aldosterone	SERMS	Selective estrogen-receptor modulators	TMP-SMX	Trimethoprim-sulfamethoxazole (Bactrim)
RADT	Rapid antigen detection test	SG	Specific gravity	TNF	Tissue necrosis factor
RAH	Right atrial hypertrophy	SI	Small intestine	TnI	Troponin I
RAS	Renal artery stenosis	SIADH	Secretion of inappropriate antidiuretic hormone	TnT	Troponin T
RASTs	Radioallergosorbent assay tests			ToF	Tetralogy of Fallot
		SIRS	Systemic inflammatory response syndrome	ToV	Transposition of vessels
RBBB	Right bundle branch block			TPN	Total parenteral nutrition
RCA	Right coronary artery	SLE	Systemic lupus erythematosus	TR	Tricuspid regurgitation
RCM	Restrictive cardiomyopathy	SLN	Sublingual nitroglycerin	TRALI	Transfusion-related acute lung injury
RF	Rheumatoid factor or Rheumatic fever	SMA	Superior mesenteric artery		
		SN	Substantia nigra	TRUS	Transrectal ultrasound
Rh	Rhesus group	SNS	Sympathetic nervous system	TS	Tricuspid stenosis
RHD	Rheumatic heart disease	SOB	Shortness of breath	TSE	Treadmill stress echocardiogram
RHF	Right-sided CHF	SP	Senile plaques		
RhIg	Rho immune globulin	SPECT	Single photon emission CT	TSH	Thyroid stimulating hormone
RIND	Reversible ischemic neurologic deficit	SS	Sjögren's syndrome	TTE	Transthoracic echocardiogram
		SS-A/Ro	Antibodies to antigen A	TTP	Thrombocytic purpura
RLD	Restrictive lung defect	SS-B-La	Antibodies to antigen B	TVS	Transvaginal sonography
RNA	Ribonucleic acid	SSRI	Selective serotonin reuptake inhibitor	TxC	Type and cross
RNS	Repetitive nerve stimulation			TZ	Transitional zone
ROM	Range of motion	StAR	Steroidogenic acute regulatory deficiency	UA	Urine analysis
RPGN	Rapidly progressive glomerulonephritis			UC	Ulcerative colitis
		STd	ST depression	UDCA	Ursodeoxycholic acid
RPR	Rapid plasma reagin	STD	Sexually transmitted disease	UE	Upper extremity
RS	Reiter's syndrome or Reed-Sternberg cells	Ste	EKG ST elevation	UFS	Urinary free cortisol test
		SV	Stroke volume	UGT	Diphosphate glucuronosyltransferase
RSI	Repetitive stress injury	SVC	Superior vena cava		
RT	Radiation beam therapy	SVR	Systemic vascular resistance	URI	Upper respiratory infection
RTA	Renal tube acidosis	SVT	Supraventricular tachycardia	US	Ultrasound
RTI	Respiratory tract infection	T3	Triiodothyronine	UTI	Urinary tract infection
RV	Residual volume	T4	Tetraiodothyronine (thyroxine)	V/Q	Ventilation-perfusion
RVH	Right ventricular hypertrophy			VC	Vital capacity
SA	Sinoatrial node	TAHBSO	Total abdominal hysterectomy with bilateral salpingo-oophorectomy	VF	Ventricular fibrillation
SAAG	Serum-ascites albumin gradient			VHL	Von-Hippel-Landau disease
				VIP	Vasoactive intestinal peptide
SACD	Subacute combined degeneration	TAS	Transabdominal sonography	VLDL	Very low density lipoprotein
		TB	Tuberculosis	VSD	Ventricular septal defect
SBE	Subacute bacterial endocarditis	TCA	Tricyclic antidepressant	VT	Ventricular tachycardia
		TEE	Transesophageal echocardiogram	vWD	Von Willebrand disease
SBP	Systolic blood pressure			vWF	Von Willebrand factor
SC	Subcutaneously	THC	delta-9-tetrahydrocannabinol	VZV	Varicella zoster virus
SCA	Sickle cell anemia	THRH	Thyrotropin-releasing hormone	WBC	White blood cell
SCC	Squamous cell carcinoma			WNL	Within normal limits
SCD	Sequential compressive device	TIA	Transient ischemic attack	WPW	Wolf-Parkinson-White syndrome
SCID	Severe combined immunodeficiency disease	TIPS	Transjugular intrahepatic portacaval shunt		
				ZE	Zollinger-Ellison syndrome
SCLC	Small cell lung cancer	TLC	Total lung capacity		

DEDICATION

This book is dedicated to my son, for whom I will always strive to be a superman.

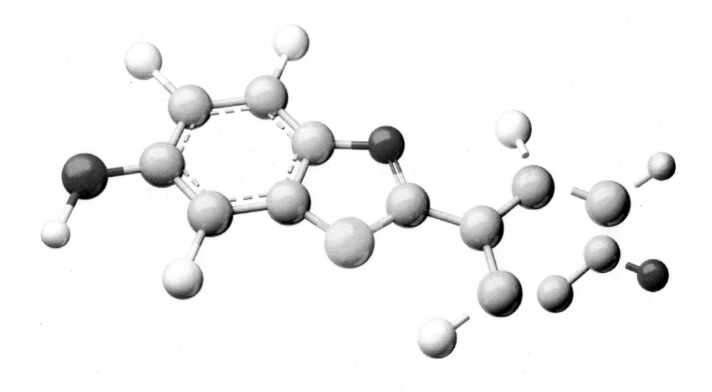

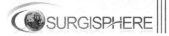

SYMBOLS

	Essential topic for the modern practice of surgery. Commonly tested on both written and oral exams.
	High-yield information that frequently appears on exams.
	Practice question covering a commonly tested concept.
	Detailed question explanation and ancillary information.
	The drug of choice for a particular disease process.
	Important property of a particular medication.

FOREWARD

The American Board of Surgery In-Training Examination is taken yearly by surgery residents around the country. It is used by residency programs as one measure of the caliber of their residents and often plays a role in promotion.[1] It is widely considered to be a prognostic indicator of your ability to pass the qualifying exam and become a board certified general surgeon. As a result, poor performance on the ABSITE over multiple years often leads to corrective action by the residency program.

This textbook and its accompanying online course and printed question book were created to improve the quality of surgical education and thereby help to improve the quality of care our patients receive. While there can be no substitute for studying the reference textbooks in the field, there are numerous moments during surgery residency to quickly review and understand high-yield topics. The focus of this program is to provide a high-yield review of topics commonly tested on the ABSITE and the surgery qualifying exam.

This material is derived from the major surgery reference textbooks and covers topics that have appeared on recent ABSITE and surgery qualifying exams. The overall organization of this textbook reflects the content outline of the surgery qualifying exam to ensure that every subject area is given due consideration. Surgery residents who have used this program in recent years have reported a 10-20% increase[2] in their scores. Surgery residency programs that use our program report a significant increase in resident ABSITE scores and clinical performance. The online program available last year was used by residents from nearly every residency program across the nation.[3] Based on their feedback and our proven approach to education, this is our solution for preparing for the ABSITE.

---

[1] Numerous residency programs use the ABSITE score as one element in promoting residents during their annual evaluations. Scores below a certain threshold often lead to corrective action, usually a focused study program. Repeatedly poor performance is predictive of poor performance on the qualifying and certifying exams, leading to a failure of the residency program to graduate board-certified residents.

[2] When comparing the group of residents who used this material to prepare for their ABSITE compared to residents who used third party material. 10-20% increase reflects the improvement in their base score when comparing their scores in prior years to current score. This is not a randomized control study and no p-values are presently available. A small retrospective case-control study is underway for this year and the results will be reported at www.Surgisphere.com.

[3] Residents around the country used this review program from 2006-2008 to prepare for the ABSITE. These residents were from surgery residency programs throughout the United States and nearly every residency program was represented.

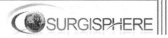

INTRODUCTION

CHAPTER CONTENTS

SECOND EDITION

Since the publication of the first edition, we have actively sought feedback from our readers on what we did well and what we could do better. After listening to your thoughts, we have made a number of improvements to our textbook and online review course. New to this edition are sections on Pediatric Surgery and Plastic Surgery. Transplant surgery has been completely rewritten and expanded. We have revised and expanded every subject, either reducing or entirely eliminating sections that are no longer covered on the ABSITE or surgery qualifying examination while expanding in other areas. Nearly a hundred new topics covering all areas of surgical care and management have been added throughout the textbook. We have added dozens of new tables and figures to more clearly illustrate various topics. New high-yield blurbs appear throughout the text to highlight topics that frequently appear on examinations. A new section at the end of the book makes a list of all high-yield topics – a worthwhile review before the examination. A feature that many readers will appreciate is the addition of particularly high-yield questions at the end of each section. These questions are meant to augment your knowledge in particular areas while helping you practice and retain what you have already learned. These high-yield questions complement those found in our question review book and cover concepts commonly found on surgery examinations.

We are pleased to bring you this second edition – the culmination of effort from residents and surgeons from leading surgery programs around the country. As always, we would be delighted to hear your thoughts. Contact us anytime.

OVERVIEW OF TOPICS

The surgery qualifying examination and the ABSITE cover a broad array of disciplines that spans both basic science and clinical medicine. Questions are derived from nearly every basic science subject and field of medicine, with the junior version of the ABSITE focusing on mostly basic science questions. Topics include Head and Neck Surgery, Breast Surgery, Gastrointestinal Surgery, Hepatopancreatobiliary Surgery, Vascular Surgery, Endocrine Surgery, Trauma Surgery, Critical Care Medicine, Transplant Surgery, Pediatric Surgery, Thoracic Surgery, Gynecology, Urology, Orthopedic Surgery, Plastic Surgery, Surgical Oncology, Anesthesia, and Medical Ethics.[4] The ABSITE covers all of these subjects.[5]

Within each of these clinical disciplines, questions are derived from both basic science and clinical topics. Of the 225 questions on the ABSITE, 60% of the questions are derived from basic science topics for the junior ABSITE and 20% of the questions are derived from basic science topics for the senior ABSITE.[5] Table 1 shows the breakdown of questions for both versions of the ABSITE.

---

[4] This information is based on the annual publication by the American Board of Surgery. It is derived from *http://home.absurgery.org/xfer/GS-QE.pdf*

[5] The ABSITE covers roughly the same information presented on the qualifying exam, hence the reason why it is predictive of performance on this exam. This information is extrapolated from *http://home.absurgery.org/default.jsp?certabsite*

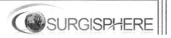

Table 1 Breakdown of the ABSITE Exam by Post-Graduate Year

	Junior ABSITE (PGY 1 and 2)	Senior ABSITE (PGY 3+)
Basic Science	60% (135)	20% (45)
Clinical Medicine	40% (90)	80% (180)
Total	100% (225)	100% (225)

The ABSITE focuses topics in a number of different categories. The breakdown is presented in Table 2.

Table 2 Breakdown of the ABSITE Exam by Category

	Junior ABSITE	Senior ABSITE
General Surgery and Critical Care Medicine	66.6%	25%
Gastrointestinal Tract	10%	25%
Cardiothoracic Surgery	7.8%	16.7%
Head and Neck Surgery, Gynecology, and Orthopedic Surgery	7.8%	16.7%
Endocrine Surgery, Hepatopancreatobiliary Surgery, Surgical Oncology, and Breast Surgery	7.8%	16.7%

Combining Table 1 and Table 2 yields an estimate of the number of questions per subject area.

Table 3 Breakdown of the ABSITE Exam by Number of Questions

	Junior ABSITE		Senior ABSITE	
General Surgery and Critical Care Medicine	Basic Science	90	Basic Science	10
	Clinical Medicine	60	Clinical Medicine	45
Gastrointestinal Tract	Basic Science	15	Basic Science	10
	Clinical Medicine	9	Clinical Medicine	45
Cardiothoracic Surgery	Basic Science	11	Basic Science	8
	Clinical Medicine	6	Clinical Medicine	30
Head and Neck Surgery, Gynecology, and Orthopedic Surgery	Basic Science	11	Basic Science	8
	Clinical Medicine	6	Clinical Medicine	30
Endocrine Surgery, Hepatopancreatobiliary Surgery, Surgical Oncology, and Breast Surgery	Basic Science	11	Basic Science	8
	Clinical Medicine	6	Clinical Medicine	30

While six questions covering clinical topics in cardiothoracic surgery may not seem like much, missing those six questions amounted to an 8-10 percent difference in score between test takers on the 2007 ABSITE. Every subject area is important and worth the time taken to review in detail.[6]

ORGANIZATION OF TEXT

This textbook and its corresponding online review program cover all of the major topics that appear on the surgery qualifying exam and the ABSITE. High-yield topics are covered with an emphasis on understanding the key information and every attempt is made to highlight the tested material. All of the surgical disciplines are covered and the appropriate emphasis is placed on basic science topics and clinical medicine topics. While all of the topics that appear in the outline for the surgery qualifying examination are covered, for the sake of clarity, the topics have been rearranged to improve the flow of the material.

Within each surgical discipline, topics are organized into one of six areas including Congenital and Structural Disorders, Metabolic and Degenerative Disorders, Inflammatory and Infectious Disorders, Vascular Disorders, Trauma, and Cancer. Where appropriate, a review of the relevant basic science is presented in a General Concepts section. The majority of the basic science topics are presented in the first two chapters of the book, Topics in Basic Science and Clinical Topics in Surgery. Following each section are pertinent questions to help you further your knowledge in additional areas while practicing what you have learned.

STUDY PLAN

How you study for the ABSITE depends on how much time you have available. Motivated residents who prepare in advance will benefit the most from the online review program and the enormous body of information available on the website. Regardless of how much time you have available, this entire review program is designed to be done piecemeal using the short periods of time you have available on call nights and in between cases. Each topic is designed to be covered in just a few minutes, and many residents report making good progress on the question bank by doing a few questions over lunch each day. Those who are on night float rotations or taking call report making good progress on the high-yield PowerPoint reviews.

Based on resident feedback, our recommendation is to keep the pocket version of the book with you at all times. It is a handy book to go through whenever a few minutes are available. This larger book is seen more and more in the hospital as the exam draws closer, but most residents recommend spending an hour every evening months in advance to review this book. While each individual study plan will be different, there are a few trends that we have noticed with high scorers:

1) Use this book in conjunction with the online questions and your existing reference books

2) Do at least a dozen questions and read through several topics every night

3) Review the high-yield PowerPoint presentations a week in advance of your exam

4) Take note of your strengths and weaknesses and focus on them accordingly

5) Keep your notes and review material from year to year

Whether you are preparing for the junior ABSITE or the senior ABSITE, we recommend going through this resource in its entirety. Topics that have appeared on one exam more than another are marked appropriately. Topics that have appeared

---

[6] Extrapolation based on analysis of resident exams and score outcomes from the 2007 and 2008 ABSITE.

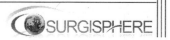

on recent exams or more than once are marked by stars. In addition, topics that the reviewers have deemed to be particularly worthwhile are also highlighted. It is important to reiterate that the purpose of this book is to help you become a better doctor and surgeon – your score on this exam should reflect your mastery of basic science and clinical medicine, and their application to the field of surgery.

FEEDBACK

We are always searching for ways to improve our products. If you have any comments or suggestions, we would love to hear from you. We would be happy to acknowledge your efforts by a free subscription to our review course for the next ABSITE.

Contact us at **Support@ClinicalReview.com** any time.

TOPICS IN BASIC SCIENCE

CHAPTER CONTENTS

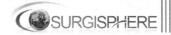

EPIDEMIOLOGY

According to the 2005 National Division of Vital Statistics, the overall top ten causes of death for both males and females are heart disease, cancer, cerebrovascular disease, chronic obstructive pulmonary disease, unintentional injuries / accidents, diabetes mellitus, influenza and pneumonia, Alzheimer disease, nephritis, nephrotic syndrome and nephrosis, and septicemia. Together, these top ten causes of death account for nearly 80% of all death in the United States of America.

Top 10 Causes of Death

- 1) Heart disease (29%)
- 2) Cancer (23%)
- 3) CVA (7%)
- 4) COPD
- 5) Accidents
- 6) Diabetes
- 7) Influenza and pneumonia
- 8) Alzheimer disease
- 9) Nephritis, nephrotic syndrome, nephrosis
- 10) Sepsis

CANCER STATISTICS

TOP 3 CANCERS BY INCIDENCE

- Prostate / Breast Cancer ← *better screening .... therefore less death/higher incidence*
- Lung Cancer
- Colorectal Cancer

TOP 3 CANCERS BY DEATH

- Lung Cancer
- Prostate / Breast Cancer
- Colorectal Cancer

> Prostate and breast cancer have the highest incidence. Lung cancer has the highest rate of death.

PREVENTIVE HEALTH CARE

PRIMARY PREVENTION

- Prophylaxis for disease (i.e. education and vaccinations)

SECONDARY PREVENTION

- Diagnosis of disease (i.e. EKG, CXR, Pap smear)

TERTIARY PREVENTION

- Treatment of disease (i.e. ACE-inhibitors for CHF, beta-blockers for HTN)

SCREENING GUIDELINES

INTRODUCTION

Preventive medicine deals with the branch of medicine dedicated to avoiding disease and promoting sound and healthy practices for well-being. Preventive medicine is responsible for the eradication of small pox in 1977, vaccines for typhoid, diphtheria, and cholera, and a treatment for rabies in the late 1800s. Preventive medicine has three levels of prevention: primary prevention is to avert the onset of illness in healthy people; secondary

Primary prevention: avoid disease (*vaccines*)
Secondary prevention: prevent disease progression (*MGM, Pap Smear, Colonoscopy*)
Tertiary prevention: decrease morbidity from disease (*medical therapy*)

prevention is to prevent the progression of a disease in people who are already afflicted; and tertiary prevention is directed towards reducing disability from a disease.

Table 4 Preventive Medicine

Preventive Medicine	
Primary level	Avert onset of illness in healthy people.
Secondary level	Prevention of progression of disease in already afflicted.
Tertiary level	Reducing disability from a disease.

ROUTINE SCREENING

Routine screening tests should be carried out at every visit to a physician. Generally, young adults should receive physical exams every 3-5 years, blood pressure and weight measurements every 2 years, cholesterol measured every 5 years, glaucoma screens at least once, and a Pap smear in women every 1-3 years. The screening guidelines in middle-aged adults (defined here as those between 40 and 65) should continue with the screening recommendations for young adults and start having fasting blood sugars measured every 3 years, **mammography yearly for women**, and **colonoscopy every 10 years**. Those over 65 should receive yearly physical exams, periodic hearing tests, and vision screening yearly. A **digital rectal exam should be done yearly after age 50** with tests for occult bleeding.

Table 5 Routine Screening Schedule

Routine Screening Schedule	
Young adults (Under 40)	Physical exams every 3-5 years,; BP and weight every 2 years; cholesterol levels every 5 years; glaucoma and pap tests every 1-3 years.
Middle age (40-65)	Same as young adults plus fasting blood sugars every 3 years, mammography yearly in women, colon cancer screen every 5 years, vision every 3 years. Digital, yearly rectal exam after 50.
Older adults (over 65)	Yearly physicals, periodic hearing tests, yearly vision test.

(1) MGM   40+   yearly
(2) Colonoscopy   50+   q10 years
(3) PSA/DRE   50+   yearly
(4) Skin exam   40+   yearly
     <40   q3yr
(5) Testicular exam   yearly

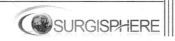

CANCER SCREENING

BREAST CANCER

2nd to heart ds

Breast cancer is the second most common cause of death in women. Screening tests recommend self breast exams every month about a week after the onset of menses. Annual exams by a physician should be made at least once a year, but even this examination is controversial up until the age of 40 or 50. The American Cancer Society recommends clinical breast exams every three years, then yearly after the age of 40. **Mammograms are recommended every 1-2 years from ages 40-49, then yearly**. The data to conduct mammograms in the 40's is currently controversial. Mammograms should not be conducted earlier than age 35 due to the density of the breast shadow and limited clinical utility of this test in younger women. However, a large multicenter trial with 40,000 women completed in 2005 suggests that mammograms using digital imaging might be appropriate for younger women. It is believed that as digital imaging solutions replace current x-ray film technology, more and more women would be eligible for the diagnostic benefits of mammography.

CERVICAL CANCER

Screening for cervical cancer is done with Papanicolaou (Pap) smears. Cervical cancer is commonly associated with certain human papillomavirus (HPV) types. Screening is generally recommended with yearly Pap smears starting at the age of 18 or when sexual activity begins, whichever is sooner. Pap smears may be performed every 3 years following 3 normal smears one year apart. Pap smears typically continue until the age of 70 in any woman who has a cervix.

COLORECTAL CANCER

Colorectal cancer screens are somewhat controversial. Most groups recommend fecal occult blood testing (FOBT) with digital rectal exams (DRE) every year after the age of 50. Flexible sigmoidoscopy should be done every 5 years or **colonoscopy every 10 years**. Some physicians recommend conducting colonoscopy in lieu of sigmoidoscopy, and some studies have discounted the benefits of FOBT. **DRE should be done in all patients as up to 50% of all colon cancers may lay within reach of the clinician's finger**.

OVARIAN CANCER

Ovarian cancer is the fourth most common cause of death in women. Risk factors include positive family history and having a pregnancy later in life. **There are no screening tests for ovarian cancer**.   *CA-125*

PROSTATE CANCER

Adenocarcinoma of the prostate is the third leading cause of death in men. Most groups prefer to individualize the screening process, but generally recommend **yearly DRE and prostate specific antigen (PSA) tests in individuals over the age of 50**. Significant elevations in PSA should be tested with a transrectal ultrasound (TRUS) of the prostate gland to confirm the clinical suspicion. Due to the increased risk of prostate cancer in African American males, some clinicians may choose to begin screening for prostate cancer earlier in this population.

SKIN CANCER

Screening for skin cancer has little backing in the medical literature. However, the ACS recommends physical exams of the skin every 3 years until the age of 40, then yearly. Individuals with particular risk factors should always get personalized schedules for screening exams.

TESTICULAR CANCER

Testicular cancer screening tests also have little supporting evidence in the literature. The ACS recommends testicular exams with every physical exam for cancer screening.

Table 6 Cancer Screening

	Cancer Screening
Breast	Self exam every month, clinical breast exam every 3 years until 40. Mammograms every 1-2 years between 40-49., *then annually*
Cervical	Yearly Pap smear starting at 18 or when sexually active. May be performed every 3 years following 3 normal smears one year apart. Typically continue until 70.
Colorectal	FOBT with DRE every year after 50. Sigmoidoscopy every 5 years or colonoscopy every 10 years.
Ovarian	No screening tests. Family history important as is late in life pregnancy.
Prostate	DRE and PSA yearly after 50. African American males earlier than 50.
Skin	Physical exam of skin every 3 years until age 40, then yearly.
Testicular	With every physical exam.

BIOSTATISTICS

STATISTICAL TESTING

- Sample size = n
  - o Sample size is the total number of patients enrolled in a particular study
- Standard deviation:

$$\sigma = \sqrt{\frac{\sum_{i=1}^{n}(x_i - \bar{x})^2}{n}}$$

- Standard error of the mean:

$$\frac{\sigma}{\sqrt{n}}$$

PREVALENCE AND INCIDENCE

- Prevalence

  - o **The number of cases of a particular disease at a point in time**

  - o Example: there are 2,000 cases of influenza at this moment in the United States

Prevalence: number of cases at a point in time
Incidence: new cases over a period of time

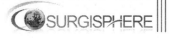

- Incidence

  o **The number of new cases of a particular disease within a span of time**

  o There were 3,200 cases of diabetes reported between January and June of last year

SENSITIVITY

- $Sensitivity = \dfrac{TP}{TP+FN}$

- Once a very sensitive test identified a patient as not having a disease, she or he is effectively **ruled out**
- A very sensitive test has a **low rate of false negatives**. Hence, you can trust a true negative result, indicating that if a test result is negative, the patient does not have a disease and is effectively ruled out.
- This permits sensitive tests to be used on a population as a **screening test**. Positive results are confirmed with a specific test.

Sensitivity: Screening test, rules out disease
Specificity: Confirmatory test, rules in disease

SPECIFICITY

- $Specificity = \dfrac{TN}{TN+FP}$

- A specific test is used to confirm a positive test result obtained from an initial screening test.
- A specific test has a very **low rate of false positives**, so a true positive is considered to be trustworthy.
- If a patient obtains a positive result on a specific test, it is considered to be indicative of having a disease (i.e. **ruling in**).

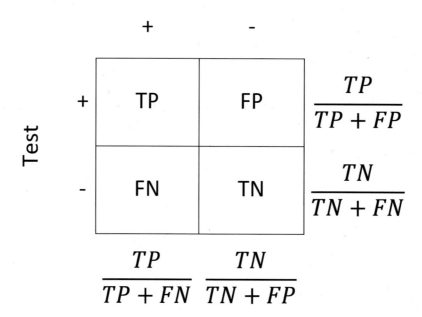

POSITIVE PREDICTIVE VALUE

> $Positive\ Predictive\ Value = \dfrac{TP}{TP+FP}$

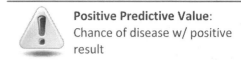

Positive Predictive Value:
Chance of disease w/ positive result

- A positive predictive value is used to determine the **chance of having a disease given a positive test result**
- A test with a very low false positive rate will have a more meaningful positive result
- Remember that the positive predictive value is always used in conjunction with the pretest probability to determine the chance the patient truly has a disease

NEGATIVE PREDICTIVE VALUE

> $Negative\ Predictive\ Value = \dfrac{TN}{TN+FN}$

- The negative predictive value determines the **chance of not having a particular illness given a negative test result**
- The negative predictive value is also used in conjunction with pretest probability and clinical suspicion

ODDS RATIO

> $Odds\ Ratio = \dfrac{TP \times TN}{FP \times FN}$

- The odds ratio is used in retrospective studies to determine the **particular effect of a risk factor on disease**
- The odds ratio is calculated using a table similar to that for sensitivity and specificity

RELATIVE RISK

> $Relative\ Risk = \dfrac{\frac{TP}{TP+FP}}{\frac{FN}{FN+TN}} = \dfrac{PPV}{NPV}$

- Relative risk is used to determine the **chance of a particular exposure leading to disease**
- It is used in cohort or prospective studies

ATTRIBUTABLE RISK

> $Attributable\ Risk = \dfrac{TP}{TP+FP} \times \dfrac{FN}{FN+TN}$ $PPV \times NPV$

- A variation of relative risk, attributable or absolute risk is used to determine the **actual number of cases** that can be attributed to a particular cause

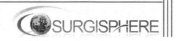

GAUSSIAN DISTRIBUTION

- A bell-shaped distribution with three

    distinct standard deviations

    - First standard deviation = 68%

        of all values

    - Second standard deviation =

        95.5% of all values

    - Third standard deviation =

        99.7% of all values

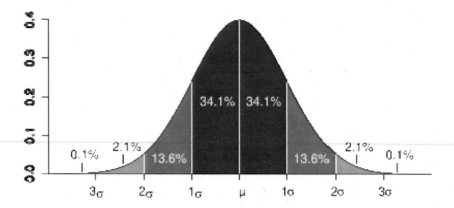

MEAN, MEDIAN, AND MODE

- Mean = Median = Mode

    - **Mean = average of all values**

    - **Median = middle value when all values are in ascending order**

    - **Mode = most common value**

Mean: average value
Median: middle value
Mode: most common value

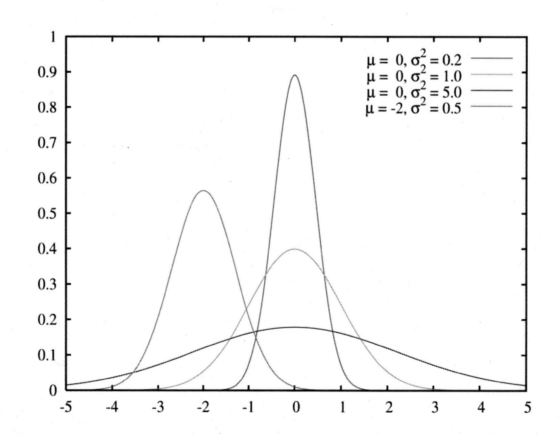

OTHER DISTRIBUTIONS

- Left-skewed distribution
  - Mean < Median < Mode
- Right-skewed distribution
  - Mode < Median < Mean
- Bimodal distribution
  - Two modes, 1 median, 1 mean
- Best descriptors of non-parametric distribution—median and quartiles

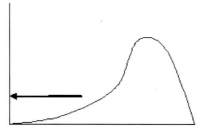
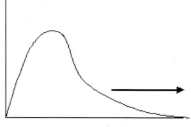

Negative Skew
Elongated tail at the **left**
More data in the left tail than would be expected in a normal distribution

Positive Skew
Elongated tail at the **right**
More data in the right tail than would be expected in a normal distribution

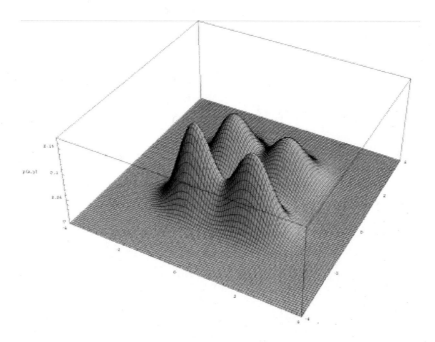

HYPOTHESIS TESTING

- Null hypothesis

  - **Assumes that a particular treatment has no effect**

  - This is the default assumption

- Alternative hypothesis

  - **Assumes that a particular treatment has the desired effect**

  - This is the assumption that is being tested

  - The assumption is accepted if it meets a particular statistical criterion

    - i.e. p<0.05 on T-test

Null hypothesis: treatment has no effect
Alternative hypothesis: treatment has effect
Type I error: treatment falsely believed to have effect (repeat study)
Type II error: treatment falsely believed **NOT** to have effect (increase sample size / power)

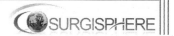

TYPE I ERROR

- **Accepting that a particular treatment has a desired effect when it really does not**
- Occurs when you reject the null hypothesis
- Repeating a study is important to determine whether a type I error has occurred
- Decreasing the p value in very important studies is also an important step, as this decreases the likelihood of making a type I error
  - o The p-value is an estimate of the chance of making a type I error
  - o Less than 5% is typically considered allowable – $p < 0.05$

TYPE II ERROR

- **Deciding that a particular treatment has no effect when it really does**
- Occurs when you falsely accept the null hypothesis
- Avoided by increasing the power of a study

POWER

- **Power is directly related to sample size:** Increasing sample size increases power
- Power is also dependent on measurement fidelity
  - o An improved ability to measure differences increases power of a study
- **Lack of power may lead to false acceptance of the null hypothesis (type II error)**
  - o The study was unable to find a difference when one really existed
  - o The power of a study is determined by the need to estimate expected differences

CORRELATION

- X-axis has one variable and the Y-axis has another variable mapped. A best-fit line is drawn.
- A correlation coefficient of 0 means that there is no direct or inverse correlation between the two variables. However, the two variables might still be otherwise related.
- A correlation coefficient between 0 and 1 means a direct correlation exists – as one goes up, the other variable generally goes up. This does not mean that one variable is causative, the other dependent. A negative correlation implies an inverse relationship.

STATISTICAL TESTS

- **T-test**
  - o Used to determine whether two quantified variables are sufficiently different based on their distributions and standard deviations
  - o Calculates a p value, which can be used to accept or reject the null hypothesis

- **ANOVA**
    - Used to determine whether three or more variables are different
    - Similar to T-test except with **more than 2 groups**
- Chi-squared
    - Used to determine whether any number of groups are different, but does so using qualitative terms
- The difference between T-tests and ANOVA vs. chi-squared is that chi-squared tests use categorical outcomes such as "yes" and "no"

> **T-test:** Two group analysis for significance
> **ANOVA:** Test for significance with more than 2 groups

PRECISION AND ACCURACY

- Precision
    - The ability to reproduce a test result
    - A finely calibrated machine will always return the same value
    - Reproducibility and reliability are key elements. Low susceptibility to random variation is also important.
- Accuracy
    - The ability to obtain a result close to the Truth
    - A test that always positively diagnosis people with a disease would have very high accuracy
    - Validity is the key element.

STUDY DESIGN

- A study must be designed to yield a practical outcome within a reasonable span of time with a minimum susceptibility to confounding
- Randomization, blinding, minimizing bias, using placebos, internal controls, and a wide sample size should be used whenever possible

CASE-CONTROL TRIAL

- **Retrospective trial** that takes a group of patients with known disease and looks into the past to determine the effect of various measured risk factors
- Susceptible to recall bias as patients with knowledge of their disease are likely to recall being subjected to a particular risk (i.e. high tension power lines)
- Very useful study when attempting to analyze risk factors leading to a rare disease

COHORT STUDY

- **Prospective study** that uses two groups of patients – one with a known exposure to a risk factor, and a control group known not to be exposed to the risk factor
- Sometimes requires a long span of time, during which loss of patients is likely to occur
- Useful when examining the effect of various risk factors on the development of disease

CLINICAL TRIAL

- **Randomized** – minimizes selection bias
- **Double-blind** – minimizes investigator and patient bias (measurement bias)
- **Multi-centered** – reduces confounding from a narrow sample
- Placebo **control** – helps ensure the trial is double-blind and reduces measurement bias

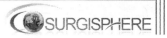

- Crossover control – patient receives treatment for half of the trial, then placebo for the remainder
    - Also reduces measurement bias
- The "best" study design in that the outcomes can typically be trusted if all tenets of study design are faithfully followed
- The major detriment is high cost
- In order for a randomized study to be properly evaluated, **the sample size must be known**

META-ANALYSIS

- Uses advanced statistical methods to **compare similar published studies** by pooling their numbers together and attempting to see whether this increased power is sufficient to identify differences
- Limitations are that it relies on work done by other investigators, which may not always be accurate or precise

CASE STUDY

- Examining the outcome of a single patient with a disease who received a particular treatment and its outcome
- Useful to note interesting or odd effects of treatment, or to note an off-label use of a medication
- May spur more rigorous clinical studies

BIAS

- Late-look bias – re-examination of the collected data after the study has been unblinded
- Lead time bias – earlier examination of patients with a particular disease lead to earlier diagnosis, giving the false impression that the patient will live longer
- Measurement bias – an investigator familiar with the study does the measurement and makes a series of errors towards the conclusion s/he expects
- Recall bias – patients informed about their disease are more likely to recall risk factors than uninformed patients
- **Sampling bias** – the sample used in the study is not representative of the population and so conclusions may not be relevant
- Selection bias – lack of randomization leads to patient's choosing their experimental group and introduces confounding

MEDICAL ETHICS

AUTONOMY

Autonomy is defined as the recognition that **patients are individuals** with their own preferences, and that the physician should make efforts to honor the patient's right to request or refuse medical care whenever possible. Autonomy is tested on the exam by testing the limits of when it is appropriate to listen to a patient and follow their requests or when ancillary measures must be taken, such as receiving parental permission or a court order in order to take action. For example, minors (those less than eighteen years of age) have autonomy in treatment for sexually transmitted diseases. No parental consent is required, and minors have the right to refuse care for their illness. Minors also have autonomy in treatment for substance abuse, birth control, and prenatal care. However, parental permission must be obtained before conducting an abortion.

Table 7 Minor Autonomy

Minor Autonomy	
Sexually transmitted disease	Substance abuse
Birth control	Prenatal care

NONMALEFICENCE

Nonmaleficence is more colloquially known as "**do no harm**." This is obviously a relative consideration, as certain therapies for cancer may cause a number of dangerous treatment-related side effects, but the therapy should proceed as scheduled as not treating the patient at all is almost certainly going to lead to death.

BENEFICENCE

Beneficence is a related concept in which physicians are required to **act in the patient's best interest** when no contradictory decision otherwise exists. This is the default action a physician should always take in the absence of other information. In this manner, the physician is acting as a fiduciary for the patient. Patient autonomy supersedes beneficence in almost every situation and it is very difficult ethically and legally to institute positive treatment for a patient against her will. The few exceptions to this are when the patient is a danger to themselves or to others.

ILLNESS IN MINORS

Discussing illnesses with children should always be done after a thorough **discussion with the parent**. The physician must first understand what the parent has told the child, and inform the child in accordance with the parent's wishes. Although minors are autonomous with regard to treatment for STDs, birth control, prenatal care, and treatment for substance abuse, they are not permitted to have an abortion without permission of the parent except in an emergency.

NONCOMPLIANCE

In situations where the patient is noncompliant with his medical care, such as not taking a necessary prescription, the best course of action is to identify the basic issue that prevents compliance. In response to most case-scenarios, the best way to proceed is to work to **improve the trust in the physician-patient relationship**. In situations where the patient is attempting to be compliant but has difficulty with maintaining the proper schedule, written directions should be provided to the patient. If appropriate, and within the patient's wishes, additional help may be solicited with family members and other health caretakers.

HIPPA GUIDELINES

As discussed previously, information flow between patients, family members, and health care team members should follow HIPPA guidelines. The health care issues involved with a patient should not be discussed with anybody except health care personnel immediately involved with care of that patient. With permission from the patient, information can be provided to family members. According to HIPPA guidelines, this discussion should take place in a private place that protects the privacy of the information; hence, discussions regarding specific patients should be undertaken only if their privacy can be protected. Identifying information should be avoided, and discussion in public places should be limited.

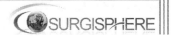

DEMANDING PATIENTS

Patients may occasionally make uncomfortable demands on the physician. Patients who request unnecessary procedures that are not medically indicated, or refuse to undertake a necessary procedure deserve to have an honest discussion with the physician. Understanding the patient's thinking is the key to resolving these types of problems. A common course of action with patient's requiring unnecessary cosmetic surgery is to alleviate the underlying psychological insecurity issues. Unnecessary procedures should not be performed in the interest of nonmaleficence. In this same vein, providing euthanasia to any patient is contraindicated. Physician-assisted suicide is not medically acceptable. However, in the interest of beneficence, the physician may provide strong pain relieving medications when medically indicated, even though their administration will coincidentally lead to a decreased life span.

ANGRY PATIENTS

Patients also get angry for a number of reasons in a health care setting. Anger over the amount of time spent waiting to see the doctor should be handled by apologizing to the patient for the wait. The physician is not obligated (and should not) attempt to explain the reasons for the delay. A patient upset with another physician or the level of care she has received elsewhere should be handled carefully. It is not professionally appropriate to discuss this situation with the patient; instead, the patient should be encouraged to speak directly with the individual that caused his grievance. In cases where the patient is upset with a member of your staff, the patient should be told that you will personally speak with that individual and address the patient's concerns.

PATIENT-PHYSICIAN RELATIONSHIPS

Finally, patients may state that they find you attractive and that they are interested in a romantic relationship with you. While standards on this vary from place to place (and are often left to the discretion of the physician but never advisable from a legal standpoint), for the purposes of the exam, romantic relationships are never appropriate between a physician and patient. In this situation, direct, close-ended questions should be used and the presence of a chaperone may be indicated. Another situation in which a chaperone is indicated is when a male physician does a breast or pelvic exam on a female.

INFORMED CONSENT

Informed consent is the practice of documenting that the patient requests that you perform an invasive procedure. Informed consent is traditionally in the written form and can serve as a legal document. Most procedures require informed consent except when the procedure must be performed on an emergency basis and consent cannot be acquired or is impractical (treat the latter situation carefully). In order for informed consent to be successfully obtained, the patient must be educated in a clear and simple manner regarding the benefits of the procedure, the risks of the procedure, alternatives to the procedure, and the consequences of not having any procedure performed. The legal standards are further met by obtaining this consent with a discussion of the pertinent information, establishing written consent stating the patient's agreement to the procedure offered, and gaining this consent in a manner free from coercion.

Table 8 Informed Consent

Informed Consent
Patient must be educated in a clear and simple manner about:
Benefits and risks of procedure.
Alternatives to procedure.
Consequences of not having procedure.
Pertinent information.
Obtaining written consent without coercion.

EXCEPTIONS TO INFORMED CONSENT

Informed consent is not practically obtained in a number of circumstances, and being familiar with the exceptions to this rule are likely to be tested. Informed consent does not need to be obtained in cases where emergency treatment is required to alleviate a life-threatening condition and there is no time to discuss the benefits and alternatives; in cases where therapeutic privilege is instituted, in which information must be withheld from the patient to prevent even greater harm than would occur with the therapy (but make this decision very carefully, as therapeutic privilege is often successfully challenged in a court); when the patient lacks the cognitive or physical ability to competently make an informed decision; and in cases where the patient signs a waiver to obtaining informed consent. It is important to note that family members cannot require that a physician not inform the patient regarding their illness. In this case, the appropriate course of action is to discuss the situation in a private room with the family members first, determine whether informing the patient would create even greater harm, and if it does not, then moving forward to inform the patient regarding their illness.

Table 9 Exceptions to Informed Consent

Exceptions to Informed Consent
Informed consent is NOT needed when:
Required to alleviate a life-threatening condition and there is no time to discuss the benefits and alternatives.
Where therapeutic privilege is instituted, in which information must be withheld from the patient to prevent even greater harm than would occur with the therapy (note caution in text above).
When the patient lacks the cognitive or physical ability to competently make an informed decision.
Where the patient signs a waiver to obtaining informed consent.

COMPETENCY

A patient's competence is established through their sound decision-making capability. Elements of a good decision-making ability include informing the patient regarding the intervention, the patient's decision does not repeatedly change over time, the decision appears to be consistent with other choices the patient would make, the patient does not have any psychosocial issues that complicate their ability to make an informed decision, and if the patient communicates a clear choice to the physician.

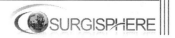

Table 10 Patient Competency

Patient Competency
Patient competency is established:
Through the patient's sound decision-making capability.
When patient is informed regarding the intervention.
When patient's decisions do not repeatedly change over time.
When the decision appears to be consistent with other choices patient would make.
When the patient communicate a clear choice to the physician.

ORAL ADVANCED DIRECTIVES

Advanced directives are a guide to providing treatment to a patient when she is otherwise unable to make a choice due to an intervening medical illness. In this case, a patient's prior **oral directives take precedence**, especially if the patient was able to make an informed, clear choice and communicate this lucidly to the physician ahead of time. The decision is considered valid if it is repeated over time.

 Oral advanced directives take precedence with regard to patient care.

WRITTEN ADVANCED DIRECTIVES

Written advanced directives are used in cases where an oral directive was not established. There are two major types of written advanced directives, including living wills and durable power of attorney. Living wills direct the physician to employ only certain life-saving measures and dictate if and when they can be withheld or withdrawn. Living wills take precedence only when there is no prior oral directive. Living wills are not flexible and are being replaced with durable power of attorney, in many cases.

DURABLE POWER OF ATTORNEY

Durable power of attorney is the designation of a surrogate, usually a spouse or other family member, who makes the judgment on behalf of the patient regarding medical decisions. The legality of durable power of attorney is predicated on the designated person making a decision similar to what the patient would choose if she were competent. A durable power of attorney incorporates elements of a living will in that the patient can designate that certain measures be taken in various clinical situations. Written advanced directives can be revoked at any time by the patient.

CONFIDENTIALITY

Confidentiality is an important cornerstone to providing medical care in a secure environment while protecting the privacy of patients. Recent regulations instituted via the Health Information Privacy Protection Act (HIPPA) dictate when and how confidentiality should operate. Generally, disclosing information about the patient to anybody except members of the health care team directly involved with the patient is disallowed. Information can be disclosed only on a need to know basis, although family members can be informed regarding the patient's condition if it is compatible with what the physician believes the patient would desire. Waivers to confidentiality can be signed by the patient.

EXCEPTIONS TO CONFIDENTIALITY

Confidentiality also has its own exceptions. Informing others regarding a patient's condition is allowed in situations where the potential harm to others is serious, as can occur if the patient is a danger to society. Confidentiality is also waived in situations where the patient is a danger to himself and the physician may make decisions to protect the patient from himself or others as deemed medically necessary. Physicians are required by law to inform people who may be harmed by the patient, thus breaching confidentiality. Other exceptions to confidentiality include informing health officials and people at risk for infectious diseases, situations involving abuse of children or elders, patients who are at risk of harming others due to inability to operate a motor vehicle or operate in a safe manner in their vocation, and in patients prone to suicide or homicide.

Table 11 Exceptions to Confidentiality

Exceptions to Confidentiality
When the potential harm to others is serious, as when a patient is a danger to society.
When the patient is a danger to himself or others.
When others are at risk of an infectious disease.
In situations involving child or elderly abuse
When patients are at risk of harming others due to inability of operate a motor vehicle or work in a safe manner at their jobs.
In patients prone to suicide or homicide.

MALPRACTICE

- Malpractice lawsuits often take place in civil court. The burden of proof is lower than in a criminal court.

- Civil court convictions require demonstration of breach of duty such that health care obligations to a patient are not met, and that the patient suffers harm from the breach of duty.

- The most common cause of malpractice lawsuits is poor physician communication.

PHARMACOLOGY

PHARMACOKINETICS

- Michaelis-Menten reaction

  - Used to model enzyme behavior
  - A free enzyme binds to a free substrate to form an enzyme-substrate complex
  - The enzyme-substrate complex is catalyzed to reform the enzyme and generate a product
  - Steady state is reached when the addition of a new substrate equals formation of new product

$$E + S \overset{k_1}{\underset{k_{-1}}{\leftrightarrow}} ES \xrightarrow{yields\ k_{cat}} E + P$$

- Enzyme is always conserved in reactions

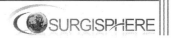

- The velocity of product formation is directly dependent on the maximum velocity of the reaction and inversely dependent on the affinity of the enzyme and amount of substrate

$$v_i = \frac{V_{max}[S]}{K_m + [S]}$$

- The **volume of distribution (V_D) quantifies the amount of drug found in the body**

 V_D = ratio of total drug to plasma concentration in body

- If the volume of distribution is known for a drug, then the amount of drug that must be given to achieve a therapeutic plasma concentration can be given

- **High lipid solubility means high volume of distribution.** This is similar with drugs that have a low plasma protein binding and high tissue binding affinities.

$$V_D = \frac{total\ drug\ in\ body}{drug\ concentration\ in\ blood}$$

- Clearance refers to the rate of elimination of a drug from the body as compared to its plasma concentration

- Clearance at steady-state is the ratio of mass generation and plasma concentration

$$CL = \frac{drug\ elimination}{plasma\ drug\ concentration}$$

$$CL = k \times V_D$$

- Half-life
  - The time it takes to clear the body of ½ of the current amount of drug
  - Approximately 4 t½ are required to achieve 95% clearance

$$t_{1/2} = \frac{0.7 \times V_D}{CL} \approx \frac{0.7}{k}$$

- Zero-order elimination
  - Proceeds linearly with a **fixed amount** of drug eliminated per unit time
  - Typically due to saturation of the elimination enzymes
- First-order elimination
  - Proceeds as exponential decay with **fixed ratio** of drug eliminated per unit time
  - Enzymes are functioning below saturation levels

 Zero-order: Fixed **amount** of drug is cleared
First-order: Fixed **ratio** of drug is cleared

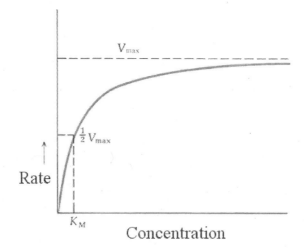

🌟 Loading dose
   o The amount of drug that may be given initially to reach a target plasma concentration more quickly

$$LD = C_P \times \frac{V_D}{F}$$
$$LD = loading\ dose$$
$$C_P = plasma\ concentration$$
$$V_D = volume\ of\ distribution$$
$$F = bioavailability$$

🌟 Maintenance dose

   o The amount of drug that is given to achieve a steady-state concentration between drug plasma concentration and drug elimination

$$MD = C_P \times \frac{CL}{F}$$
$$MD = maintenance\ dose$$

PHARMACODYNAMICS 🌟

🌟 Competitive antagonist

   o If the left graph is the agonist, the right graph is the
      agonist plus the competitive antagonist

   o The right graph also reflects the new potency of the left
      graph following tolerance

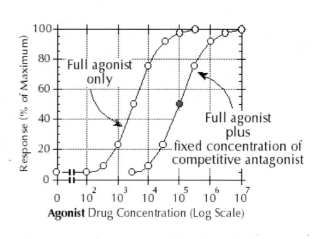

- Partial agonist

    o A partial agonist decreases the efficacy of a particular

        medication

- Noncompetitive antagonist

    o A noncompetitive antagonist would be similar to the

        partial agonist in the graph to the right

- The therapeutic index of a particular drug is shown in the graph on

    the right

    o At ED50 for the drug, half of all patients will respond

    o As the dose is increased, more and more patients will

        enter the range of the lethal dose and risk succumbing to

        the lethal side effects of the drug

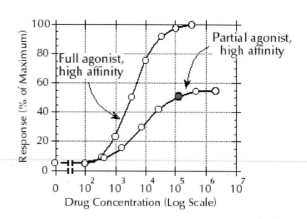

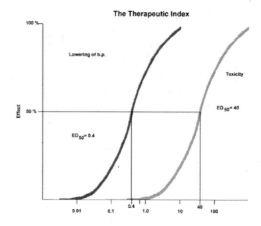

EFFICACY AND POTENCY

- Efficacy
    o Two drugs that reach the same maximum
       desired effect are equally efficacious
    o Heroin and morphine have approximately
       the same efficacy in that both can lead to
       100% analgesia. Codeine is less efficacious
       than either of these drugs.

- Potency
    o Potency refers to the minimum dose
       needed to achieve a desirable therapeutic
       effect.
    o Heroin is more potent than morphine in
       that a lower dose is needed to achieve
       100% analgesia.

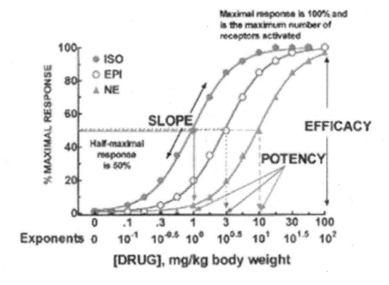

DRUG DEVELOPMENT

 Involves hundreds of millions of dollars in capital with dozens of potential drug candidates

 After extensive testing, a few prototypic drugs are chosen for further analysis

 Based on early trials in patients, the number of potential drugs is narrowed

 Approval is submitted for the best drugs, a process that takes nearly 10 years

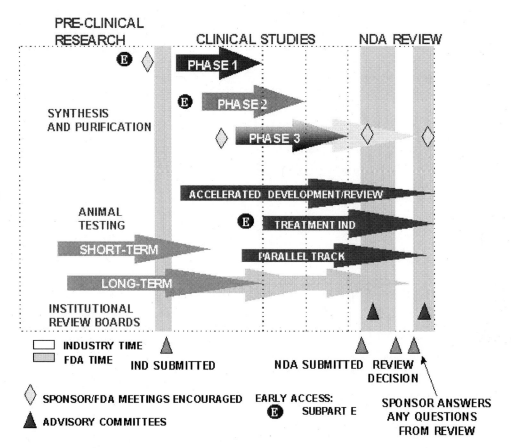

PRACTICE QUESTIONS

 A physician requests a specific test that will ensure that a positive result confirms his already high clinical suspicion. Which of the following defines specificity?

A. True negatives divided by the sum of true negatives and false negatives

B. True negatives divided by the sum of true negatives and false positives

C. True negatives divided by the sum of true negatives and true positives

D. True positives divided by the sum of true positives and false negatives

E. True positives divided by the sum of true positives and false positives

The best answer is <u>True negatives divided by the sum of true negatives and false positives</u>. The physician is asking for a specific test that will confirm a positive test result; the correct formula for specificity is the number of true negatives divided by the sum of true negatives and false positives.

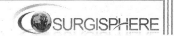

Which of the following best describes a type II error?

A.   A study that does not find a difference when one really does not exist
B.   A study that does not find a difference when one really exists
C.   A study that finds a difference when one really does not exist
D.   A study that finds a difference when one really exists
E.   Making an error even with sufficiently powered studies

The best answer is <u>A study that does not find a difference when one really exists</u>. Lack of power may lead to false acceptance of the null hypothesis. Being unable to therefore find a difference when one really exists leads to a type II error. Increasing power via increasing sample size can help to avoid this type of error.

What is the definition of sensitivity?

A.   FP / (FP+FN)
B.   FP / (FP+TN)
C.   TP / (TP+FN)
D.   TP / (TP+TN)

The best answer is <u>TP / (TP+FN)</u>. Sensitivity is the proportion of true positives to the sum of true positives and false negatives (all patients with disease). A very sensitive test has a low rate of false negative. Hence, you can trust a true negative result, indicating that if a test result is negative, the patient does not have a disease and is effectively ruled out. This permits sensitive tests to be used on a population as a screening test. Positive results are confirmed with a specific test.

CLINICAL TOPICS IN SURGERY

CHAPTER CONTENTS

INFECTION AND ANTIBIOTICS

SURGICAL PROPHYLAXIS

Use of cefazolin or cefuroxime is preferred for most clean general surgery procedures. Upper GI procedures or hepatobiliary procedures receive ciprofloxacin or ceftizoxime with metronidazole. Large bowel resections are prepared with erythromycin with ceftizoxime, bisacodyl, and a clear liquid diet (CLD). GoLytely is often used. Appendectomy receives ceftizoxime or cefotetan with the addition of metronidazole. Cefazolin is commonly used in numerous other types of procedures. Vancomycin is used with procedures dealing with the pancreas or kidneys. **Antibiotics must be given at least 30 minutes prior to incision** for maximal effectiveness. Most practitioners will **continue prophylactic antibiotics for at least 24 hours** post-surgery. Of note, the most common hospital-acquired infection and the **most common infection** in patients with diabetes is a **urinary tract infection**.

Preoperative antibiotics must be given 30 minutes prior to incision. Continue for 24 hours following surgery.

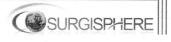

Table 12 Surgical Prophylaxis

Prophylaxis	
Surgery Type	**Prophylaxis**
General Surgery	Cefazolin or cefuroxime.
Upper GI procedures or hepatobiliary	Ciprofloxacin or ceftizoxime with metronidazole.
Large bowel resections	Erythromycin with ceftizoxime, bisacodyl, CLD. GoLytely is often used.
Appendectomy	Ceftizoxime or cefotetan with the addition of metronidazole.
Pancreas or kidneys	Vancomycin

WOUND CONTAMINATION

ETIOLOGY

The rate of postoperative wound infections is highly dependent on a number of factors inherent to both the patient and the operation. The most important is the type of operation and how contaminated the field becomes as a result of surgery. Adequate skin preparation is essential in order to limit the size of the initial bacterial inoculation into the incisional plane. Wound infections tend to become more common with operations over two hours long and with extensive tissue damage, such as following coagulation of dermal or fascial planes instead of cutting through them. Seromas and hematomas dramatically increase the risk of infection. Patient factors include the elderly, the presence of chronic illness, cardiovascular instability, malnutrition (especially an **albumin < 2.5**), and the presence of immunosuppressants. As discussed below, the most common cause of postoperative wound infection in non-gastrointestinal and non-biliary procedures is due to skin flora: **Staphylococcus and Streptococcus** spp. With **GI and biliary procedures, gram negative and anaerobic organisms** are more common.

An albumin < 2.5 is the largest perioperative risk factor.

Table 13 Classification of Wound Contamination

Classification of Wound Contamination		
Clean	1.5% infection rate	An elective operation with an incision made under ideal conditions. No entry into gastrointestinal tract or respiratory tract.
Clean-Contaminated	8% infection rate	An elective operation with an incision made under ideal conditions. Controlled entry into the gastrointestinal tract or respiratory tract with no spillage of contents and no infectious process present (i.e. abscess).
Contaminated	18% infection rate	Emergent operations with entry into the gastrointestinal tract or urinary tract with gross spillage or presence of infection. Trauma operations.
Dirty	40% infection rate	Entry into a perforated viscus or wounds with frank pus, old trauma wounds, or grossly contaminated wounds. Open fractures are an example.

TREATMENT

Contaminated wounds are typically defined as those that have an overall bacterial count less than 100,000 and satisfactorily intact host responses to infection. Once the host response is overwhelmed and bacteria start to proliferate, the wound status becomes infected. Contaminated wounds are typically debrided thoroughly during surgery with satisfactory hemostasis to prevent the formation of a hematoma. Tissues should be approximated and no open spaces should be left (i.e. Halstead principles for wound management). Copious irrigation is also commonly used to ensure the removal of all foreign bodies and detritus. Pulse irrigation is more effective at reducing the rate of infection than other methods. Once thoroughly prepared, the tissue should be closed in layers. If these criteria cannot be met, the fascia should be closed and the overlying tissues permitted to close secondarily. The use of a wound V.A.C. device has shown to reduce the time needed for wound closure. The rate of infection of such open wounds is less than 15%.

COMMON ANTIBIOTICS

ANTIMICROBIALS

PENICILLINS

Table 14 Antimicrobials: Penicillin

DRUG	INDICATIONS	MECHANISM OF ACTION	COMPLICATIONS	CONTRAINDICATIONS	NOTES
Penicillin G	GPC (Streptococcus, meningococcus, enterococcus) GPR, GNC Spirochetes	Inhibits cross-linking of cell wall leading to bacterial lysis → bactericidal	Hypersensitivity (anaphylaxis?), hemolytic anemia	Do not use in bacteria with beta-lactamases or w/ known hypersensitivity (common rxn is skin rash,	Especially effective against *Neisseria spp.*, *C. perfringens*, *Fusobacteria*, and *Treponema* IV formulation Used for syphilis.
Amoxicillin	GPC, GPR, GNR *E. coli, H. influenzae, L. monocytogenes, P. mirabilis, Salmonella*	Inhibits cross-linking of cell wall leading to bacterial lysis → bactericidal	As above plus pseudomembranous colitis. Seizures at high doses.	Do not use if hypersensitivity to penicillins.	Use with clavulanic acid or sulbactam to block beta-lactamases. Wide spectrum. Oral.
Piperacillin	Extended spectrum. *Pseudomonas.* GNR	Inhibits cross-linking of cell wall leading to bacterial lysis → bactericidal	Hypersensitivity, hemolytic anemia, platelet dysfunction.	Do not use if hypersensitivity to penicillins. Sodium loading.	

⚠ Resistance to penicillins comes from beta-lactamases that cleave the penicillins to make them impotent.

⚠ Penicillins bind to PBPs with subsequent inhibition of the transpeptidase step leading to cell lysis. It will not affect organisms that do not have a cell wall.

⚠ Penicillins are cleared renally, which can be slowed with the administration of probenecid

CEPHALOSPORINS – FIRST GENERATION

Table 15 Antimicrobials: First Generation Cephalosporins

DRUG	INDICATIONS	MECHANISM OF ACTION	COMPLICATIONS	CONTRAINDICATIONS	NOTES
Cefazolin	GPC *E. coli* *K. pneumoniae* *P. mirabilis*	Inhibit cell wall synthesis by preventing cross-linking. Bactericidal.	Hypersensitivity (rash). 10% penicillin cross hypersensitivity	Aminoglycosides (nephrotoxicity). Alcohol (disulfiram reaction)	Less susceptible to beta-lactamases.

⚠ Resistance to cephalosporins comes from beta-lactamases that cleave the penicillins to make them impotent.

⚠ Cephalosporins have a hexagonal ring with two functional groups. Penicillins have a pentagonal ring with one functional group. Both are susceptible to beta-lactamases.

CEPHALOSPORINS – SECOND GENERATION

Table 16 Antimicrobials: Second Generation Cephalosporins

DRUG	INDICATIONS	MECHANISM OF ACTION	COMPLICATIONS	CONTRAINDICATIONS	NOTES
Cefoxitin	GPC, *E. coli* *Enterobacter* *H. influenzae* *K. pneumoniae* *Neisseria spp.* *P. mirabilis* *Serratia spp.*	Inhibit cell wall synthesis by preventing cross-linking. Bactericidal.	Hypersensitivity (rash).	Avoid with aminoglycosides (nephrotoxicity). Avoid with alcohol (disulfiram reaction)	Less susceptible to beta-lactamases. Broader range compared to first generation.

CEPHALOSPORINS – THIRD GENERATION

Table 17 Antimicrobials: Third Generation Cephalosporins

DRUG	INDICATIONS	MECHANISM OF ACTION	COMPLICATIONS	CONTRAINDICATIONS	NOTES
Ceftriaxone	Gram-negatives. Meningitis Resistant organisms Serious infections Broad range. Low activity against gram positives.	Inhibit cell wall synthesis by preventing cross-linking. Bactericidal. Broadest range.	Hypersensitivity (rash).	Avoid with aminoglycosides (nephrotoxicity). Avoid with alcohol (disulfiram reaction)	Cross blood-brain barrier. Ceftazidime is especially good against *Pseudomonas*.

MONOBACTAMS / CARBAPENEMS

Table 18 Antimicrobials: Monobactams and Carbapenems

DRUG	INDICATIONS	MECHANISM OF ACTION	COMPLICATIONS	CONTRAINDICATIONS	NOTES
Aztreonam	GNR *Klebsiella spp.* *Pseudomonas spp.* *Serratia spp.*	Prevents synthesis of cell wall. Bactericidal. Improved activity with aminoglycosides	GI Sx.	No effect against anaerobes or gram-positive bacteria.	No cross-sensitivity with penicillins. Especially recommended in renal disease.
Imipenem	GPC, GNR Anaerobes *Enterobacter*	Beta-lactamase resistant cell wall synthesis inhibitor. Bactericidal.	GI Sx. Rash. CNS toxicity leading to seizures at high doses. Nephrotoxic. Eosinophilia.	Renal disease.	Imipenem is always given with cilastatin to avoid inactivation in kidney. Synthetic.

AMINOGLYCOSIDES

Table 19 Antimicrobials: Aminoglycosides

DRUG	INDICATIONS	MECHANISM OF ACTION	COMPLICATIONS	CONTRAINDICATIONS	NOTES
Gentamicin	Severe gram-negative infections. Aerobes only. *Pseudomonas.*	30S inhibitor. Bacteriostatic. Cause mRNA misreading by preventing formation of initiation complex → bactericidal.	Nephrotoxic. Ototoxic. Cause NMJ blockade after surgery. Possible superinfection.	Do not use with cephalosporins. Do not use with loop diuretics. Renal clearance – avoid in renal disease.	Require O2 for use → no effect against anaerobes. Given IV.

- R-factor resistance leads to drug inactivation and decreased uptake.
- May also be modified through acetylation, adenylation, or phosphorylation of the compound. Excreted unchanged by kidney.

TETRACYCLINES

Table 20 Antimicrobials: Tetracyclines

DRUG	INDICATIONS	MECHANISM OF ACTION	COMPLICATIONS	CONTRAINDICATIONS	NOTES
Doxycycline	*B. burgdorferi* Chlamydia Mycoplasma Propionibacterium Rickettsia Tularemia Ureaplasma V. cholerae	30S inhibitor prevents tRNA attachment. Bacteriostatic.	GI Sx. Tooth discoloration and stunted growth in children. Fanconi syndrome. Photosensitivity (common). Possible superinfection.	Avoid in renal patients. Avoid in children.	Do not use in CNS infections.

- R-factor resistance leads to drug inactivation and decreased uptake. Also has increased removal from cell.
- Avoid dairy foods, iron-containing preparations, and antacids with use of tetracyclines.

MACROLIDES

Table 21 Antimicrobials: Macrolides

DRUG	INDICATIONS	MECHANISM OF ACTION	COMPLICATIONS	CONTRAINDICATIONS	NOTES
Azithromycin !	Pneumonia and URTI. GPC *Mycoplasma* *Legionella* *Chlamydia* *Neisseria*	50S inhibitor prevents translocation and inhibits protein synthesis. Bacteriostatic.	GI Sx (common). Hepatitis. Eosinophilia. Skin rashes.	Avoid in hepatic patients. Macrolides are excreted in bile.	

⚖ Resistance by rRNA methylation leading to prevention of binding to 50S unit.

FLUOROQUINOLONES ⭐

Table 22 Antimicrobials: Fluoroquinolones

DRUG	INDICATIONS	MECHANISM OF ACTION	COMPLICATIONS	CONTRAINDICATIONS	NOTES
Ciprofloxacin !	**GNR** *Pseudomonas* *Neisseria spp.* Gram-positives (MRSA) UTI, TB GI infections	**Prevents action of topoisomerase II**. Bactericidal.	GI Sx. Tendon rupture. **Theophylline** levels increase in plasma.	Avoid in pregnancy and children due to cartilage damage. Avoid in renal patients.	Very potent drugs. Broad spectrum except against anaerobes and some GPC. Renal secretion.

⚖ Resistance by change in DNA gyrase. Drug penetration may also change. No plasmid-resistance.

SULFONAMIDES / TRIMETHOPRIMS ⭐

Table 23 Antimicrobials: Sulfonamides and Trimethoprims

DRUG	INDICATIONS	MECHANISM OF ACTION	COMPLICATIONS	CONTRAINDICATIONS	NOTES
Sulfamethoxazole !	Gram-positives Gram-negatives *Nocardia* *Chlamydia* Recurrent otitis media UTI	Inhibits DHP synthase by PABA metabolites. Bacteriostatic.	Allergic reactions. Nephrotoxicity, kernicterus, changes volume of other medications. Rash, anemia, crystalluria.	G6PD deficiency, avoid in infants, use with care with other drugs. Avoid in pregnancy.	Combined with TMP. Resembles PABA. Penetrate CNS.
Trimethoprim	UTI Prostatitis *Shigella* *Salmonella* *P. carinii* Nocardiosis HIB	Prevents the use of DHFR in bacteria. Bacteriostatic. Additive with SMX.	Megaloblastic anemia, pancytopenia. BMS.		Give with folate to avoid anemia. Used for recurrent UTIs. TMP-SMX used for *P. carinii* pneumonia.

⚖ Resistance by modification of DHP synthase, increased synthesis of PABA, or decreased uptake of drug.

OTHER ANTIMICROBIALS

Table 24 Antimicrobials: Other Drugs

DRUG	INDICATIONS	MECHANISM OF ACTION	COMPLICATIONS	CONTRAINDICATIONS	NOTES
Chloramphenicol	Meningitis	50S inhibitor to decrease tRNA binding to A site. **Bacteriostatic.**	Aplastic anemia, gray baby syndrome.	Avoid in pregnancy and infants (low UDP-glucuronyl transferase).	Crosses BBB.
Metronidazole	Protozoa. *G. vaginalis.* Anaerobes. Bacteroides. *Clostridium spp.*	Formation of toxic products. Bactericidal.	GI sx	Avoid with alcohol due to disulfiram reaction.	Used for numerous STDs.
Vancomycin	Serious infections Gram-positive bacteria resistant to other agents *S. aureus / MRSA / PRSP C. difficile*	Prevents cell wall formation through D-ala D-ala binding and sequestration.	Nephrotoxic. Ototoxic (deafness). DVTs. Red man syndrome.	Renal disease. Renally cleared agent.	Avoid red man syndrome with antihistamines and gradual administration.
Clindamycin	Anaerobic infections. *B. fragilis. C. perfringens.*	50S inhibitor. Bacteriostatic.	Pseudomembranous colitis	Renal and hepatic clearance.	PO. Treat pseudomembranous colitis with flagyl. A lincosamide.

⚠ Resistance to vancomycin comes from mutation of D-ala D-ala to D-ala D-lac. Plasmid-mediated.
⚠ R-factor resistance for chloramphenicol leads to drug inactivation by acetyltransferase inactivation and decreased uptake.

ANTIFUNGALS

ANTIFUNGALS

Table 25 Antifungals

DRUG	INDICATIONS	MECHANISM OF ACTION	COMPLICATIONS	CONTRAINDICATIONS	NOTES
Amphotericin B	Systemic infections. Meningitis *Cryptococcus Aspergillus Histoplasma Candida Mucor*	Sequesters ergosterol and has detergent-like effect on cell wall. Fungicidal at high doses.	F/C. Hypotension. Nephrotoxicity. Arrhythmias.	Avoid in renal disease.	Does not cross BBB. Must be given intrathecally for meningitis. Given slowly via IV.
Nystatin	*Candida*	Sequesters ergosterol, disrupts cell wall.			Oral candidiasis. Topical only.
Fluconazole	Systemic infections. Cryptococcal meningitis. *Candida.*	Block formation of ergosterol by lanosterol. Fungistatic.	Gynecomastia, hepatitis, F/C.	Avoid in hepatic disease.	Good absorption and CNS penetration.

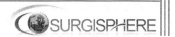

ANTIVIRALS

ANTIVIRALS ⭐

Table 26 Antivirals

DRUG	INDICATIONS	MECHANISM OF ACTION	COMPLICATIONS	CONTRAINDICATIONS	NOTES
Acyclovir !	HSV VZV EBV	Inhibits viral DNA polymerase, guanine analog.	Tremor, nephrotoxicity.	Avoid in renal patients.	Also treated with vidarabine (adenosine analog)
Ganciclovir	CMV in IC EBV in IC	Inhibits viral DNA polymerase.	Pancytopenia, especially with WBCs.	Use with care due to BMS.	Like ACV.

! Phosphorylation by the virus of DNA polymerase permits DNA polymerase binding and subsequent inhibition of DNA synthesis.

ANTIPARASITICS

ANTIPARASITICS

Table 27 Antiparasitics

DRUG	INDICATIONS	MECHANISM OF ACTION	COMPLICATIONS	CONTRAINDICATIONS	NOTES
Metronidazole	*Giardia, Entaboeba histolytica, Gardnerella vaginalis, Trichomonas*	Targets DNA.	Disulfiram-like reaction.		Does not eliminate cysts.

COMMON INFECTIONS

GENERAL CONCEPTS ⭐

Staphylococcus aureus is best treated with nafcillin or cloxacillin. An alternative to penicillin is cefazolin in methicillin-sensitive species (MSSA). For methicillin resistant species (**MRSA**), **vancomycin** is used. An alternative regimen is TMP-SMX or minocycline with rifampin. Coagulase-negative organisms are treated with vancomycin or nafcillin, if sensitive; alternative treatment includes cefazolin or clindamycin. GAS and GBS are treated with clindamycin, with backups including benzylpenicillin and cefazolin. Enterococci infections are treated with ampicillin and gentamicin, and vancomycin is the alternative treatment. *E. coli and Proteus spp.* are treated first with ampicillin, then cefazolin, gentamicin, or levofloxacin, if the first treatment fails.

Potent exotoxins are made generally by gram positive organisms. These include *S. aureus, C. perfringens, E. coli*, and *V. cholerae*. *C. botulinum* generally has the most potent exotoxin, with 1mg sufficient to kill thousands of people. Bacterial lipopolysaccharides (LPS) are formed from the outer membrane of gram negative bacteria. This endotoxin leads to septic shock when released in significant amounts. The O-antigen is the major source of antigenicity and consists of polysaccharides. LPS induces septic shock by activating TNF and IL1, leading to cascade activation of IL6, IL8, GM-CSF, and other immunomodulators.

Table 28 General Antibiotics

General Antibiotics	
S. Aureus	Nafcillin or cloxacillin. An alternative to penicillin is cefazolin for MSSA.
MRSA	Vancomycin. An alternative regimen is TMP-SMX or minocycline with rifampin.
Coagulase -organisms	Vancomycin or nafcillin. Alternative treatment includes cefazolin or clindamycin.
GAS & GBS	Clindamycin, with backups including benzylpenicillin and cefazolin.
Enterococci infections	Ampicillin and gentamicin, and vancomycin is the alternative treatment.
E. coli & *Proteus spp.*	Ampicillin, then cefazolin, gentamicin, or levofloxacin, if the first treatment fails.

SOFT TISSUE INFECTIONS

Cellulitis is the infection of skin and underlying tissues commonly following local trauma. Cellulitis presents with local pain and swelling, numerous constitutional symptoms, and lymphadenopathy. The affected region is red and warm. Hypotension is common. Areas of necrosis may be found in the area. Common causes include S. pyogenes, S. aureus, S. pneumoniae, and more exotic causes in IC patients. Cellulitis by *Streptococcus* or *Staphylococcus* is treated with nafcillin or clindamycin. Penicillin G is the choice for documented Streptococcal infection. Decubitus ulcers are treated with amoxicillin and clavulanate, ampicillin and sulbactam, clindamycin and ciprofloxacin, ceftizoxime, or piperacillin and tazobactam with tobramycin. Necrotizing fasciitis is treated with penicillin with clindamycin and aminoglycosides, ampicillin with sulbactam and aminoglycosides, or imipenem; aggressive surgical debridement is also required. **Vancomycin** is used with resistant organisms and in patients with numerous risk factors for more severe disease.

Table 29 Soft Tissue Infections

Soft Tissue Infections	
Cellulitis by *Streptococcus* or *Staphylococcus*	Nafcillin or clindamycin. Penicillin G is the choice for documented Streptococcal infection.
Decubitus ulcers	Amoxicillin and clavulanate, ampicillin and sulbactam, clindamycin and ciprofloxacin, ceftizoxime, or piperacillin and tazobactam with tobramycin.
Necrotizing fasciitis	Clindamycin and aminoglycosides, ampicillin with sulbactam and aminoglycosides, or imipenem

TOXIC SHOCK SYNDROME

ETIOLOGY AND PATHOPHYSIOLOGY

Toxic shock syndrome (TSS) is an erythema with systemic manifestations due to *S. aureus*. The formation of a superantigen known as TSS toxin-1 (TSST-1) leading to cytokine release throughout the body leads to the diffuse injury and systemic symptoms. Shock can occur.

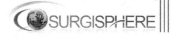

PRESENTATION AND DIAGNOSIS

TSS presents with symptoms include fever, hypotension, organ involvement, and distal extremity desquamation. Erythema is present with a scarlatiniform eruption. The tongue is cherry red, and hyperemia of mucous membranes is common. Several organs may be involved leading to serious systemwide damage and complications. Diagnosis is made by culture.

TREATMENT

Supportive therapy is used with TSS, including IVF, pressors, antibiotics, and draining the affected regions. Silver sulfadiazine cream is contraindicated; mupirocin ointment is used instead. Standard antistaphylococcus antibiotics are used as previously discussed.

TOXIC EPIDERMAL NECROLYSIS / STEVENS JOHNSON SYNDROME

Causes of toxic epidermal necrolysis include dilantin and bactrim. Biopsy of the skin will indicate nondisjunction of the dermal and epidermal interface.

BITES

Following a human bite, an incision and drainage should be done. Augmentin should be given to the patient. Tetanus vaccination should also be verified and IgG should be considered. Human bites lead to infection with *S. aureus* and *Eikenella corrodens*. Wounds are typically left open following irrigation and debridement. Bites from animals are treated in a similar fashion. Cat bites are more likely to be infected than dog bites due to the presence of *Pasteurella multocida*. Bites from most animals (and humans) can be safely treated with Augmentin or Bactrim. A bite from a brown recluse spider can be treated with dapsone.

TETANUS

Tetanus is caused by neurotoxin release by C. tetani, leading to a 30% mortality rate if not treated early. Tetanus infection must be especially considered in the presence of dirty wounds contaminated by soil or feces, puncture wounds, burns, and frostbite. For clean, minor wounds, children under 7 should be treated with a DPT (*Diphtheriae*, *Pertussis*, and *Tetanus*) vaccination as prophylaxis. Children over 7 can be treated with the Td (tetanus toxoid) vaccination for similar wounds. Adults should receive a Td if the most recent vaccination is over 10 years ago. All dirty or major wounds receive a Td unless the full immunization schedule has been followed and the most recent vaccination is less than 5 years ago.

MUSCULOSKELETAL INFECTIONS

Osteomyelitis is best treated with nafcillin and rifampin or nafcillin with an aminoglycoside. Diabetic foot ulcers are treated with piperacillin and tazobactam or ampicillin and sulbactam with an aminoglycoside. Gonococcal septic arthritis is treated with ceftriaxone, or ciprofloxacin with doxycycline. GAS or *S. aureus* infection is treated with nafcillin and gentamicin, or nafcillin with ciprofloxacin. Prosthetic joints automatically get vancomycin with rifampin and a cephalosporin.

Table 30 Musculoskeletal Infections

Musculoskeletal Infections	
Osteomyelitis	Nafcillin and rifampin or nafcillin with an aminoglycoside.
Diabetic foot ulcers	Tazobactam or ampicillin and sulbactam with an aminoglycoside.
Gonococcal septic arthritis	Ceftriaxone, or ciprofloxacin with doxycycline.
GAS or *S. aureus*	Nafcillin and gentamicin, or nafcillin with ciprofloxacin.
Prosthetic joints	Vancomycin with rifampin and a cephalosporin.

PNEUMONIA

Community acquired pneumonia, with *Mycoplasma* or *Chlamydia* as the likely source, is treated with ceftriaxone or cefuroxime and erythromycin, clarithromycin,, or azithromycin. Quinolones can also be used. In ICU patients, ampicillin and sulbactam or piperacillin and tazobactam are used. With aspiration, ciprofloxacin with clindamycin or metronidazole is used or ampicillin and sulbactam. Bronchiectasis is treated in a similar fashion. Hospital acquired pneumonia with *E. coli, Enterobacter, Pseudomonas*, or *Klebsiella* is treated with piperacillin and tazobactam with tobramycin, or clindamycin and ciprofloxacin, or ceftazidime, or imipenem with an aminoglycoside. Infection with *Staphylococcus aureus* is treated with nafcillin if MSSA; otherwise, vancomycin is used for MRSA.

Table 31 Pneumonia

Pneumonia	
Community acquired *Mycoplasma* or *Chlamydia*	Ceftriaxone or cefuroxime and erythromycin, clarithromycin,, or azithromycin. Quinolones can also be used.
ICU patients	Ampicillin and sulbactam or piperacillin and tazobactam are used.
Aspiration & Bronchiectasis	Ciprofloxacin with clindamycin or metronidazole is used or ampicillin and sulbactam
Hospital acquired-- *E. coli, Enterobacter, Pseudomonas*, or *Klebsiella*	Piperacillin and tazobactam with tobramycin, or clindamycin and ciprofloxacin, or ceftazidime, or imipenem with an aminoglycoside. Infection with *Staphylococcus aureus* is treated with nafcillin if MSSA; otherwise, vancomycin is used for MRSA.

GASTROINTESTINAL INFECTIONS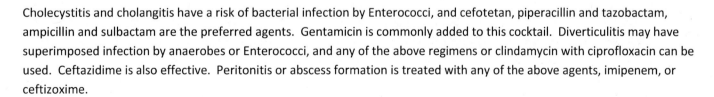

Cholecystitis and cholangitis have a risk of bacterial infection by Enterococci, and cefotetan, piperacillin and tazobactam, ampicillin and sulbactam are the preferred agents. Gentamicin is commonly added to this cocktail. Diverticulitis may have superimposed infection by anaerobes or Enterococci, and any of the above regimens or clindamycin with ciprofloxacin can be used. Ceftazidime is also effective. Peritonitis or abscess formation is treated with any of the above agents, imipenem, or ceftizoxime.

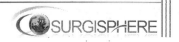

Table 32 GI Infections

GI Infections	
Enterococci	Cefotetan, piperacillin and tazobactam, ampicillin and sulbactam are the preferred agents. Gentamicin is commonly added to this cocktail.
Anaerobes	Any of the above or clindamycin with ciprofloxacin. Ceftazidime is also effective.
Peritonitis or Abscess	Any of the above and imipenem, or ceftizoxime.

GENITOURINARY INFECTIONS

Cystitis is treated with TMP-SMX, cephalexin, or nitrofurantoin. Pyelonephritis with *E. coli* or *Proteus* is treated with TMP-SMX, aminoglycosides, ceftriaxone, or ciprofloxacin. Gram-negative pyelonephritis, or infection with *Pseudomonas* or *Enterococci* is treated with ampicillin and gentamicin, piperacillin and tazobactam with tobramycin, or ciprofloxacin with ampicillin. Prostatitis is treated with ceftriaxone, or ciprofloxacin with doxycycline if the infectious agent is *Neisseria gonorrhea* or *Chlamydia*. Enterobacteriaceae infection is treated with TMP-SMX or ciprofloxacin. Chronic prostatitis is treated in a similar manner.

Table 33 Genitourinary Infections

Genitourinary Infections	
Cystitis	TMP-SMX, cephalexin, or nitrofurantoin.
Pyelonephritis with *E. coli* or *Proteus*	TMP-SMX, aminoglycosides, ceftriaxone, or ciprofloxacin.
Gram-negative pyelonephritis, or infection with *Pseudomonas* or *Enterococci*	Ampicillin and gentamicin, piperacillin and tazobactam with tobramycin, or ciprofloxacin with ampicillin.
Prostatitis Enterobacteriaceae	*Neisseria gonorrhea* or *Chlamydia*--- ceftriaxone, or ciprofloxacin with doxycycline TMP-SMX or ciprofloxacin.

CNS INFECTIONS

Meningitis is commonly treated with a third generation cephalosporin such as ceftriaxone. Ampicillin is often added if the patient is in a high-risk category. Following neurosurgery, vancomycin and ceftazidime are used. Immunosuppressed patients receive ampicillin and ceftriaxone. Recall that Listeria monocytogenes, fungal, mycobacteria, and community acquired infections are especially common in this group. For encephalitis, ACV is likely the only successful regimen. Brain abscesses are treated with ceftriaxone and metronidazole with penicillin G.

Table 34 CNS Infections

CNS Infections	
Meningitis	Third generation cephalosporin such as ceftriaxone. Ampicillin is often added if the patient is in a high-risk category.
Following neurosurgery	Vancomycin and ceftazidime.
Immunosuppressed patients	Ampicillin and ceftriaxone.
Encephalitis	ACV
Brain abscesses	Ceftriaxone and metronidazole with penicillin G.

HEAD AND NECK INFECTIONS

Acute sinusitis is commonly the result of *S. pneumoniae* (TMP-SMX), *H. influenzae* (cefuroxime), or *Moraxella catarrhalis* (amoxicillin and clavulanate). Chronic sinusitis receives amoxicillin with clavulanate. Pharyngitis with GAS (exudative pharyngitis) is treated with penicillin. Ulcerative pharyngitis due to HSV or Coxsackie virus is treated with ACV. Membranous pharyngitis due to EBV or *Diphtheria* receives either no treatment in the former case, or erythromycin for the latter cause. Epiglottitis due to GAS or *H. influenzae* receives cefuroxime or ceftriaxone. Orbital cellulitis can be treated with either cefuroxime or ampicillin with sulbactam. Acute mastoiditis is treated with either dicloxacillin or cefuroxime; cefuroxime is the preferred agent with *S. pyogenes* and *S. aureus*. Chronic mastoiditis is treated with tobramycin with piperacillin and tazobactam. All cases of mastoiditis will likely require surgery.

Table 35 Head and Neck Infections

Head and Neck Infections	
Acute sinusitis	*S. pneumoniae* ---TMP-SMX. *H. influenzae* ---cefuroxime. *Moraxella catarrhalis* ---amoxicillin and clavulanate.
Chronic sinusitis	Amoxicillin with clavulanate.
Pharyngitis with GAS	Penicillin
Epiglottitis due to GAS or *H. influenzae*	Cefuroxime or ceftriaxone.
Acute Mastoiditis	Dicloxacillin or cefuroxime; cefuroxime is the preferred agent with *S. pyogenes* and *S. aureus*. Surgery.
Chronic Mastoiditis	Tobramycin with piperacillin and tazobactam. Surgery.

SEXUALLY TRANSMITTED DISEASES

Urethritis, cervicitis, and prostatitis due to *N. gonorrhea* or *Chlamydia* are treated with ceftriaxone, ciprofloxacin with doxycycline, or ciprofloxacin with azithromycin. Disseminated gonococcal infection is treated with ceftriaxone followed by ciprofloxacin. PID is treated with ceftriaxone with doxycycline or cefotetan with doxycycline. HSV receives ACV or VCV. *Haemophilus ducreyi* leading to chancroid is treated with ceftriaxone, erythromycin, or azithromycin. LGV due to *Chlamydia* is treated with doxycycline. Syphilis due to *Treponema pallidum* is treated with benzathine penicillin or penicillin G if neurosyphilis is present.

Table 36 STDs

STDs	
STD	**Treatment**
Urethritis, cervicitis, and prostatitis due to *N. gonorrhea* or *Chlamydia*	Ceftriaxone, ciprofloxacin with doxycycline, or ciprofloxacin with azithromycin
Disseminated gonococcal infection	Ceftriaxone followed by Cipro.
PID	Ceftriaxone with doxycycline or cefotetan with doxycycline.
HSV	ACV or VCV.
Haemophilus ducreyi	Ceftriaxone, erythromycin, or azithromycin.
LGV due to *Chlamydia*	Doxycyline

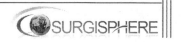

FUNGAL INFECTIONS

Blastomycosis and histoplasmosis are treated with itraconazole or amphotericin B. *Cryptococcus* is treated with amphotericin B with 5-flucytosine (5-FC). Superficial *Candida albicans* infection is treated with fluconazole, 5-FC, miconazole, clotrimazole, or ketoconazole. Fluconazole is used for esophageal infections. Invasive or disseminated Candida infection is treated with amphotericin B or fluconazole. Other fungal infections are commonly treated with amphotericin B, especially if they are life-threatening or rapidly progressing.

Table 37 Fungal Infections

Fungal Infections	
Blastomycosis and histoplasmosis	Itraconazole or amphotericin B
Cryptococcus	Amphotericin B with 5-FC
Superficial *Candida albicans*	Fluconazole, 5-FC, miconazole, clotrimazole, or ketoconazole.
Esophageal infections	Fluconazole
Other fungal infections	Amphotericin B

COMMON ORGANISMS

BACTERIA

GRAM POSITIVE COCCI

STAPHYLOCOCCUS

Table 38 Gram Positive Cocci: Staphylococcus

ETIOLOGY	FEATURES	PATHOPHYSIOLOGY	PRESENTATION	TREATMENT
Staphylococcus aureus	Exotoxin	Superantigen with IL-1/IL-2 synthesis. Toxic shock syndrome from TSS toxin-1 that leads to cytokine release. Scaled skin syndrome from exfoliative toxin release – exotoxins ET-A and ET-B that breakdown tight junctions. Preformed toxin leads to rapid onset of food poisoning.	Toxic shock syndrome – fever, hypotension, distal extremity desquamation, hyperemia. Scalded skin syndrome – exfoliative dermatitis in infants and children leading to sepsis and death Acute bacterial endocarditis Osteomyelitis	Methicillin Vancomycin Cefazolin Clindamycin TMP-SMX Linezolid Dalfopristin Quinopristin

 Staphylococcus spp. form a **biofilm** that protects bacteria from antibiotics. This is the reason why line infections are difficult to treat and may require a line change.

STREPTOCOCCUS

Table 39 Gram Positive Cocci: Streptococcus

ETIOLOGY	FEATURES	PATHOPHYSIOLOGY	PRESENTATION	TREATMENT
Streptococcus pneumoniae	**IgA protease. Encapsulated.**	#1 cause of meningitis in children and elderly, otitis media, and pneumonia.	Meningitis Neonatal conjunctivitis. Otitis media. Pneumonia	Penicillin Ampicillin
Streptococcus pyogenes	GAS Bacitracin sensitive. Exotoxin	Erythrogenic toxin (superantigen) and streptolysin O (ASO titers; hemolysin). M protein antibody. Gas production in necrotizing fasciitis (other causes include *C. perfringens* and *Vibrio*). Superantigen SSA expression may lead to systemic symptoms.	**Pharyngitis** **Cellulitis / Necrotizing fasciitis** **Impetigo / Erysipelas** **Scarlet fever** – erythema, fever, strawberry tongue, desquamation **Toxic shock syndrome** **Rheumatic fever** – erythema marginatum, mitral valve damage **Acute glomerulonephritis (PSGN)**	Penicillin Ampicillin Clindamycin and vancomycin for necrotizing fasciitis

⚐ IgA protease permits organisms to colonize mucosal surfaces and cause infection.

⚐ Encapsulated bugs that cause infection following splenectomy: *S. pneumoniae, N. meningitidis, H. influenzae B., K. pneumoniae.*

GRAM NEGATIVE COCCI

NEISSERIA

Table 40 Gram Negative Cocci: Neisseria

ETIOLOGY	FEATURES	PATHOPHYSIOLOGY	PRESENTATION	TREATMENT
Neisseria meningitidis	**IgA protease.** Maltose and glucose fermenter. **Encapsulated**	Common cause of meningitis.	Meningitis Waterhouse-Friderichsen syndrome.	Vaccination available. Ceftriaxone

GRAM POSITIVE RODS

NON-SPORE FORMERS

Table 41 Gram Positive Rods: Non-Spore Formers

ETIOLOGY	FEATURES	PATHOPHYSIOLOGY	PRESENTATION	TREATMENT
Actinomyces israelii	Obligate anaerobe. Draining sulfur granules (yellow flecks).		**Oral / facial abscess.** **IUD infection.**	Penicillin *(SNAP)*

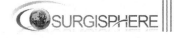

SPORE FORMERS

Table 42 Gram Positive Rods: Spore Formers

ETIOLOGY	FEATURES	PATHOPHYSIOLOGY	PRESENTATION	TREATMENT
Clostridium difficile	Obligate anaerobe	Caused by clindamycin, neomycin, broad-spectrum antibiotics.	**Pseudomembranous colitis** – diarrhea, fever, sepsis.	Vancomycin. Metronidazole.
Clostridium perfringens	Exotoxin Obligate anaerobe.	Lecithinase with gas production.	**Myonecrosis** – gas gangrene with severe infection. **Food poisoning** from reheated meat.	Surgical debridement and IV antibiotics

Serious exotoxin production occurs with Clostridial spp., which can lead to the development of necrotizing fasciitis as soon as six hours following an operation. The clostridial group function as gram positive rods, and are obligate anaerobes. C. perfringens in particular produces several toxins, including a necrotizing, hemolytic Lecithinase (alpha toxin), a hemolysin (theta toxin), a collagenase (kappa toxin), a hyaluronidase (mu toxin), and a deoxyribonuclease (nu toxin). An endotoxin is also produced by this potent bacterium. Rapid spread requiring surgical intervention and serial debridement may be required in the worst cases, and may lead to death even with aggressive therapy. C. difficile produces a potent exotoxin that leads to pseudomembranous colitis leading to diarrhea. Metronidazole or vancomycin are orally given with infection. Cholestyramine can be given to bind toxin. C. tetani produces a neurotoxin that leads to rigidity and muscular spasms, culminating in asphyxiation and death. Treatment is wound debridement and penicillin. C. botulinum produces a neurotoxin leading to GI symptoms, diplopia, and finally paralysis.

GRAM NEGATIVE RODS

AEROBES

Table 43 Gram Negative Rods: Aerobes

ETIOLOGY	FEATURES	PATHOPHYSIOLOGY	PRESENTATION	TREATMENT
Pseudomonas aeruginosa	Blue-green pigment. Lactose nonfermenter. Oxidase positive. **Encapsulated**	Eschar formation in burn patients with secondary infection.	**Burn infections** **Pneumonia in CF** **Sepsis** **Otitis externa** **UTI**	Ampicillin and gentamicin Ceftazidime Ciprofloxacin

FACULTATIVE ANAEROBES

Table 44 Gram Negative Rods: Facultative Anaerobes

ETIOLOGY	FEATURES	PATHOPHYSIOLOGY	PRESENTATION	TREATMENT
Helicobacter pylori	Spirals	Uses urease to breakdown mucus layer and lead to ulcer formation in stomach and duodenum	**Gastritis** **Duodenal ulcer** **Gastric ulcer**	**Bismuth, metronidazole, amoxicillin, clarithromycin, omeprazole.**

ENTEROBACTERIACEAE

Table 45 Gram Negative Rods: Enterobacteriaceae

ETIOLOGY	PATHOPHYSIOLOGY	PRESENTATION	TREATMENT
Enterobacter		Bacteremia, lower **respiratory tract** infection. **Most common cause of liver abscess in a patient with diverticulitis**	Imipenem, cilastatin, Meropenem, Cefepime, Ciprofloxacin.
Escherichia coli	Heat-labile toxin with adenylate cyclase production through ADP ribosylation of Gs protein; heat-stable works on guanylate cyclase.	**Food poisoning** from undercooked meat; watery diarrhea (ETEC). **Bloody diarrhea** (EIEC, EHEC, EHEC O157:H7). **Meningitis** in elderly. **Bacteremia in biliary tract** (most common)	Symptomatic Ampicillin and gentamicin Meropenem Ciprofloxacin
Klebsiella pneumoniae		**Pneumonia** with currant jelly sputum. Cholecystitis (uncommon).	Cefotaxime, Ceftriaxone, Gentamicin, Amikacin, Piperacillin / tazobactam.
Proteus mirabilis	Ammonium magnesium phosphate stones.	**Struvite stones** in UTI.	Ceftriaxone, Gentamicin, Imipenem / cilastatin. Surgical stone removal.
Salmonella enteritidis	Invasive. 10,000 required for disease.	**Food poisoning** from poultry, meat, eggs with bloody diarrhea	Permit natural course as antibiotics will worsen disease. Consider TMP-SMX for systemic disease.

- antigen – polysaccharide of endotoxin; K antigen – capsular antigen (virulence factor); H antigen – found in motile varieties
- Glucose fermenter

ANAEROBES

Table 46 Gram Negative Rods: Anaerobes

ETIOLOGY	FEATURES	PATHOPHYSIOLOGY	PRESENTATION	TREATMENT
Bacteroides fragilis			Normal bowel flora	Neomycin, Clindamycin.

- Obligate anaerobes lack catalase and are foul smelling gas formers.
- B. fragilis is the most common bacterium within the intestine

ATYPICAL BACTERIA

Table 47 Atypical Bacteria

ETIOLOGY	PATHOPHYSIOLOGY	PRESENTATION	TREATMENT
Mycobacterium tuberculosis	Found in the apex of the lung due to the highest PO2.	Tuberculosis – night sweats, fever, anorexia, hemoptysis. Primary: Ghon complex in lower nodes with fibrotic healing and caseating granulomas, progressive disease, bacteremia, or allergic reaction. Secondary: Fibrocaseous cavitation with secondary spread in body.	Rifampin, Isoniazid, Streptomycin, Pyrazinamide, Ethambutol, Cycloserine

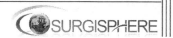

FUNGOLOGY

TOPICAL INFECTIONS

Table 48 Cutaneous Fungal Infections

ETIOLOGY	PATHOPHYSIOLOGY	PRESENTATION	TREATMENT
Candida albicans ⚠	Budding yeast with pseudohyphae and germ tube formation. Water soluble toxin leads to pain.	Oral thrush. Infectious esophagitis. Diaper rash. Vaginal infection.	Nystatin topical therapy. Fluconazole or amphotericin B for systemic infection or vaginal infection. Selenium sulfide for diaper rash.

SYSTEMIC INFECTIONS

Table 49 Systemic Fungal Infections

ETIOLOGY	PATHOPHYSIOLOGY	PRESENTATION	TREATMENT
Aspergillus fumigatus ⚠	Allergic reaction to a septate, monomorphic, hyphae mold. Methenamine silver / PAS +.	Lung cavitary lesions with fungus balls followed by disseminated cutaneous infection. Papules, ulcers, eschars.	Amphotericin B
Coccidioidomycosis ⚠	Hyphal filaments with arthroconidia becoming spherules with endospores.	Primary – flu-like illness and erythema nodosum common in kids and travelers. Systemic – African Americans and other groups with an HLA predisposition leading to skin, tissue, bone, and meningeal infection. Also affects third trimester pregnancy, immunocompromised.	Local: fluconazole Systemic: amphotericin B
Cryptococcus neoformans	Encapsulated yeast, monomorphic. From pigeon droppings. Latex agglutination test. India ink	Meningitis or acute pulmonary infection in IC.	Amphotericin B
Pneumocystis carinii ⚠	Yeast. Methenamine silver stain.	Diffuse pneumonia in IC.	Pentamidine CD4<200 TMP-SMX Dapsone

⚠ Mold form outside body. Yeast form, in warmer temperatures, inside body.

OSTEOMYELITIS ❋

Table 50 Causes of Osteomyelitis

EPIDEMIOLOGY	MOST COMMON	OTHER CAUSES
All persons	*S. aureus*	
Sexually-active	*S. aureus*	*N. gonorrhea*
IVDA	*S. aureus*	*Pseudomonas*
Sickle cell	***Salmonella***	*S. aureus*

PHARYNGITIS

Table 51 Causes of Pharyngitis

EPIDEMIOLOGY	MOST COMMON
Bacterial	GAS, *N. gonorrhea*, HIB, *Mycoplasma*,
Viral	Adenovirus, Influenza, EBV, HSV

PNEUMONIA

Table 52 Causes of Pneumonia

EPIDEMIOLOGY	MOST COMMON	OTHER CAUSES
All patients	*S. pneumoniae*	*Klebsiella, H. influenza, E. coli, Pseudomonas*
Asthma, COPD, smoking, IC	*H. influenzae*	*Klebsiella, E. coli, Pseudomonas, Enterobacter, Serratia*
Alcoholics, DM, COPD	*Klebsiella*	*E. coli, Pseudomonas, Enterobacter, Serratia*
IVDA	*S. aureus*	*E. coli, Pseudomonas, Enterobacter, Serratia*
Outbreaks	*Legionella*	

URINARY TRACT INFECTION

Table 53 Causes of Urinary Tract Infections

EPIDEMIOLOGY	MOST COMMON	OTHER CAUSES
Most persons	*E. coli*	*Klebsiella, S. saprophyticus*
Hospital	*E. coli*	*Proteus, Klebsiella, Serratia, Pseudomonas*

PERIOPERATIVE MANAGEMENT

INDICATORS OF MORBIDITY AND MORTALITY

The most significant perioperative risk factor is an albumin of less than 2.5. According to the Golden criteria, the next most significant criterion is the presence of an **S3 gallop**.

HYPOTHERMIA

Hypothermia is a drop in the core body temperature below 35°C leading to a destabilization in the ability of the body to produce and maintain a normal body temperature. Hypothermia presents with chills, dyspnea, nausea, dizziness, stiffness, weakness, shivering, and ataxia. More severe hypothermia has J waves on EKG, slow reflexes, cold diuresis, delirium, cessation of shivering, and eventually, ventricular fibrillation, hypotension, pulmonary edema, and coma. Treatment of hypothermia is to start ACLS, O2, NG tube, warm hydration, external warming, and core rewarming.

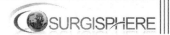

HYPERTHERMIA

Hyperthermia is the result of uncontrolled heat buildup in the body leading to end-organ damage. Several thousand people die every year from hyperthermia, and mortality is high. Hyperthermia evolves after symptoms of heat exhaustion occur, which include constitutional symptoms, headache, dizziness, irritability, myalgia, and muscle cramps. Sudden onset of CNS symptoms and psychosis herald hyperthermia; diaphoresis is as common as anhidrosis. Orthostatic hypotension is present along with piloerection and tachycardia. With heat exhaustion, the body temperature is less than 41°C. With hyperthermia, the temperature is typically more than 41°C (106°F). DIC may be present. Treatment involves cooling the patient with tepid water and large fans after ABCs and IVF.

IMAGING STUDIES

MRI

 The use of gadolinium dye may lead to dizziness and hyperventilation in patients. Using contrast MRI via gadolinium in patients with a creatinine of less than 1.5 may lead to **systemic nephrogenic sclerosis** with systemic fibrosis and ultimately death.

ULTRASOUND

 Imaging of flow is possible when using color in a Doppler ultrasound.

LYMPHOSCINTIGRAPHY

Lymphoscintigraphy is needed for the confirmation of unilateral non-pitting edema.

PRACTICE QUESTIONS

A patient is taking medications that are eliminated via first order kinetics. Which of the following best describes first order kinetics for drug elimination?

A. Elimination cannot be increased by inducing liver function enzymes
B. Half life of the drug is a fixed amount and not related to rate of elimination
C. Rate of elimination is proportional to the concentration of drug in the body
D. Rate of elimination occurs at a certain level independent of drug concentration
E. Volume of distribution is directly related to plasma concentration

The best answer is <u>Rate of elimination is proportional to the concentration of drug in the body</u>. First order kinetics for drug elimination refers to a rate of elimination of drug that is directly proportional to the concentration of drug in the body. As a result, a constant fraction of drug is eliminated per unit of time, and is dependent only on drug concentration. A fixed amount is not eliminated (i.e. 10 mg / min) as in zero order kinetics. Therefore, drug half life is equal to the rate of elimination. Other relationships: loading dose is equal to volume of distribution times the desired steady state plasma concentration; volume of distribution is equal to dose divided by plasma concentration.

A patient on vancomycin is found to have a high trough level. What is the next best step?

A. Decrease the dose and increase the interval
B. Decrease the drug dose
C. Increase the drug dose
D. Increase the interval of dosing
E. Skip the next dose

 The best answer is Increase the interval of dosing. A high vancomycin trough level should lead to an increase in interval, i.e. from 12 hours to 24 hours. A high peak should lead to a decrease in dose.

 An ICU patient being treated for multifactorial sepsis develops erythema multiforme. What is the most likely antibiotic leading to this allergic reaction?

A. Augmentin
B. Cefoxitin
C. Fluconazole
D. Isoniazid
E. Trimethoprim-sulfamethoxazole

 The best answer is Trimethoprim-sulfamethoxazole. Bactrim has been associated with both frequent mild allergic reactions and serious adverse effects including Stevens-Johnson syndrome (and its precursor, erythema multiforme), myelosuppression, mydriasis, agranulocytosis, as well as severe liver damage (cholestatic hepatosis, hepatitis, liver necrosis, fulminant liver failure). Due to displacement of bilirubin from albumin there is an increased risk of kernicterus in the newborn during the last 6 weeks of pregnancy. Also renal impairment up to acute renal failure and anuria has been reported. These side-effects are seen especially in the elderly and may be fatal. The folic acid is likely not the best option for the treatment of some adverse effects with associated with TMP-SMX, a better treatment is probably administration of folinic acid.

 What is the most common bacterium in the colon?

A. B. fragilis
B. E. coli
C. Peptostreptococcus
D. Staphylococcus
E. Streptococcus

 The best answer is B. fragilis. The most common colonic bacteria is the bacteroides species, specifically B. fragilis. The next most common bacterium is E. coli. The most common bacterium of the skin is staphylococcus.

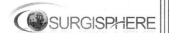

A 27 year old recently postpartum female develops significant right upper quadrant pain. She recalls taking antibiotics for an unrelated condition recently. Ultrasound of the right upper quadrant detects sludge within the gallbladder, but no pericholecystic fluid, no significant stones, and no obstruction. Which of the following antibiotics can lead to sludge formation within the gallbladder?

A. Cefoxitin
B. Ceftriaxone
C. Ciprofloxacin
D. Erythromycin
E. Metronidazole

The best answer is <u>Ceftriaxone</u>. One of the side effects of ceftriaxone, a treatment for gonorrhea, is the formation of biliary sludge. Other causes of sludge formation within the gallbladder include pregnancy, fasting after a gastrointestinal surgery, trauma, TPN, and organ transplantation. Biliary sludge formation is a reversible process.

 Which of the following antibiotics is bactericidal?

A. Chloramphenicol
B. Ciprofloxacin
C. Clindamycin
D. Doxycycline
E. Sulfamethoxazole

The best answer is <u>Ciprofloxacin</u>. The bacteriostatic antibiotics include tetracyclines, clindamycin, sulfa drugs, trimethoprim, chloramphenicol, dapsone, INH, and macrolides. The bactericidal antibiotics include fluoroquinolones, rifampin, and aminoglycosides.

 Which of the following is not an accepted method of decreased the incidence of surgical site infection?

A. 100% FiO2 during the operation
B. 100% FiO2 for six hours in the PACU
C. Decreased temperature in the operating room
D. Preoperative antibiotics
E. Preservation of the sterile field

The best answer is <u>Decreased temperature in the operating room</u>. Decreased body temperature during an operation leads to a dramatic increase in the incidence of infection. The other options are necessary means of minimizing the incidence of surgical site infections.

HEAD AND NECK SURGERY

CHAPTER CONTENTS

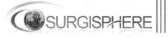

GENERAL CONCEPTS

BRACHIAL PLEXUS

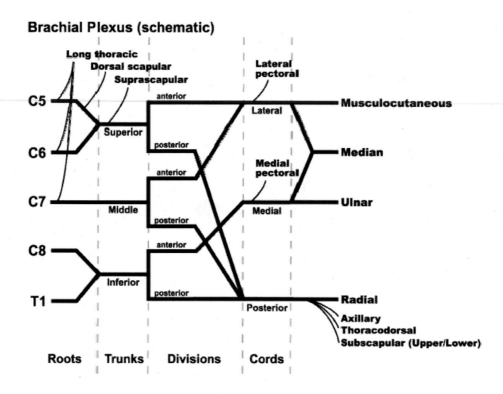

Brachial Plexus (schematic)

- C5 – Shoulder abduction, extension, and external rotation; some elbow flexion

- C6 – Elbow flexion, forearm pronation and supination, some wrist extension

- C7 – Diffuse loss of function in the extremity without complete paralysis of a specific muscle group, consistently supplies the latissimus dorsi

- **C8 – Finger extensors, finger flexors, wrist flexors, hand intrinsics**

    o The ulnar nerve is responsible for innervations to the intrinsic muscles of the hand. Transection of this nerve is not repaired primarily.

- T1 – Hand intrinsics

REFLEXES

- Biceps – C5,C6 (MC nerve)
- Triceps – C6, C7 (radial nerve)
- Knee Jerk – L3, L4 (femoral and common peroneal nerves)
- Ankle Jerk – L5, S1 (tibial nerve)

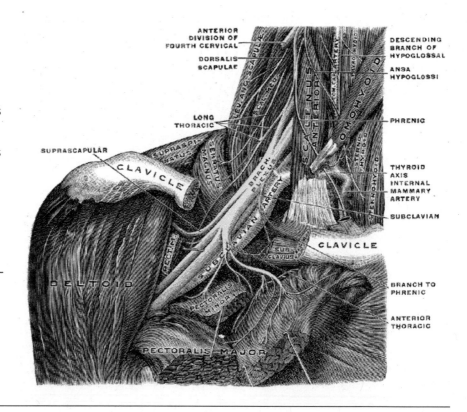

NERVE REGENERATION

- The rate of peripheral nerve regeneration following injury is approximately 1cm per month.

CEREBRAL PERFUSION PRESSURE

Cerebral perfusion pressure is the difference between the mean arterial pressure and intracranial pressure. Normal perfusion pressure is between 80 and 100 mmHg. A decrease in cerebral perfusion pressure occurs with an increase in intracerebral pressure or a drop in systemic pressure. A drop below 60mmHg can lead to significant ischemia.

$$CPP = MAP - ICP$$

METABOLIC AND DEGENERATIVE

DELIRIUM

OVERVIEW

Delirium is characterized by changes in attention and cognition due to a particular medical condition or substance. The most common substance-induced causes of delirium include alcohol or benzodiazepine withdrawal and toxicity from anticholinergic drugs. Delirium predominantly affects hospitalized, post-surgical patients, especially those over 65 and in intensive care units (ICUs). Delirium is hallmarked by a disturbance of consciousness leading to deficits in attention and arousal, an alteration in cognition and memory, relatively rapid development over a period of hours, and a distinct medical condition or substance-related trigger. In delirium, the sleep-wake cycle is disturbed, and profound psychomotor agitation may be present. There may be difficulty separating delirium from dementia, especially since dementia is a positive predictor for the onset of delirium. The key differences are that delirium is reversible, develops relatively quickly, and the presence of an obvious, immediate precipitating factor. Major causes of delirium can be remembered with the mnemonic HIDE, for hypoxia, infection (especially urinary tract infections), drugs (especially anticholinergics), and electrolyte disturbances.

TREATMENT

Delirium carries with it a 50% chance of mortality in one year. Treatment of delirium includes mostly supportive therapy while addressing the cause of the delirium. Haloperidol has been used as an antipsychotic to reduce agitation. Benzodiazepines can also be used as needed. Brightly lit rooms, plenty of cues to help orient the patient, and the presence of health care personnel and family can help reassure a delirious patient.

Table 54 Delirium

Delirium	
Etiology	Alcohol or benzodiazepine withdrawal, anticholinergics drugs.
Presentation	Disturbance of consciousness leading to deficits in attention and arousal, an alteration in cognition and memory, relatively rapid development over a period of hours, and a distinct medical condition or substance-related trigger profound psychomotor agitation.
Differential diagnosis	Delirium is reversible, develops relatively quickly, and the presence of an obvious, immediate precipitating factor, dementia does not.
Treatment	Address cause, supportive therapy, haloperidol, benzodiazepines.

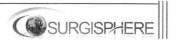

MULTIPLE SCLEROSIS

ETIOLOGY AND PATHOPHYSIOLOGY

Multiple sclerosis (MS) is a progressive, inflammatory, demyelinating disorder of the CNS that leads to various manifestations. Physical disability is inevitable over time and occurs due to the formation of plaques and sclerosis. MS can present as a progressive disorder, relapsing disorder, or a remitting disorder. It is more common in Caucasians in the northern latitudes but the precise environmental factor responsible for MS remains unelucidated. MS leads to infiltration of lymphocytes and macrophages into the nervous tissue followed by expression of various inflammatory cytokines. MS affects some 350,000 patients and they have a decreased lifespan. Males are affected more than females, and a genetic predisposition is apparent in some patients.

PRESENTATION AND DIAGNOSIS

MS presents with intermittent attacks with overall progression to disability. Some patients have mostly intermittent relapses, while others progress more continuously. After a point in the disease, the deterioration progresses more rapidly and neurodegeneration occurs. Weakness and fatigue are universal, and optic nerve dysfunction may occur leading to transient blindness. Cognitive changes occur in some, ataxia in others, along with hemiparesis, depression, and psychomotor changes. Psychiatric changes occur later in life. Color desaturation and patchy vision loss can occur. Bilateral facial weakness and trigeminal neuralgia are strongly indicative of MS. Incontinence and sexual dysfunction are common. CSF examination often indicates oligoclonal banding, normal glucose, normal or high protein, and high WBC count with a high IgG index. MRI is used to localize the regions of sclerosis. Evoked auditory and visual potentials are somewhat sensitive in diagnosis.

TREATMENT

Treatment of MS involves primarily supportive care while minimizing the effects of intercurrent illness and psychomotor stressors. Amantadine or modafinil are beneficial for fatigue mitigation. Disease progression can be slowed with interferon beta-1a, interferon beta-1b, and glatiramer acetate. Acute exacerbations can be minimized with methylprednisone, and high-dose IV steroids may be beneficial in certain situations. Surgical options are available as part of supportive therapy. Medications used for the treatment of MS are effective in delaying the progression, reducing relapses, maintaining a baseline function for a greater period of time, and decreasing the incidence of lesions detected by imaging studies.

Table 55 Multiple Sclerosis

Multiple Sclerosis (MS)	
Etiology	Unknown
Presentation	Weakness and fatigue, optic nerve dysfunction leading to transient blindness. Cognitive changes occur in some, ataxia in others, along with hemiparesis, depression, and psychomotor changes. Bilateral facial weakness and trigeminal neuralgia are strongly indictors. Incontinence and sexual dysfunction are common.
Diagnosis	CSF examination indicates oligoclonal banding, normal glucose, normal or high protein, and high WBC count with a high IgG index. MRI.
Treatment	Supportive care while minimizing the effects of intercurrent illness and psychomotor stressors. Surgical options are available as part of supportive therapy. Medications used for the treatment of MS are effective in delaying the progression, reducing relapses, maintaining a baseline function for a greater period of time, and decreasing the incidence of lesions detected by imaging studies.

MYASTHENIA GRAVIS

ETIOLOGY AND PATHOPHYSIOLOGY

Myasthenia gravis is an autoimmune disorder that leads to weakness and fatigue due to **antibodies versus the acetylcholine receptor (AChR)** and neuromuscular junction (NMJ). MG is very rare, and mortality has decreased significantly with modern therapy. MG can occur at any age and affects females decades before it affects males. MG is typically idiopathic, but exposure to **penicillamine** can cause this disorder. MG is exacerbated by a number of drugs.

 Myasthenia gravis results from antibodies against the nicotinic acetylcholine receptor. First sign is eye muscle weakness.

PRESENTATION AND DIAGNOSIS

MG presents as variable weakness worsened on exertion and improved with rest. **Extraocular muscles (EOM) are weak** and ptosis may be present in many patients. Facial muscle weakness is obvious on physical exam, along with weakness in the bulbar muscles, extremities, respiratory muscles, and ocular muscles. Antibodies against the AChR can be readily demonstrated in most patients. A false positive may be found with SCLC, thymoma, Lambert-Eaton syndrome, RA, and spontaneously in a minority of the population. Antibodies to striated muscle (anti-SM) are found in some patients with MG. CXR is used to rule out thymoma. Electromyography (EMG) is diagnostic, along with repetitive nerve stimulation (RNS).

TREATMENT

MG has no clear treatment. Inhibitors of AChE have been used with some effect; **medications include pyridostigmine and neostigmine**. Plasmapheresis and thymectomy are somewhat beneficial. Plasma exchange (PE) is useful in minimizing exacerbations. Immunomodulation with prednisone, azathioprine, and cyclosporine A (CsA) have some benefit.

Table 56 Myasthenia Gravis

Myasthenia Gravis (MG)	
Etiology	Autoimmune disorder.
Presentation	Weakness worsens on exertion and improves with rest. EOM are weak and ptosis maybe present
Diagnosis	EMG and RNS, facial muscle weakness is obvious on physical exam, along with weakness in the bulbar muscles, extremities, respiratory muscles, and ocular muscles, antibodies against the AChR.
Treatment	No clear treatment. Inhibitors of AChE have been used with some effect; medications. Plasmapheresis and thymectomy are somewhat beneficial. PE is useful in minimizing exacerbations. Immunomodulation with prednisone, azathioprine, and CsA have some benefit.

PSEUDOBULBAR PALSY

A significant finding in pseudobulbar palsy is aspiration due to failure of deglutination.

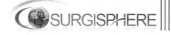

INFLAMMATORY AND INFECTIOUS

BACTERIAL MENINGITIS

ETIOLOGY AND PATHOPHYSIOLOGY

Bacterial meningitis is commonly the result of infection of the pia and arachnoid membranes by *Streptococcus pneumoniae* (over half of all cases), *Neisseria meningitidis, Listeria monocytogenes,* gram-negative rods, *Haemophilus influenzae,* and group B streptococcus (GBS). Young adults are likely to have meningitis from *N. meningitidis*; IC patients are more likely to suffer from *L. monocytogenes*; neonates are likely to acquire GBS perinatally. Infection may occur through the bloodstream, direct invasion, or from otitis or sinusitis.

PRESENTATION AND DIAGNOSIS

Meningitis presents with headache, neck stiffness, fever, and photophobia. Mental status changes leading to worsening Glasgow coma scale scores is common. Seizure is present in some patients. Kernig's sign is typically positive with extension of the knee and thigh leading to pain in the back. Brudzinski's sign is positive demonstrating neck flexion and leads to knee and hip flexion. CBC indicates a leukocytosis with PMNs. Blood cultures are positive in about half of all individuals. Lumbar puncture indicates increased neutrophils, increased protein, low glucose, and high opening pressure. CSF culture is more sensitive than blood culture. The presence of numerous monocytes indicates infection by *L. monocytogenes*.

TREATMENT

Treatment of bacterial meningitis is empirical and typically includes vancomycin plus cefotaxime or ceftriaxone. This is also the standard treatment for *Streptococcus pneumoniae*. If *N. meningitidis* is the identified cause, treatment can proceed with penicillin G or ceftriaxone. *L. monocytogenes* infection is treated with ampicillin and gentamicin.

Table 57 Bacterial Meningitis

Bacterial Meningitis	
Etiology	Infection of the pia and arachnoid membranes by *Streptococcus pneumonia, Neisseria meningitidis, Listeria monocytogenes*, gram-negative rods, *Haemophilus influenzae*, and GBS.
Presentation	Headache, neck stiffness, fever, and photophobia. Seizure is present in some patients.
Diagnosis	Worsening GCS scores. Kernig's and Brudzinski's signs are typically positive. CBC indicates a leukocytosis with PMNs. Blood cultures are positive in about half of all individuals. LP indicates increased neutrophils, increased protein, low glucose, and high opening pressure. CSF culture.
Treatment	Vancomycin plus cefotaxime or ceftriaxone. If *N. meningitidis* is the identified cause, treatment can proceed with penicillin G or ceftriaxone. *L. monocytogenes* infection is treated with ampicillin and gentamicin.

VIRAL MENINGITIS

ASSESSMENT AND MANAGEMENT

Table 58 Viral Meningitis

Viral Meningitis	
Etiology	Virus
Presentation	Similar to bacterial meningitis.
Diagnosis	LP with high WBCs, normal protein and glucose, normal or high opening pressure.
Treatment	Supportive

BRAIN ABSCESS

ASSESSMENT

A brain abscess may develop insidiously or following trauma, surgery, or with spread from a nearby infection such as sinusitis or otitis media. The incidence has increased with AIDS, and mortality is very high if the abscess ruptures. Common causes are *S. aureus*, *S. intermedius*, *Bacteroides*, *Prevotella*, *Fusobacterium*, Enterobacteriaceae, *Pseudomonas*, and other infectious agents. Brain abscess is typically present for only a few weeks prior to diagnosis. Symptoms of neurologic impingement occur, including headache, neurologic changes and deficits, fever, seizures, nuchal rigidity, and papilledema. Rupture may lead to rapid decompensation. Abscess in the cerebellum may lead to defects in motor balance and subsequent ataxia and nystagmus. Abscess in the brainstem may lead to auditory and facial nerve defects. Frontal abscess may lead to mental status changes. Temporal lobe abscess may lead to visual defects. CT is the preferred test to determine the extent of disease.

MANAGEMENT

Surgical excision with long-term antibiotic use is the standard of care following precise planning of the surgical approach with the aid of CT. Penicillin is a good choice against streptococci and staphylococci. Metronidazole is used against gram-negative bacilli. Ceftazidime is used against Pseudomonas. A third generation cephalosporin with metronidazole is commonly used with otitis, mastoiditis, and sinusitis. Dental infections get penicillin and metronidazole. Vancomycin plus a cephalosporin is used following trauma or surgery.

Table 59 Brain Abscess

Brain Abscess	
Etiology	Common causes are *S. aureus*, *S. intermedius*, *Bacteroides*, *Prevotella*, *Fusobacterium*, Enterobacteriaceae, *Pseudomonas*, and other infectious agents.
Presentation	Neurologic impingement, headache, fever, seizures, nuchal rigidity, papilledema.
Diagnosis	CT
Treatment	Surgical excision with long-term antibiotic use is the standard of care following precise planning of the surgical approach with the aid of CT.

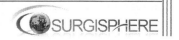

SUPPURATIVE PAROTIDITIS

It most commonly occurs in the elderly following surgery, and is due to obstruction of Stenson's duct leading to retrograde transit of oral flora. It presents with worsening pain and swelling with edema. The most common cause of suppurative parotiditis is by **S. aureus**. The treatment is hydration and appropriate antibiotic coverage. It sufficient therapy is not started soon, Ludwig's angina can develop leading to significant morbidity and mortality.

OTITIS MEDIA

Table 60 Otitis Media

Otitis Media	
Etiology	Dysfunction of the Eustachian tube due to infection.
Presentation	Pain in middle ear. Serous otitis in anyone with a significant history of smoking or alcohol abuse deserves a nasopharyngoscopy as a screening test for cancer.
Treatment	Primarily with amoxicillin or TMP/SMX for a duration of ten days. A beta-lactamase may also be added to the regimen as dictated by resistance, tubes in some children.

VASCULAR

CEREBROVASCULAR ACCIDENTS

EPIDEMIOLOGY

Cerebrovascular accidents (CVA) affect more than 400,000 patients a year with a rapid increase projected over the next 50 years. Stroke is the third leading cause of death; overall, it is the second leading cause of death worldwide. Men are at more risk than women, and up to ¼ of all strokes affect individuals under the age of 65.

ETIOLOGY

Cerebrovascular disease (CVD) and cerebrovascular accidents present with acute focal neurologic deficits commonly due to loss of circulation to a portion of the brain. Also known as a stroke, there are numerous types of CVAs. Broadly, CVA is categorized as either hemorrhagic or ischemic. Ischemic strokes are commonly secondary to embolism from elsewhere in the body or intracranial thrombosis. Disruption of the blood flow leads to neuronal death and infarction of the brain. Common sources of the embolism include valvular or mural thrombi, carotid circulation, and occasionally, the right heart in the presence of a right to left shunt. About 20% of all strokes lead to lacunar infarcts (which involve the subcortical cerebrum and brainstem). Lacunar infarcts are most common in patients with DM and HTN. Lacunar infarcts lead to pure sensory deficit, a pure motor deficit, or a hemiparetic stroke with ataxia. Sources of thrombus formation include the branch points within the circle of Willis and near the internal carotid artery (ICA). Stenosis, atherosclerosis, and platelet defects are common causes of arterial blockade; other causes are hypercoagulable states, polycythemia, and sickle cell anemia. Overall, other causes of stroke include vascular dissection, hypotension, and excessive hemorrhage. Risk factors that increase CVA include increasing age, HTN, smoking, CHD, LVH, atrial fibrillation, hypertriglyceridemia, oral contraceptive use, pregnancy, and hypercoagulable states. Thrombotic strokes are typically slower in onset, while embolic strokes are sudden in onset.

Table 61 Stroke Etiology

Stroke Etiology	
Ischemic	Commonly secondary to embolism from elsewhere in the body, thrombus, stenosis, platelet defect.
Lacunar infarct	DM, HTN.
Hemorrhagic	Excessive bleeding, vascular dissection.
Risk factors	HTN, smoking, CHD, LVH, atrial fibrillation, hypertriglyceridemia, oral contraceptive use, pregnancy, and hypercoagulable states.

ISCHEMIC STROKE

The brain is highly sensitive to disruption in blood supply. An ischemic cascade begins almost immediately following loss of perfusion and eventually leads to irreversible infarction. The area of the brain that still receives some transient blood flow is a region of reversible ischemia; this region forms a sort of penumbra (think of the sun during a full eclipse) around the area of the stroke. The result of ischemia is a failure of membrane transport, large calcium influx, large quantities of neurotransmitter release with additional calcium influx, and local oxidative and ischemic injury. Large amounts of inflammatory mediators are created and free radical injury occurs. Degradation of the cell membrane occurs, and necrosis and apoptosis take place. The region that has infarcted has little chance of restoration. Current medical efforts attempt to save the region of the ischemic penumbra through limitation of toxic free radical formation, reducing the duration of ischemia, and protecting the neurons from additional insults. Reperfusion must take place within 3 hours to avoid permanent damage to the penumbra.

HEMORRHAGIC STROKE

Hemorrhagic stroke is categorized as either subarachnoid bleeds or intracerebral bleeds. Subarachnoid bleeds most commonly occur as the result of head trauma, AV malformations, and aneurysms. Intracerebral bleeds may occur in HTN, bleeding diatheses, and amyloidosis. Hypoperfusion may also lead to stroke and affect especially the parasaggital strips of the cortex (a region known as the watershed area where the end points of the circulation to the brain are located). Hemorrhagic stroke leads to direct injury to neurons by the toxic effects of blood. Compressive injury and electrolyte imbalances worsen the injury. Hemorrhagic strokes worsen with rising in the morning and evolve over a period of minutes.

Table 62 Types of Strokes

Types of Strokes	
Stroke in evolution	Progressive, ongoing injury.
Completed stroke	Irreparable harm to particular region of brain & has been stable for a few days.
Transient ischemic attack	Stroke that resolves within 30 minutes to 24 hours.
Reversible ischemic neurologic deficit	TIA that lasts 24 hours but less than 3 weeks.

PRESENTATION OF STROKE

CVAs present as an acute neurologic deficit or an altered state of consciousness. Numerous constitutional symptoms are typically present in addition to one or more of the following: abrupt onset of paresis, visual deficits, vestibular or hearing

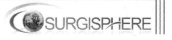

deficits, aphasia, dysarthria, and ataxia. Physical exam may uncover cardiac or vasculature abnormalities or evidence of trauma that can be used to pinpoint the cause of the stroke. A full neurologic exam is required and together with diagnostic testing, can be used to identify the precise site of neurologic injury.

DIAGNOSIS OF STROKE

Noncontrast CT is the initial preferred test and is mandatory for distinguishing the various types of stroke and identifying the particular location of injury. Patients with acute ischemic stroke may entirely bypass this diagnostic study and be taken for immediate therapy. CT has normal findings in the first 6 hours; however, edema over this time leads to changes in the form of a hypodense region. Lumbar puncture should be done in all patients suspected of having a subarachnoid hemorrhage, as CT changes are sometimes nonspecific in this particular etiology. Carotid duplex scanning is done in patients who may have stenosis of the carotid artery, leading to possible endarterectomy in some patients. Echocardiography and other diagnostic studies are also used if particular causes of stroke are suspected. MRI is useful in patients that have a cerebellar or lacunar defect. Angiography is the definitive study that precisely identifies even subtle occlusion.

Table 63 Imaging Tests

Imaging Tests	
Noncontrast CT	Distinguishes various types of strokes; earliest diagnostic test.
Lumbar puncture	Patients suspected of having subarachnoid hemorrhage.
Carotid duplex scanning	Patients who may have stenosis of the carotid artery.
Echocardiography	If particular causes of stroke are suspected.
Angiography	Precisely identifies occlusions.

TREATMENT OF STROKE

GENERAL TREATMENT

Treatment of stroke depends on the particular type and severity of stroke. Basic emergency management includes establishing airway, breathing, and circulation (ABCs), especially with a GCS of less than 9 or dropping GCS scores. Endotracheal intubation may be necessary with increased intracranial pressure (ICP). Hyperventilation is the key to decreasing ICP and cerebral blood flow. Hydration status should be assessed and overhydration prevented. Lowering BP is necessary with HTN, and commonly used agents include nitroprusside and labetalol. Antipyretics should be used with fever, and cerebral edema prevented.

TREATMENT OF STROKE

Use of calcium-channel blockers such as lubeluzole may be beneficial very early in the evolution of stroke to avoid calcium influx. Free-radical scavengers such as tirilazad and citicoline and stabilizers of neuronal membranes such as citicoline are useful later in the ischemic cascade. Antibodies against leukocyte adhesion molecules, such as enlimomab, may serve a neuroprotective role. Anticoagulation with heparin may have some protection in progressive stroke and especially with occlusion affecting the vertebrobasilar artery. However, anticoagulation for stroke has up to a 4% risk of hemorrhage. Contraindications for anticoagulation include concomitant HTN, bleeding diatheses, and intracranial hemorrhage. Tissue-plasminogen activators (t-PA) can be used to restore cerebral blood flow and help resolve an evolving neurologic defect. However, the use of t-PAs such as streptokinase, urokinase, or alteplase can increase mortality in some groups through increased intracranial bleed (which can lead to death in up to half of all patients). Overall, 1 in 8 patients had full recovery with t-PA treatment, 1 in 17 had intracranial bleeds, and 1 in 40 died from complications of therapy. Of all the medications available for t-PA, only alteplase is recommended and approved for therapy; streptokinase is not recommended. t-PA therapy should be given within 3 hours in order to be effective.

TREATMENT OF TIA

TIAs should be treated with antiplatelet agents including aspirin and clopidogrel. Anticoagulation may be necessary with heparin and warfarin. Carotid endarterectomy should be considered if the carotid artery is implicated as a causative agent. Any patient with a stroke that has a contraindication for anticoagulation needs an **IVC filter** if they have additional comorbidities. This includes pathologies such as GI bleed or a DVT. Most practitioners will not begin to heparinize for at least ten days.

Table 64 Treatment of Stroke

	Treatment of Stroke
Emergency	ABCs. Intubation with increased ICP. Hyperventilation to decrease ICP and cerebral blood flow. Avoid overhydration. Lower BP with HTN, antipyretics with fever, and cerebral edema prevented.
Early in evolution	Calcium-channel blockers.
Later in evolution	Free-radical scavengers, antibodies against leukocyte adhesion molecules, anticoagulation.
Treatment of TIA	Antiplatelet agents, possibly carotid endarterectomy.

EPIDURAL HEMORRHAGE

- Etiology: Temporal bone fracture
- Pathophysiology: Middle meningeal artery rupture (branch of maxillary artery)
- Presentation: **Lucid interval followed by rapid deterioration**
- Imaging tests: Mass does not cross suture lines
- **Management: Treated surgically with immediate evacuation**

 Epidural hemorrhage: Lucid interval, needs <u>surgical evacuation</u>
Subdural hemorrhage: Progressive symptoms. <u>Do not evacuate</u> surgically

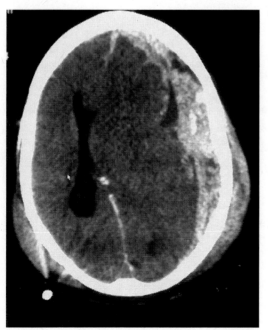

SUBDURAL HEMORRHAGE

- Etiology: Elderly, alcoholics, trauma
- Pathophysiology: Bridging vein rupture with venous bleeding
- Presentation: **Delayed symptoms** followed by progressive deterioration
- Clinical imaging: Crosses suture lines
- **Management: Typically not treated surgically due to continuing bleeding**
- A subdural hematoma is associated with a high mortality rate due to the underlying brain contusion that likely accompanies this presentation.

SUBARACHNOID HEMORRHAGE

- Etiology: APKD, Ehlers-Danlos, Marfan
- Pathophysiology: Berry aneurysm rupture, which may occur at the Circle of Willis bifurcation point especially at the anterior communicating artery.
- Presentation: Worst HA of the patient's life

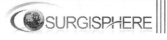

ANTERIOR CEREBRAL ARTERY INFARCTION

- Changes in mental status, impaired judgment, apraxia, and weakness of the contralateral lower extremities, incontinence & personality or behavioral changes.

MIDDLE CEREBRAL ARTERY INFARCTION

- Contralateral hemiparesis and hemiplegia with sensory loss.
- Contralateral hemianopsia, contralateral hemianesthesia.
- Agnosia and aphasia may occur (Wernicke more common), especially if the dominant hemisphere is affected.
- Upper extremity deficits are typically prominent.

POSTERIOR CEREBRAL ARTERY INFARCTION

- Changes in vision, agnosia, defects in memory, and altered mental status.
- Weber (CN III palsy leading to contralateral hemiplegia) & Benedikt (contralateral ataxia) syndromes.
- Contralateral homonymous hemianopia with macular sparing due to occipital lobe injury.

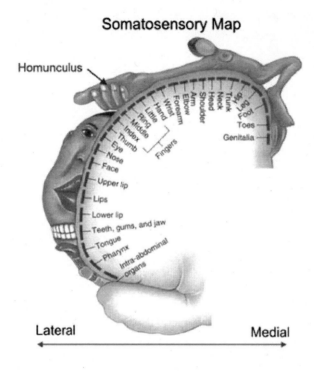

ANTERIOR SPINAL ARTERY INFARCTION

Anterior spinal artery infarction is rare and leads to flaccid paralysis followed by spastic paresis through ischemic damage to the spinal cord. Vibration and proprioception remain intact, but pain and temperature are lost. The presence of anterior spinal syndrome manifests with hyper-reactive deep tendon reflexes.

Table 65 Anterior Spinal Artery Infarction

Anterior Spinal Artery Infarction	
Etiology	Trauma, dissecting aortic aneurysm, aortography, polyarteritis nodosa, hypertensive crisis
Presentation	Flaccid paralysis followed by spastic paresis, loops of pain and temperature.
Diagnosis	Imaging studies
Treatment	Symptomatic

VERTEBROBASILAR ARTERY INFARCTION

Vestibular effects, visual effects, motor defects, and loss of pain and temperature on the ipsilateral face and contralateral body. Mostly affects the pons and leads to locked-in-syndrome

TRAUMA

HEAD TRAUMA

Following severe head trauma, spinal cord function may remain intact with brisk deep tendon reflexes in patients who are brain dead. A patient with a closed head injury who has hypernatremia and a urine osmolarity greater than 300 should receive DDAVP for the treatment of DI. The Cushing response involves bradycardia, hypertension, and irregular respirations, and is a sign of a head injury. Hypotension in the setting of head trauma requires urgent fluid resuscitation. Head trauma with a fracture deviation greater than the width of the skull requires operative intervention for a washout followed by antibiotics. Patients with fractures with limited deviation can be treated conservatively. Most patients with head injury will receive 24 hours of seizure prophylaxis.

GLASGOW COMA SCALE

The Glasgow coma scale is used for rapid neurologic assessment following acute head injury or stroke. It is closely tied to outcome and is often used to dictate therapy in certain instances. The GCS ranges between 3 and 15, with 3 being the worst. Three responses are gauged, including eye response, verbal response, and motor response. The eye responses range from 1-4, and include no eye opening (1 point), eye response to pain (2), eye response to verbal command (3), and spontaneous eye response (4). No verbal response gets 1 point, incomprehensive sounds (2), inappropriate words (3), confused (4), and oriented gets 5 points. Motor responses range from no response (1), extension to pain (2), flexion to pain (3), withdrawal from pain (4), localizing pain (5), and obeying commands (6). A range of 13 or more correlates with mild or nonexistent brain injury. Between 9 and 12 is considered a moderate injury, and less than 9 is a severe injury. **The motor element is the most important response.** An unstable trauma patient with gross peritoneal signs and a widened mediastinum should receive an exploratory laparotomy first. An unstable trauma patient with a light pink diagnostic peritoneal lavage and a pelvic fracture should receive an external fixation of the fracture first.

Table 66 Glasgow Coma Scale (GCS)

Glasgow Coma Scale (GCS)	
Eye response	No eye opening (1 point), eye response to pain (2), eye response to verbal command (3), and spontaneous eye response (4).
Verbal response	No verbal response gets 1 point, incomprehensive sounds (2), inappropriate words (3), confused (4), and oriented gets 5 points.
Motor response	No response (1), extension to pain (2), flexion to pain (3), withdrawal from pain (4), localizing pain (5), and obeying commands (6).
Interpretation	>13 mild or nonexistent brain injury; 12-9 moderate injury; <9 is severe and may require intubation

UNCAL HERNIATION

- Ipsilateral pupilllary dilation with a sluggish reaction suggests uncal herniation. This suggests compromise of the ipsilateral oculomotor nerve.

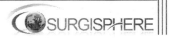

OCULOMOTOR NERVE

- All muscles of eye except superior oblique and lateral rectus
- **Internuclear Ophthalmoplegia**
    - o Signs of right or left eye loss of conjugate gaze
    - o Impaired adduction during lateral gaze of the affected eye
    - o Leads to nystagmus of the affected eye
    - o **MS is the most common cause, and this is often the initial presenting sign**

VAGUS NERVE

- Vagus nerve
    - o Sensory to laryngopharynx
    - o Superior branch is motor to arch IV muscles
    - o PNS
    - o **Damage presents with hoarseness; tends to occur with CEA**
- Recurrent laryngeal branch
    - o Motor to arch VI muscles
    - o Sensory to larynx

HYPOGLOSSAL NERVE

- Motor to tongue

SPINAL CORD COMPRESSION

- Cord compression is commonly the result of tumor, disk herniation, abscess, or hematoma formation – especially in the thoracic levels
- Disturbances to the upper central cord lead to loss of sensory and motor function in the distal upper extremities with sparing of the lower extremities

BROWN-SEQUARD SYNDROME

- Etiology: Brown-Sequard syndrome, CNS trauma, ALS
- Pathophysiology
    - o Damage to CNS with **hemisection of the spinal cord**
    - o Seen in general brain defects, stroke, central tract lesions
- **Presentation: Hemiparesis with some limb drift, hyperreflexia, spasticity, Babinski; loss of contralateral pain and temperature sensation**
- **Damage above T1 leads to Horner syndrome (miosis, ptosis, anhidrosis)** – especially common in lung CA

SPINAL SHOCK

Injuries to the spinal cord are most likely to occur at the cervical level (55%), followed by the thoracic (30%) and lumbar (15%) regions. Intervention requires **methylprednisone** to avoid edema and additional injury. It is continued to 48 hours. Spinal shock may occur with injuries above T5, leading to loss of background excitability from loss of lower pathways, decreased reflex function for at least 1 week and perhaps permanently, and loss of vestibulospinal and reticulospinal pathways. This leads to **bradycardia, vasodilation, and hypotension**. Treatment of spinal shock is with **fluids and pressors**.

PERIPHERAL NERVE INJURIES

ERB-DUCHENNE PALSY

Occurs due to injury to the superior roots of the brachial plexus, **C5 and C6**, leads to paralysis of the following muscles: deltoid, biceps, brachialis, coracobrachialis, brachioradialis, supraspinatus, infraspinatus, teres minor, and subscapularis. The upper limb is adducted at shoulder, medially rotated, and extended at the elbow. Erb-Duchenne palsy is the result from too much traction on the neck, or forcible lateral neck bending, as can occur during delivery. The Moro reflex is absent in an infant.

KLUMPKE PALSY

Klumpke palsy is due to **lower brachial plexus injury**. It occurs when a person grabs something to break a fall or a baby's arm is pulled too much during delivery. The dorsal and ventral roots of the spinal nerves that form the inferior trunk of the brachial plexus (C8 and T1) may be avulsed. As a result, the short muscles of the hand are affected. It presents as claw hand.

SATURDAY NIGHT PALSY

Saturday night palsy is due to injury to the **radial nerve** as a result of a mid-shaft humerus fracture. It leads to wrist drop. The deep branch of the radial nerve can be injured by deep puncture wounds to the forearm, leading to extension of the thumb and the MP joints. Superficial damage leaves a coin-shaped area distal to the bases of the 1st and 2nd metacarpals without sensation.

LARYNGEAL NERVE

- Damage to the superior laryngeal nerve affects the timber of the voice. This frequently leads to loss of high-pitched speech.
- The superior laryngeal nerve is sensory to the supraglottis region.
- Bilateral recurrent laryngeal nerve injury requires permanent tracheostomy to prevent loss of the airway.
- **Damage to a recurrent laryngeal nerve typically requires medialization of the vocal folds to help protect the airway and avoid hoarseness.**

CRICOTHYROIDOTOMY

A cricothyroidotomy is an incision through the cricothyroid membrane and into the trachea. In this procedure, the thyroid cartilage is clearly identified via palpation. Just below the thyroid cartilage is the cricothyroid membrane. Just below this membrane is the cricoid cartilage. **The incision is made through the cricothyroid membrane** (below the thyroid cartilage and above the cricoid cartilage). **Needle cricothyroidotomy can be done for children under 12 years of age and can be used for up to 45 minutes before intubation becomes necessary.**

OTORRHEA

Basilar skull fractures may present with otorrhea. The treatment for traumatic otorrhea is elevation of the head above 30 degrees and observation. Antibiotics are not usually indicated.

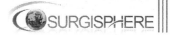

CANCER

SARCOMA

The prognosis with sarcoma is made based off **tumor grade**. Kaposi sarcoma is due to the loss of tumor suppressor genes. Following the diagnosis of a soft tissue sarcoma, a core biopsy should be obtained to evaluate the tissue for staging. A fine needle aspiration is insufficient. Excisional biopsies with 2cm margins are done for tumors less than 5cm. An incisional biopsy is required for all tumors larger than 5cm, and radiotherapy may be required. The most common site for metastasis is the lung. Chemotherapy is used to control metastatic disease.

NECK MASS

A neck mass of less than 4 cm deserves a fine needle aspiration as the initial step in diagnosis. A soft tissue mass **larger than 4 cm receives an incisional biopsy** along the longitudinal plane. Radiotherapy is mandatory for masses larger than 5 cm. The presence of a palpable cervical lymph node in the elderly is the result of metastatic cancer until proven otherwise.

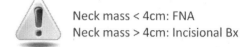

Neck mass < 4cm: FNA
Neck mass > 4cm: Incisional Bx

PAROTID TUMOR

The most common benign parotid tumor is a **pleomorphic adenoma**, which can be treated with a **superficial parotidectomy**. A mobile parotid tumor (typically a low grade acinar tumor) can also be treated with a superficial parotidectomy with sparing of the facial nerve. This is also the treatment of choice when an indeterminate fine needle aspiration results on cytology. 80% of parotid tumors are benign in nature. The most common **malignant** tumor of the parotid is a **mucoepidermoid tumor**, which may elicit a **total parotidectomy**. Every attempt is made to spare the facial nerve unless tumor is it is invaded by tumor.

PRACTICE QUESTIONS

Which of the following is the most common site of an intervertebral disc herniation?

A. L2-L3
B. L3-L4
C. L4-L5
D. L5-S1
E. T12-L1

The best answer is L4-L5. L4-L5 is the most common site of an intervertebral disc herniation, which most commonly presents as a posterolateral herniation. Chronic back pain is common, and loss of big toe dorsiflexion may be a presenting sign with nerve impingement. Foot drop is another presenting sign, along with pain on a straight leg raise. Herniation along L3-L4 leads to a weak knee jerk reflex. Herniation at L5-S1 prevents the patient from standing on their tiptoes, weak ankle jerk, and weak plantar flexion. Treatment is typically with NSAIDs. Lifestyle alterations and physical findings with symptoms over 1-2 months are treated with surgery.

A 32 year old patient involved in an ATV accident presents with a displaced skull fracture of approximately 2cm. What is the next best course of action?

A.   Antibiotics only
B.   Drain placement and observation
C.   Observation
D.   Seizure prophylaxis
E.   Washout, primary closure, and antibiotics

 The best answer is <u>Washout, primary closure, and antibiotics</u> . As this patient has a displaced skull fracture greater than the width of the bone, they should be taken to the OR for a washout and primary closure. Antibiotics are necessary. Skull fractures without significant displacement can be treated with observation only. Seizure prophylaxis is typically required in all circumstances.

 A 59 year old female who recently had a modified radical mastectomy with axillary lymph node dissection reports difficulty with getting herself out of a sitting position. She has difficulty pulling on things with her arm. Which of the following nerves is most likely to have been injured?

A.   Intercostobrachial nerve
B.   Lateral pectoral nerve
C.   Long thoracic nerve
D.   Posterior cord of the brachial plexus
E.   Thoracodorsal nerve

 The best answer is <u>Thoracodorsal nerve</u>. The thoracodorsal nerve supplies the latissimus dorsi, which is responsible for arm and shoulder adduction, a muscle maneuver used to help people get out of sitting positions. The long thoracic nerve leads to winged scapula. The intercostobrachial nerve is a purely sensory nerve to the medial aspect of the upper arm and chest. Injury to the pectoral nerves is uncommon. The posterior cord of the brachial plexus should never be injured in an axillary dissection.

 Which of the following nerves can be injured leading to the inability to make high pitched sounds?

A.   External superior laryngeal nerve
B.   Hypoglossal nerve
C.   Internal superior laryngeal nerve
D.   Recurrent laryngeal nerve
E.   Vagus nerve

 The best answer is <u>External superior laryngeal nerve</u>. The external superior laryngeal nerve travels with the vagus and superior thyroid artery and supplies the cricothyroid muscle. Damage to this nerve prevents the formation of high pitched sounds. The internal superior laryngeal nerve is a sensory nerve that also controls secretions from the larynx.

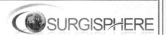

Which of the following is not one of the changes that occur in neurogenic shock?

A.   Decreased CO

B.   Decreased PCWP

C.   Decreased SVO2

D.   Decreased SVR

E.   Increased CVP

The best answer is <u>Increased CVP</u>. In neurogenic shock, injury to the central nervous system and spinal cord may present as warm extremities with hypotension and bradycardia. Fluid resuscitation is required. Presenting signs include a decrease in CVP, CO, SVO2, SVR, and PCWP. Early treatment of spinal shock is pressors.

THORACIC SURGERY

CHAPTER CONTENTS

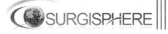

GENERAL CONCEPTS

ANATOMY AND PHYSIOLOGY

LUNG

ALVEOLI

Type I alveoli form the structure of the alveolar wall. **Type II alveoli secrete surfactant** to decrease the surface tension of water and permit gas exchange. Type III alveoli are immune cells that destroy foreign invaders.

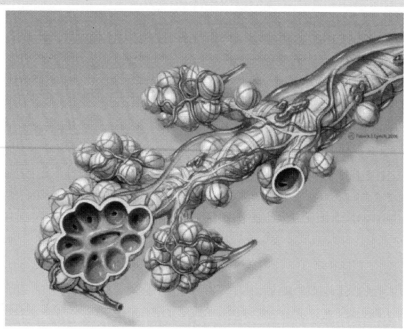

ESOPHAGUS

The layers of the esophagus include the innermost mucosa (which includes the lamina propria), muscularis mucosa, submucosa, muscularis propria (between the inner circular and outer longitudinal muscle layers), then the adventitia. The submucosal plexus is also known as Meissner plexus; the muscular propria plexus is also known as Auerbach plexus.

PULMONARY FUNCTION TESTING

Pulmonary function tests (PFTs) are a mainstay for diagnosis of various pulmonary etiologies. PFTs measure different aspects of lung volume, including the total lung capacity (TLC), residual volume (RV), forced expiratory volume over 1 second (FEV_1), forced vital capacity (FVC), and midmaximal forced expiratory flow (FEF). The permeability of the alveoli is tested with the diffusability of carbon monoxide (D_{LCO}). Bronchial hyperreactivity is tested with a methacholine challenge test, and is contraindicated in asthmatics. Pulmonary vascular resistance increases with hypoxia. **PFTs are required before lung surgery and must have a predicted post-op FEV1 greater than 0.8. FEV1 must be** at least 2L prior to a pneumonectomy, 1L prior to a lobectomy, and 0.6L prior to a wedge resection.

> ⚠️ FEV1 > 0.8L required prior to lung surgery. FEV1 > 2L prior to pneumonectomy.

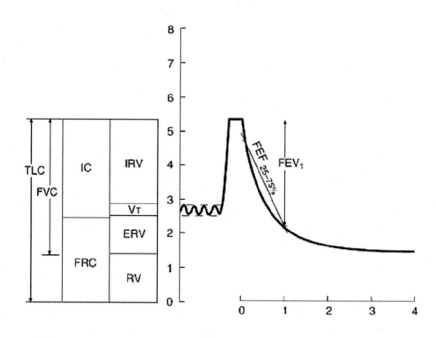

LUNG VOLUMES

The TLC is the entire volume of air that the lung can retain with maximal inspiration. **RV is the remaining volume after maximum expiration**, and is a volume of air that is always present. The vital capacity (VC) is the difference in volume between the TLC and RV. The **functional reserve capacity (FRC) is the volume that remains after a normal breath**, in addition to the RV. The inspiratory capacity (IC) is the maximum inspiratory volume that can be taken in with a normal breath. The IC and FRC add up to the VC, and, as stated above, the VC plus the RV equal the TLC. With a normal breath, the inspiration is known as the tidal volume (V_T). The additional volume that is available for inspiration is known as the inspiratory reserve volume (IRV), while the additional volume available for expiration is the expiratory reserve volume. The IRV plus V_T plus ERV equal the VC. With a normal breath, the ERV is equal to the FRC.

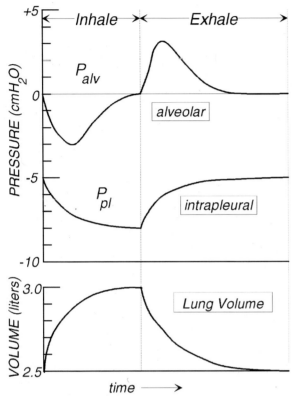

$$TLC = RV + VC = RV + FRC + IC = RV + ERV + V_T + IRV$$

$$VC = FRC + IC = ERV + V_T + IRV$$
$$VC = TLC - RV$$
$$FRC = ERV \text{ (normal breath)}$$

$$\text{Expiratory flow rate} = \frac{FEV_1}{FVC} = FEF$$

The diffusing capacity of the alveoli (D_{LCO}) is generally decreased with interstitial lung disease and emphysema.

⚠ Improving oxygenation in a patient who is already on 100% oxygen with adequate ventilation can be done by improving recruitment of the lung. This is done by increasing the PEEP, which in turn increases FRC.

⚠ Increased ventilation leads to a drop in CO2.

OXYGENATION AND DELIVERY

Disorders with gas exchange can lead to impaired oxygen delivery to vital tissues and present with symptoms of hypoxia. Oxygen transport relies on sufficient cardiac output and hemoglobin of sufficient saturation and quantity. In patients with poor CO or Hgb, giving the patient 100% oxygen does little to improve the oxygenation. Calculating oxygenation can be done with the alveolar-arteriolar gradient:

$$PAO2 = 150 - \frac{PaCO_2}{0.8}$$

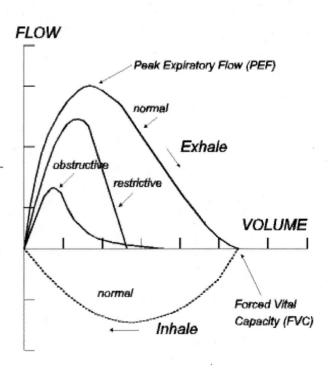

$$A - a \text{ gradient} = P_A O_2 - P_a O_2$$

Faulty gas exchange can manifest as hypoxia. Causes of hypoxia can be attributed to poor ventilation-perfusion (V-Q) mismatch leading to poorly ventilated alveoli or ventilation of poorly perfused alveoli; a right to left cardiac shunt that moves poorly oxygenated blood into the systemic circulation; anemia that leads to decreased oxygen carrying capacity in the blood and subsequent poor oxygenation; poor perfusion from MI or shock; increased oxygen demand with poor increases in supply; impairment in oxygen delivery due to cyanide or carbon monoxide poisoning; and low inspired oxygen at higher altitudes.

Table 67 Causes of Hypoxia

Causes of Hypoxia	
Poor ventilation-perfusion mismatch; and low inspired oxygen at higher altitudes.	A right to left cardiac shunt that moves poorly oxygenated blood into the systemic circulation.
Anemia that leads to decreased oxygen carrying capacity.	Increased oxygen demand with poor increases in supply.
Impairment in oxygen delivery due to CN or CO poisoning.	Poor perfusion from MI or shock.
Low inspired oxygen at higher altitudes.	

The most significant contributor to **oxygen carrying capacity is hemoglobin**. Increasing PO2 over 100 increases oxygen only slightly via increased dissolved oxygen in the blood. Fe^{3+} improves oxygen delivery **Oxygen delivery is defined as the amount of oxygen made available to the body in one minute**. It is equal to the cardiac output times the arterial oxygen content. This is approximately 1,000mL O2 per minute. Oxygen consumption is the amount of oxygen used every minute. Approximately 25% of the arterial oxygen is used every minute (95%+ saturation of blood leaving the heart, ~70% saturation of venous blood returning to the heart). Oxygen extraction decreases with the volume of oxygen, as it becomes harder to remove oxygen from insufficiently populated hemoglobin molecules. SVO2 increases with an increase in cardiac output.

OXYGEN-HEMOGLOBIN DISSOCIATION CURVE

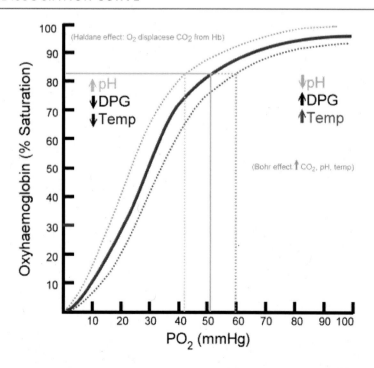

Table 68 Oxygen-Hemoglobin Dissociation Curve Factors

Variable	Right Shift	Left Shift
Temperature	High	Low
2,3 DPG	High	Low
PCO2	High	Low
PCO	Low	High
pH	Acidosis	Alkalosis
Hemoglobin	Adult hemoglobin	Fetal hemoglobin

ARTERIAL BLOOD GAS

The arterial blood gas is used to measure oxygenation of the blood and to determine the nature of any potential hypoxia. ABG measures six values, including pH, PaCO2, PaO2, HCO3, O2 saturation, and base excess. The normal range of pH is 7.35-7.45; PaCO2 ranges from 35 to 45; PaO2 ranges from 80-100; HCO3 ranges from 21-27; O2 saturation ranges from 95-100; and base excess ranges from -2 to +2. Acidosis or alkalosis is determined by the pH. Hypoxemia is determined by the PaO2. Compensation for any potential acidosis or alkalosis is measured by PaCO2 and HCO3. There are certain relationships found in acidosis and alkalosis, depending on the particular etiology:

Acute respiratory acidosis: $\Delta \text{pH} = 0.08 \times \dfrac{(\text{PaCO}_2 - 40)}{10}$

Chronic respiratory acidosis: $\Delta \text{pH} = 0.03 \times \dfrac{(\text{PaCO}_2 - 40)}{10}$

Acute respiratory alkalosis: $\Delta \text{pH} = 0.08 \times \dfrac{(40 - \text{PaCO}_2)}{10}$

Chronic respiratory alkalosis: $\Delta \text{pH} = 0.03 \times \dfrac{(40 - \text{PaCO}_2)}{10}$

A corrected HCO3- is calculated to determine whether there is additional variation in the bicarbonate that was not initially detected due to a changed anion gap. This correction is relatively straightforward:

$$\text{Corrected HCO3-} = \text{measured HCO3-} + (\text{anion gap} - 12)$$

The normal corrected HCO3 should be approximately 24. Significant variation indicates a complex metabolic disturbance – HCO3 more than 24 indicates a coexisting metabolic alkalosis, while an HCO3 less than 24 indicates a coexisting non-anion gap metabolic acidosis.

Finally, the expected respiratory compensation for a metabolic disturbance can be calculated. This is due to a linear relationship between changes in HCO3 and compensation by the lung to change PaCO2. This formula is known as Winter's formula:

$$\text{Expected PaCO2} = (1.5 \times \text{HCO3-}) + (8 \pm 2)$$

A simple metabolic acidosis would lead to a drop in PaCO2 as respiratory compensation. Variation outside of the range specified by Winter's formula indicates a concurrent respiratory disturbance. Winter's formula can only be used for metabolic acidosis; it does not predict the respiratory compensation in response to a metabolic alkalosis. With metabolic alkalosis, the respiratory response will typically lead to a PaCO2 above 40 but less than 50, and alkalotic pH above 7.42.

In short, metabolic acidosis is the abnormal gain in hydrogen ions or loss of bicarbonate. The compensation is increased respiratory ventilation. Changes in lab values include a drop in pH, a drop in PaCO2, and a drop in HCO3. Metabolic alkalosis is the opposite. Respiratory acidosis is abnormal hypoventilation leading to compensation by the body to generate bicarbonate. The changes in lab values are a drop in pH, increase in PaCO2, and an increase in HCO3. Respiratory alkalosis is due to hyperventilation leading to consumption of bicarbonate, with changes in lab values such as a drop in pH and a drop in PaCO2.

Table 69 Arterial Blood Gas (ABG)

Arterial Blood Gas (ABG)	
Measures	Oxygenation of the blood and to determine the nature of any potential hypoxia
Metabolic acidosis	Abnormal gain in hydrogen ions or loss of bicarbonate. Lab values include a drop in pH, a drop in PaCO2, and a drop in HCO3.
Metabolic alkalosis	Abnormal loss in hydrogen ions or gain of bicarbonate. Lab values include a rise in pH, a rise in PaCO2, and a rise in HCO3.
Respiratory acidosis	Abnormal hypoventilation leading to compensation by the body to generate bicarbonate. Lab values indicate a drop in pH, increase in PaCO2, and an increase in HCO3.
Respiratory alkalosis	Due to hyperventilation leading to consumption of bicarbonate, with changes in lab values such as a drop in pH and a drop in PaCO2.

Table 70 Arterial Blood Gas Interpretation

Variable	Normal Range	Notes
pH	7.35 - 7.45	Determines acidosis vs. alkalosis and helps determine the presence of mixed disorders and compensation.
pCO2	35 - 45	PCO2 is determined by ventilation. A high PCO2 with low pH indicates respiratory acidosis. A low PCO2 with high pH indicates respiratory alkalosis. Values above 60 may indicate the need for mechanical ventilation.
pO2	75 - 100	Values below 60 may indicate the need for mechanical ventilation.
HCO3-	22 - 30	Indicates the presence of a metabolic derangement. A low HCO3- indicates metabolic acidosis; high values indicate metabolic alkalosis.
Base excess	-2 - +2	Negative base excess indicates acidosis. Positive values indicate alkalosis.

ACID-BASE

METABOLIC ACIDOSIS

ANION GAP METABOLIC ACIDOSIS

ASSESSMENT AND MANAGEMENT

An anion gap metabolic acidosis is commonly due to **lactic acidosis**, **ketoacidosis** (but not ketone bodies), **uremia** in chronic renal failure, and ingestion of **toxins** such as aspirin, ethylene glycol, methanol, and paraldehyde. Anion gap metabolic acidosis is diagnosed by ketoacids being present (as in alcoholic ketoacidosis, diabetic ketoacidosis [DKA], paraldehyde poisoning, starvation, high-fat diet, and isopropyl alcohol poisoning) or ketoacids being absent (as in renal failure, lactic acidosis, methanol poisoning, ethylene glycol poisoning, and aspirin poisoning). The indications for dialysis include acidosis, hyperkalemia, symptomatic uremia, drug filtration, and fluid overload.

Table 71 Anion Gap Metabolic Acidosis

Anion Gap Metabolic Acidosis	
Etiology	Due to lactic acidosis, ketoacidosis, uremia in chronic renal failure, and ingestion of toxins such as aspirin, ethylene glycol, methanol, and paraldehyde.
Presentation	Decreased DTR, hypotension, paresthesia, coma, and specific EKG changes.
Diagnosis	Ketoacids being present or ketoacids being absent (see above text for discussion).
Treatment	Symptomatic treatment; treat reversible causes; hydration

NON-ANION GAP METABOLIC ACIDOSIS

ASSESSMENT AND MANAGEMENT

A non-anion gap metabolic acidosis is a disturbance common in renal tubular acidosis (**RTA**), **diarrhea**, GI tract **fistulas**, **pancreatic disease**, carbonic anhydrase inhibitors administration, acid ingestion, dilution of alkali, **ileostomy**, and various medications (beta-blockers, spironolactone). Treatment is to correct the underlying etiology but to avoid hypernatremia, fluid overload, and excessive bicarbonate infusion.

Table 72 Non- Anion Gap Metabolic Acidosis

Non-Anion Gap Metabolic Acidosis	
Etiology	RTA, diarrhea, fistulas with the pancreas, carbonic anhydrase inhibitors, acid ingestion, dilution of alkali, ileostomy, and various medications.
Treatment	Correct the underlying etiology but to avoid hypernatremia, fluid overload, and excessive bicarbonate infusion.

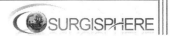

RENAL TUBULAR ACIDOSIS

ASSESSMENT

Renal tubular acidosis occurs in one of four types, of which only three are relevant to the present discussion. RTA type I is known as distal RTA, and occurs with medications such as amphotericin, lithium, and NSAIDs, in nephrolithiasis, sickle cell anemia, infection, and autoimmune disorders. RTA type I presents with inability to acidify urine with secondary hyperaldosteronism, hypokalemia, nephrolithiasis, and nephrocalcinosis. RTA type II is known as proximal RTA, and occurs with Wilson disease, Fanconi syndrome, amyloidosis, vitamin D deficiency, hypocalcemia, hepatitis, and autoimmune diseases. RTA type II leads to basic urine in the early stage until the bicarbonate is lost, then subsequent urine acidification. RTA type II also has hypokalemia, and may lead to osteomalacia and rickets. RTA type IV is known as hypoaldosteronism RTA, and is due to a decrease in aldosterone or insensitivity to angiotensin II, diabetes, Addison disease, sickle cell disease, and renal insufficiency. RTA type IV presents with hyperkalemia and hyperchloremic non-anion gap metabolic acidosis.

MANAGEMENT

RTA type I is treated with oral bicarbonate and potassium replacement. RTA type II is treated with potassium replacement and volume depletion to enhance bicarbonate reabsorption. Thiazide diuretics are also useful. RTA type IV is treated with fludrocortisone, a mineralocorticoid.

METABOLIC ALKALOSIS

ASSESSMENT

Metabolic alkalosis leads to an increase in pH, increased bicarbonate, and increase in PaCO2 (the opposite of metabolic acidosis). Chloride-responsive metabolic alkalosis has a urine chloride of less than 15, and is commonly due to **vomiting**, pyloric stenosis, **laxative** abuse, **diuretics**, and following hypercapnia. Chloride-resistant forms have a urine chloride more than 15, and are commonly a result of severe potassium or magnesium deficiency (as in diuretic abuse), increased **mineralocorticoids**, Bartter's syndrome, chewing tobacco, and licorice consumption.

MANAGEMENT

Neuromuscular excitability, hypokalemia, and hypovolemia are commonly found on exam, and treatment involves correcting the underlying disorder. KCl is sometimes given to correct significant electrolyte abnormalities. Potassium must be corrected first in chloride-resistant metabolic alkalosis.

Table 73 Metabolic Alkalosis

Metabolic Alkalosis	
Etiology	**Chloride-responsive** is commonly due to vomiting, pyloric stenosis, laxative abuse, diuretics, and following hypercapnia. **Chloride-resistant** are commonly a result of severe potassium or magnesium deficiency, increased mineralocorticoids, Bartter's syndrome, chewing tobacco, and licorice consumption.
Diagnosis	Neuromuscular excitability, hypokalemia, and hypovolemia are commonly found on exam.
Treatment	Correct underlying disorder. KCl is sometimes given to correct significant electrolyte abnormalities.

RESPIRATORY ACIDOSIS

ASSESSMENT

Respiratory acidosis is commonly due to **hypoventilation** leading to increased bicarbonate. Causes of respiratory suppression include COPD, airway obstruction, pneumothorax, myasthenia gravis, muscular dystrophy, nervous system disorders (such as Guillain-Barré syndrome [GBS]), botulism, tetanus, organophosphate poisoning, and central depression of the respiratory system (as in narcotic abuse or general endotracheal anesthesia [GETA]). Presenting signs include confusion leading to stupor and coma, and encephalopathy.

MANAGEMENT

Respiratory acidosis is managed by treating the underlying cause, and using artificial ventilation to decrease CO2 retention. Oxygenation of these patients may lead to further depression of the respiratory drive, so only the minimum amount of oxygen via nasal cannula should be provided to maintain oxygenation of the blood.

Table 74 Respiratory Acidosis

Respiratory Acidosis	
Etiology	Commonly due to hypoventilation. Causes include COPD, airway obstruction, pneumothorax, myasthenia gravis, MD, GBS, botulism, tetanus, organophosphate poisoning, and central depression of the respiratory system.
Presentation	Confusion leading to stupor and coma, and encephalopathy.
Treatment	Treating the underlying cause and using artificial ventilation. Oxygenation of these patients may lead to further depression of the respiratory drive. Only the minimum amount of oxygen via NC should be provided.

RESPIRATORY ALKALOSIS

ASSESSMENT

Respiratory alkalosis presents with elevated pH, decrease PCO2, and a decrease in bicarbonate. It is commonly a result of **hyperventilation** (as in anxiety), but may also be a consequence of **shock**, pulmonary disease, pregnancy, **cirrhosis**, **hyperthyroidism**, and **aspirin** poisoning. Presentation is with rapid, deep breathing, anxiety, chest pain, and circumoral paresthesia.

MANAGEMENT

Treatment is to minimize anxiety in the patient, breathing into a paper bag to increase PCO2, and decreasing minute volume, if the patient is artificially ventilated.

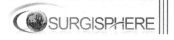

Table 75 Respiratory Alkalosis

Respiratory Alkalosis	
Etiology	Hyperventilation, shock, pulmonary disease, pregnancy, cirrhosis, hyperthyroidism, and aspirin poisoning.
Presentation	Elevated pH, decrease PCO2, and a decrease in bicarbonate, rapid, deep breathing, anxiety, chest pain, and circumoral paresthesia.
Treatment	Minimize anxiety in the patient, breathing into a paper bag, and decreasing minute volume, if the patient is artificially ventilated.

ESOPHAGUS

CONGENITAL AND STRUCTURAL

ACHALASIA

EPIDEMIOLOGY

Achalasia is due to increased LES tone and failure of normal peristalsis of the esophagus, leading to severe dysphagia with solid foods and liquids. Achalasia affects males and females equally. A study in England rated the incidence of achalasia as affecting about 1 in 100,000 patients. **Normal pressures at the LES range from 10-20mmHg with a length of 3-5cm.**

PATHOPHYSIOLOGY

Achalasia stems from a loss of conducting neurons in the esophagus. These neurons are responsible for maintaining the normal progression of peristalsis. Loss of these neurons within Auerbach's plexus is due to scarring, and the primary cause of the scarring is presently being explored. Secondary causes of this scarring can be attributed to invasive lymphoma or gastric carcinoma, scleroderma, and Chagas disease (reminder: Chagas leads to DCM, toxic megacolon, and achalasia).

PRESENTATION

Many of the signs and symptoms of achalasia are secondary to the severe dysphagia that accompanies this disease. Weight loss often results, along with dysphagia with both solids and liquids, and regurgitation of food. The denervation of the esophagus combined with difficulty with normal movements can also exacerbate a cough, and lead to a diffuse chest pain, especially after the consumption of food. Contractions of the esophagus often resemble simultaneous small waves from superior to inferior.

DIAGNOSIS

Diagnosis of achalasia is made by barium swallow, which identifies a **dilated esophagus** and a **bird-beak narrowing** at the inferior aspect. The narrowing at the inferior aspect occurs as a result of **failure of the LES to relax**. Manometry is also used to diagnose achalasia, and findings include a normal to **high pressure at the LES** with no change after swallowing.

 Achalasia: Dilated esophagus, bird-beak narrowing, failure of LES to relax → high LES pressures.

Esophagogastroduodenoscopy (EGD) is required to rule out gastric carcinoma and lymphoma, two infrequent causes of achalasia (about 1% of patients with gastric carcinoma have achalasia). The typical gastric bubble is also missing on plain films of the abdomen.

TREATMENT

Medical treatments for achalasia include: the use of nitroglycerin to relieve symptoms; injection of botulinum toxin into the LES, to block acetylcholine-induced muscle contraction; and calcium-channel blockers, to treat on a symptomatic basis. **Botulinum toxin** injections are successful in about 2/3 patients, but must be repeated over time. Achalasia is surgically treated with **pneumatic dilation** at the LES that tears the muscle fibers (and thereby decreases LES pressure), and permits the semi-normal transport of food and liquid to the stomach. Balloon dilation of the LES can cause perforation in about 1-2% of patients.

Table 76 Achalasia

Achalasia	
Pathophysiology	Loss of conducting neurons with increased LES tone; failure of normal peristalsis; severe dysphagia; weight loss; cough; diffuse chest pain.
Diagnosis	Barium swallow (bird-beak narrowing in inferior esophagus); manometry (normal to high pressure at LES), EGD to rule out gastric carcinoma; gastric bubble absent on plain film.
Treatment	Nitroglycerin to relieve symptoms, calcium channel blockers, botulinum into LES, pneumatic dilation of LES.

DIFFUSE ESOPHAGEAL SPASM

PATHOPHYSIOLOGY AND PRESENTATION

DES is a generalized spasm of the esophagus secondary to failure of activity of the inhibitory neurons within Auerbach's plexus. Spontaneous contractions of the esophagus occur that do not resemble peristalsis. The diffuse contractions in DES lead to dysphagia and chest pain.

DIAGNOSIS

Diagnosis of DES is made by barium swallow and manometry. Barium swallow indicates a **corkscrew-like pattern** due to the uncoordinated activity of various parts of the esophagus. Large waves are seen after swallowing. Manometry confirms the uncoordinated activity of the esophagus and detects high amplitude contractions that may extend into the upper 1/3 of the esophagus. The LES is typically at normal or slightly low pressure.

TREATMENT

Fewer treatments are available for DES than for achalasia due to the lack of ameliorative effect of changing the behavior of the LES. DES sometimes responds to calcium-channel blockers, nitroglycerin, and anticholinergics.

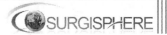

Table 77 Diffuse Esophageal Spasm

Diffuse Esophageal Spasm (DES)	
Pathophysiology	Spasm of esophagus, dysphagia, chest pain.
Diagnosis	Barium swallow (corkscrew-like pattern) & manometry (high amplitude contractions in upper 1/3 of esophagus).
Treatment	Calcium channel blockers, nitroglycerin, and anticholinergics.

NUTCRACKER ESOPHAGUS

PATHOPHYSIOLOGY AND PRESENTATION

Nutcracker esophagus is due to **high-amplitude contractions** that arise from increased activity of the neurons within the esophageal plexuses. It presents similarly to DES, with dysphagia, diffuse chest pain, and large waves of contraction.

DIAGNOSIS AND TREATMENT

Nutcracker esophagus is diagnosed by manometry, which indicates high-amplitude peristaltic contractions. Barium swallow distinguishes between nutcracker esophagus and DES, as the latter has a corkscrew appearance. Treatment is primarily symptomatic and similar to that of DES with the use of nitroglycerin, calcium-channel blockers, and anticholinergic.

Table 78 Nutcracker Esophagus

Nutcracker Esophagus	
Pathophysiology	High-amplitude peristaltic contractions, dysphagia, chest pain.
Diagnosis	Manometry (high-amplitude contractions). Barium swallow (differentiates from DES in that DES has corkscrew appearance Nutcracker does not).
Treatment	Same as with DES.

ESOPHAGEAL OBSTRUCTIONS

EPIDEMIOLOGY AND PATHOPHYSIOLOGY

Plummer-Vinson syndrome and Schatzki rings are two of the most common anatomic esophageal obstructions that can occur. Plummer-Vinson syndrome is characterized by hypopharyngeal webs in conjunction with iron-deficiency anemia. It is most common in middle-aged women. Plummer-Vinson syndrome presents with complaints of dysphagia immediately after swallowing food. Schatzki rings are narrow mucosal rings located in the lower esophagus just proximal to the LES with concomitant dysphagia. Schatzki rings affect both males and females, and appear to target individuals with pre-existing symptoms of intermittent dysphagia. Nearly 10% of Schatzki rings are asymptomatic.

DIAGNOSIS AND TREATMENT

Both Plummer-Vinson syndrome and Schatzki rings are diagnosed with barium swallow. Treatment is through balloon dilation of the rings, which is the preferred method of treating Schatzki rings. Plummer-Vinson syndrome often requires more involved surgical management. Complications of Plummer-Vinson syndrome include an elevated risk of squamous cell carcinoma.

Table 79 Esophageal Obstructions

Esophageal Obstructions	
Etiology	**Plummer-Vinson--** hypopharyngeal webs in conjunction with iron-deficiency anemia **Schatzki rings--** narrow mucosal rings located in the lower esophagus
Diagnosis/ Treatment	Barium swallow, balloon dilation, surgery
Complications	Plummer-Vinson-- elevated risk of squamous cell carcinoma

ZENKER DIVERTICULUM

ETIOLOGY AND PATHOPHYSIOLOGY

Zenker diverticulum is the presence of a **pouch** extending outside of the esophagus due to a defect in the **muscular layer** below the epithelium. It is specifically located between the thyropharyngeus and cricopharyngeus muscles. It is most common in the **posterior hypopharynx** where the muscular layer is thinner and in the upper 1/3 of the esophagus. It leads to dysfunction of the cricopharynx.

PRESENTATION AND DIAGNOSIS

Zenker diverticulum presents with halitosis, aspiration of ingested contents through **regurgitation** of food, and esophageal obstruction leading to **dysphagia**. **Noisy eating** with progressive dysphagia is a hallmark. Diagnosis is through barium swallow which identifies the outpouching as a contrast-filled region. Endoscopy and intubation should not be done due to the risk of perforation.

TREATMENT

Treatment of Zenker diverticulum is through cricopharyngeal myotomy or diverticulectomy.

Table 80 Zenker Diverticulum

Zenker Diverticulum	
Pathophysiology	Pouch extending outside of the esophagus due to a defect in the muscular layer of the epithelium. Typically in posterior hypopharynx.
Presentation/ Diagnosis	Halitosis, aspiration of food, dysphagia. Diagnose through barium swallow.
Treatment	Surgical removal.

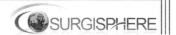

INFLAMMATORY AND INFECTIOUS

GASTROESOPHAGEAL REFLUX DISEASE

EPIDEMIOLOGY

According to a journal article in "Gastroenterology", gastroesophageal reflux disease (GERD) affects nearly 20% of the population on a weekly basis, and nearly 40% of people on a monthly basis. GERD increases the risk of developing Barrett's esophagus and subsequently, esophageal adenocarcinoma.

PATHOPHYSIOLOGY

Gastroesophageal reflux disease is predominantly due to incompetence of the lower esophageal sphincter (LES), leading to reflux of stomach contents into the esophagus. Other causes include the presence of a hiatal hernia, delayed emptying of the stomach, and decreased motility of the esophagus.

LES INCOMPETENCE

Failure of the LES to properly function may be attributed to one or more causes. The high level of progesterone in pregnancy contributes a great deal to the symptoms of heartburn and substernal burning that causes many pregnant women suffering. Consumption of acidic foods and fatty foods, in addition to chocolate, peppermint, alcohol, and coffee can exacerbate LES dysfunction and potentiate the symptoms of GERD. Smoking has also been tied to a decrease in LES tone. Finally, a variety of medications that have effects on muscle tone, such as calcium-channel blockers, β-blockers, nitrates, anticholinergics, and theophylline have been implicated as having a negative effect on maintaining the tone of the LES.

PRESENTATION

The signs and symptoms of GERD include heartburn, dysphagia, increased salivation, cough, and asthma-like symptoms. The hydrochloric acid secreted by the stomach travels up the esophagus due to LES incompetence, and leads to a burning feeling in the epigastric or substernal region, known as heartburn. This pain may occasionally present as chest pain, and so GERD should be on the differential diagnosis of angina and chest pain. Dysphagia in GERD is often a result of the formation of anatomic defects in the esophagus, such as webs and strictures. Increased salivation in GERD leads to a water brash. Cough in GERD is often dry and non-productive. GERD may also exacerbate underlying asthma or may present as symptoms of asthma in certain individuals.

DIAGNOSIS

Diagnosis of GERD is made by a careful consideration of the history and confirmed through the use of a 24-hour pH probe, barium swallow, esophagoscopy, and biopsy. The latter tests are more commonly used in long-standing cases of GERD to rule out histologic changes that may lead to the formation of adenocarcinoma and to detect any underlying anatomical defects.

TREATMENT

GERD is treated by inducing lifestyle changes in the patient in conjunction with the use of medications. In patients highly compliant with lifestyle changes, the use of medications may not be necessary. Lifestyle modifications include obese patients losing weight, promoting the consumption of smaller meals to avoid overburdening the stomach and thereby minimizing reflux, elevating the head of the bed to use gravity to keep food in the stomach, discontinuing the foods mentioned above, cessation of smoking, and eating several hours before bedtime to allow food to travel to the small intestine. A **Nissen fundoplication** can also be done as a surgical repair. Significant retching following this repair requires a gastrograffin swallow study to ensure that the wrap is not too tight. Fundoplication has an 80% success rate.

MEDICATIONS

The first line of medications that is often tried by patients is oral antacids, such as Mylanta and Tums. In GERD that is refractory to lifestyle changes and over-the-counter medications, H2 blockers and/or proton pump inhibitors are commonly used. H2 blockers tend to be curative in about half of all patients, while proton pump inhibitors are even more successful. In patients with an identified anatomical defect, or those who are refractory to medical management, Nissen fundoplication can be used to position the stomach around the lower esophageal sphincter to allow the normal contractions of the stomach and to keep the LES closed.

COMPLICATIONS

GERD is commonly thought of as a relatively benign complaint, but serious complications can develop over a long period of time, if GERD is not appropriately managed. GERD can lead to esophageal damage, which can lead to bleeding and friability. These inflammatory changes are known as **esophagitis**. In about 10% of patients, peptic **strictures** can form that further heighten the symptoms of dysphagia. **Columnar cell metaplasia** of the lower 2/3's of the esophagus can also occur in a condition known as **Barrett's esophagus**. This transformation from the normal squamous cell epithelium predisposes individuals to developing **adenocarcinoma** of the esophagus. Finally, continuing smoking in the face of GERD, in conjunction with damage to the upper 1/3 of the esophagus, can lead to the development of squamous cell carcinoma. The use of certain medications for the treatment of GERD can also lead to **decreased B12 absorption** and impaired absorption of other medications.

Table 81 Gastroesophageal Reflux Disease

Gastroesophageal Reflux Disease (GERD)	
Pathophysiology	Incompetence of LES leading to gastric reflux into esophagus (pregnancy, acidic and fatty food, smoking, medications); hiatal hernia; decreased motility of esophagus, delayed gastric emptying.
Presentation	Heartburn, dysphagia, increased salivation, cough, asthma-like symptoms.
Diagnosis	History, pH probe, barium swallow, esophagoscopy, biopsy.
Treatment	Weight loss in the obese, smaller meals, elevating the head of the bed, avoiding certain foods, medications (H2 blockers, proton pump inhibitors, oral antacids).

SCLERODERMA

ETIOLOGY AND PATHOPHYSIOLOGY

Scleroderma is the autoimmune disorder that causes significant fibrosis throughout the body with numerous systemic effects. Induction of collagen production and a general increase in the matrix (ECM) proteins leads to diffuse fibrosis that affects numerous organs.

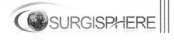

PATHOPHYSIOLOGY AND PRESENTATION

Scleroderma occasionally presents with the CREST syndrome, including calcinosis, Raynaud phenomenon, esophageal dysmotility, sclerodactyly, and telangiectasis. The esophageal dysmotility that may occur with scleroderma and the CREST syndrome is similar to achalasia in that fibrotic changes of the esophagus lead to dysphagia and defects in peristalsis. Unlike achalasia, the LES is incompetent. Esophageal dysmotility in scleroderma presents with progressive dysphagia from solids to liquids and GERD from LES incompetence. Skin changes are among the initial changes detected, and lead to a wrinkling and aged appearance in otherwise younger persons. Fibrosis of arteries can lead to malignant HTN. Pulmonary HTN occurs due to fibrosis of pulmonary vessels, which can lead to RHF. Telangiectasiae are noted throughout the body. Other causes for esophageal dysmotility include SLE, polymyositis, and dermatomyositis.

DIAGNOSIS AND TREATMENT

Esophageal dysmotility in scleroderma is diagnosed with a barium swallow, which indicates **decreased peristalsis** in the lower 2/3's of the esophagus, and decreased smooth muscle contraction on manometry and motility studies. Treatment consists of minimizing the symptoms of GERD, but there is no known treatment for avoiding the esophageal dysmotility. Diagnosis is confirmed by the presence of an **SCL-70 antibody to topoisomerase**, antibodies to centromeres and various components of the nuclei, a normocytic normochromic anemia, elevations in ESR and CRP, and restrictive lung disease (diminished VC on PFT).

Table 82 Scleroderma

Scleroderma	
Etiology	Autoimmune disorder that causes significant fibrosis throughout the body with numerous systemic effects.
Presentation	Skin changes are among the initial changes detected. Esophageal fibrosis presents with progressive dysphagia. Telangiectasiae are noted throughout the body. Scleroderma may also present as part of the CREST syndrome.
Diagnosis	The presence of an SCL-70 antibody to topoisomerase, antibodies to centromeres and various components of the nuclei, a normocytic normochromic anemia, elevations in ESR and CRP, and restrictive lung disease.
Treatment	Therapy for scleroderma includes penicillamine to decrease permanent fibrotic changes, captopril to limit the extent of renal HTN, and calcium-channel blockers to decrease Raynaud's phenomenon.

TRAUMA

ESOPHAGEAL PERFORATION

ETIOLOGY AND EPIDEMIOLOGY

Perforation or rupture of the esophagus is commonly due to trauma to the esophagus, whether through medical procedures or following severe vomiting. Common iatrogenic causes include endoscopy, esophageal dilation, the use of Blakemore tubes, intubation of the esophagus instead of the trachea, and the use of nasogastric (NG) tubes. Leakage of air and ingested contents may occur into the mediastinum, causing mediastinitis and rampant infection. Mortality following perforation or rupture occurs in up to 50% of patients, and is commonly due to uncontrolled hemorrhage. A delay in diagnosis is associated with a rapid increase in mortality. Iatrogenic causes are the most common (60%), followed by spontaneous (15%) and traumatic (20%). Treatment involves primary repair with drainage of the mediastinum and NGT decompression. A Nissen repair is done for abdominal esophagus perforations.

Table 83 Esophageal Perforation

Esophageal Perforation	
Etiology	Trauma to the esophagus (endoscopy, vomiting, dilation, NG tubes, improper intubation).
Presentation	Uncontrolled hemorrhage.
Treatment	Primary repair

BOERHAAVE SYNDROME

Boerhaave syndrome is a **full-thickness tear** of the esophagus typically located in the **left posterolateral portion of the distal 1/3 of the esophagus**. Full-thickness tears are commonly due to forceful vomiting and retching, strong and chronic cough, heavy lifting or physical labor, and direct trauma. Presentation of Boerhaave syndrome is typically with unremitting bleeding and **hematemesis** that quickly leads to death. Those patients with a Boerhaave rupture over six hours require a thoracotomy for resection.

 Boerhaave syndrome: Full-thickness tear in left posterolateral distal esophagus. Tends to kill.

Table 84 Boerhaave Syndrome

Boerhaave Syndrome	
Pathophysiology	Full thickness tear of esophagus located in left, posterolateral, distal 1/3.
Etiology	Forceful vomiting, strong cough, heavy lifting, direct trauma.
Presentation	Bleeding, hematemesis. Severe pain that radiates to the chest, back, and abdomen.
Diagnosis	CXR (identifies pleural effusion and emphysema); esophagogram; endoscopy.
Treatment	Pressure to stop hemorrhage, surgical repair.

MALLORY-WEISS SYNDROME

The most common site of the perforation in Mallory-Weiss syndrome is through the **squamocolumnar junction near the LES**. This is a **partial-thickness tear** that is commonly on the right posterolateral portion of the distal 1/3 esophagus. Presentation of Mallory-Weiss syndrome occurs with transient bleeding and is often secondary to forceful vomiting and retching.

Table 85 Mallory-Weiss Syndrome

Mallory-Weiss Syndrome	
Pathophysiology	Perforation through the squamocolumnar junction near the LES. Transient bleeding, vomiting.
Presentation	Sever pain that radiates to chest , back and abdomen, dysphagia.
Diagnosis	CXR (identifies pleural effusion and emphysema); esophagogram; endoscopy.
Treatment	Pressure to stop hemorrhage, surgical repair.

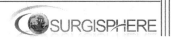

PRESENTATION

Boerhaave and Mallory-Weiss syndromes generally present with the sudden onset of severe pain that radiates to the chest, back, and abdomen. Dyspnea sometimes occurs, especially with bleeding into the pleural cavity. Subcutaneous emphysema and mediastinal emphysema are often present in Boerhaave syndrome due to the leakage of air from the esophagus into those cavities. Mediastinal emphysema presents with a rapid crunching sound known as Hammon's crunch, and is due to expansion of the pericardium with every heart beat against air trapped in the region. Mallory-Weiss syndrome may present with dysphagia. Abdominal pain with back pain after vomiting requires a gastrograffin swallow study in appropriate patients to diagnose this type of tear.

TREATMENT

Diagnosis of esophageal perforation or rupture is often done with a chest x-ray (CXR) that identifies a pleural effusion with mediastinal, pleural, or subcutaneous emphysema. An esophagogram with water-soluble contrast (Gastrograffin) can be done to identify movement of the contrast out of the esophagus and into a cavity in the thorax. Barium cannot be used due to the risk of chemical mediastinitis. Endoscopy and other studies may also be done. Endoscopy is sometimes preferred due to the ability to exert pressure on the bleeding in an attempt to stop the hemorrhage. Emergent surgical repair is required for all episodes of Boerhaave syndrome.

CANCER

BARRETT ESOPHAGUS

PATHOPHYSIOLOGY

Barrett's esophagus is the **transformation of squamous cell epithelium to mucus-producing columnar cell epithelium**. This transformation is likely secondary to an attempt by the body to protect the lower esophagus from continuing damage due to acid reflux from an incompetent LES. Barrett's esophagus occurs due to chronic reflux and over a period of time of continuing symptoms. These metaplastic changes are most common in patients with GERD, affecting some 20% of these patients. Barrett's metaplasia is a strong positive predictor of **adenocarcinoma**, carrying a relative risk of 30 times that of normal. The presence of Barrett's metaplasia plus dysplasia is known as Orringer syndrome.

DIAGNOSIS AND TREATMENT

Diagnosis of Barrett's esophagus is made by examining biopsied specimens for columnar cell epithelium superior to the LES. Treatment is to limit the symptoms of GERD, with medications if possible but surgery if the reflux is refractory to medical management. Repeated EGDs should be done after diagnosis. If no dysplastic changes are present, EGD should be repeated every 5 years. If low-grade dysplasia is present, EGD should be repeated twice a year. **High-grade dysplasia is a strong predictor of adenocarcinoma, and prophylactic esophageal resection should be done**. The risk of adenocarcinoma is

 High-grade dysplasia in Barrett esophagus = esophagectomy.

worsened with concomitant Barrett's esophagus with metaplasia extending about six inches, dysplastic changes, and a history of smoking.

Table 86 Barrett Esophagus

Barrett Esophagus	
Pathophysiology	Metaplasia (squamous cell epithelium to mucous producing columnar epithelium).
Diagnosis & Treatment	Biopsy for columnar epithelium. Limit symptoms of GERD with medications or surgery. Multiple EGDs.

LEIOMYOMA

The presence of a symptomatic esophageal **leiomyoma requires enucleation**, along with any tumor larger than 5cm. It presents as a **smooth filling defect** on a contrast study in a patient with intermittent dysphagia should have enucleation of the masses. It tends to be asymptomatic but may lead to retrosternal pain or dysphagia.

> ⚠ Smooth filling defect with leiomyoma. Treat with enucleation.

ESOPHAGEAL CANCER

EPIDEMIOLOGY AND ETIOLOGY

The most common type of esophageal carcinoma is adenocarcinoma (60-85%), which is typically associated with Barrett's esophagus and occurs more frequently in Caucasian males. Squamous cell carcinoma is more common in African American males over the age of 40 and with a history of smoking. Adenocarcinoma is more likely to occur in the distal 1/3 of the esophagus, while squamous cell carcinoma is more likely in the proximal 1/3 of the esophagus. Adenocarcinoma and squamous cell carcinoma have approximately equal incidence in the middle 1/3 of the esophagus.

PATHOPHYSIOLOGY

Squamous cell carcinoma has a number of risk factors, including a history of alcohol consumption, a long-standing history of smoking, esophageal motility disorders such as achalasia, anatomic defects such as Plummer-Vinson syndrome, and consumption of carcinogens such as foods rich in nitrates and certain spices. The largest positive predictive value of squamous cell carcinoma risk is smoking.

PRESENTATION

With squamous cell carcinoma and adenocarcinoma, the esophageal cancer spreads inward circumferentially to cause progressive dysphagia. Initially, the dysphagia is with solid foods, but it steadily progresses to affect the transport of liquids in the esophagus. The decrease in food consumption, in addition to the effects of the cancer, leads to weight loss, poor nutritional status, and referred pain substernally or to the back. Due to the nature of squamous cell carcinoma, hypercalcemia is sometimes present and can be diagnosed through laboratory tests.

DIAGNOSIS

Diagnosis of esophageal cancer is initially made through barium swallow studies, which will detect **jagged edges** inside the esophagus representing rows of cancerous cells. Biopsy through EGD is required to establish the diagnosis.

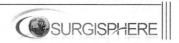

TREATMENT

The primary treatment for esophageal cancer is with **surgical resection**, a procedure that carries a high mortality rate. Indications for esophagectomy include **Barrett's esophagus with high-grade dysplasia** or locally advanced cancer. **Chemotherapy** is standard with a platinum-agent such as cisplatin, and 5-fluorouracil (5-FU). **Radiation** therapy is also used to help prevent recurrence. The majority of tumors metastasize outside of the esophagus on diagnosis, leading to a 5 year survival of less than 10%. Survival is less than 6 months if surgical intervention is not done. Unresectable cancer is followed by bronchoscopy and possible stenting to preserve the airway. Esophageal cancer spreads through the submucosal layer. Of note, 5-FU functions as a dihydrofolate reductase inhibitor leading to inhibition of purine nucleotide synthesis (similar to 6-MP, methotrexate, and cytarabine).

Table 87 Esophageal Carcinoma

Esophageal Carcinoma	
Pathophysiology	Squamous cell carcinoma risk factors: smoking, alcohol, achalasia, carcinogens.
Diagnosis	Barium swallow (detects jagged edges); biopsy through EGD.
Treatment	Surgical resection, chemotherapy (5-FU, cisplatin), radiation.

DIAPHRAGM AND MEDIASTINUM

CONGENITAL AND STRUCTURAL

PNEUMOMEDIASTINUM

ASSESSMENT

Pneumomediastinum, sometimes referred to as mediastinal emphysema, is the result of air in the mediastinum. It is commonly due to rupture of the esophagus, alveolar rupture, tracheal damage, or dissection of the neck or abdomen with an air leak. Pneumomediastinum is treated by reversing the underlying etiology.

DIAGNOSIS

This disease is often found in asthmatics, those with DKA, and those with pernicious vomiting. Hammon's sign is present in 50% of the cases. Confirmation is by radiography demonstrating gas within the mediastinal tissues.

Table 88 Pneumomediastinum

Pneumomediastinum (Mediastinal Emphysema)	
Etiology	Air in mediastinum (ruptured alveoli or esophagus, tracheal damage, surgical air leaks).
Presentation	Intense chest pain that worsens with movement
Diagnosis	Found in asthmatics, those with DKA, and pernicious vomiting. Hammon's sign is present in 50% of cases. Confirmation by radiography demonstrating gas within the mediastinal tissues.
Treatment	Reverse underlying cause.

INFLAMMATORY AND INFECTIOUS

MEDIASTINITIS

ASSESSMENT

Inflammation of the mediastinum may be due to rupture of the esophagus, anthrax infection leading to hemorrhage (nearly 100% fatal), and infection by TB or histoplasma. Mediastinitis presents with constitutional symptoms followed by hypoxia, dyspnea, hemorrhage, and death.

MANAGEMENT

Mediastinitis requires prompt medical attention. The underlying etiology is rapidly treated with antibiotics, including penicillins, fluoroquinolones, and tetracyclines and drainage as necessary.

Table 89 Mediastinitis

Mediastinitis	
Etiology	Rupture of esophagus, anthrax, TB, histoplasma.
Presentation	Hypoxia, dyspnea, hemorrhage.
Diagnosis	CT, CXR
Treatment	Antibiotics, drainage

CANCER

LYMPHOMAS

HODGKIN DISEASE

ETIOLOGY AND PATHOPHYSIOLOGY

Hodgkin lymphoma (HL) is a distinct malignant lymphoma with a **clonal B-cell population** proliferating as Reed-Sternberg (RS) cells. These cells propagate the effects of HL while numerous inflammatory cells lead to local insult and injury. HL accounts for fewer than 1% of all cancers and has a decent 5 year survival rate, if caught early. It is more common in Caucasian males. It has been postulated that infection by **EBV** is a predecessor to HL.

PRESENTATION AND DIAGNOSIS

HL presents with supradiaphragmatic lymphadenopathy (typically seen in the neck and axilla), numerous constitutional symptoms, chest pain, intermittent fever, and pruritus. Hepatosplenomegaly is typically evident on physical exam. On laboratory workup, ESR and LDH are elevated. CBC typically indicates an anemia of chronic disease. CT scans are used to identify the extent of disease, and flow cytometry is the key for diagnosis. The most common site for a single positive lymph node is the **axilla**.

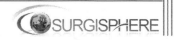

Table 90 Hodgkin Lymphoma Staging

Stage	Features
Stage I	Single lymph node or single extralymphatic site involvement
Stage II	Two or more lymph nodes on the same side of the diaphragm or one lymph node region and one contiguous extralymphatic site
Stage III	Involvement of lymph nodes on either side of the diaphragm (including spleen), or limited contiguous extralymphatic organ involvement
Stage IV	Disseminated disease in extralymphatic organs

TREATMENT

HL is treated with radiation therapy and chemotherapy. The MOPP or ABVD regimen is often used; MOPP stands for the trade names of mechlorethamine, vincristine, procarbazine, and prednisone and ABVD stands for adriamycin, bleomycin, vinblastine, and dicarbazine. Other regimens are also used for HL therapy. BMT is sometimes also used. **PET scans** are used to assess the success of the therapy. Of note, one side effect of bleomycin is pulmonary fibrosis. Adriamycin leads to DNA template disruption and the formation of free radicals. Vinblastine leads to inhibition of mitosis via tubulin binding and subsequent disruption of spindle formation. Staging of Hodgkin lymphoma when supraclavicular and mediastinal lymph nodes are positive without abdominal involvement in a symptomatic patient is stage 2B disease. Staging typically occurs with laparotomy except for stage I disease.

Table 91 Hodgkin Lymphoma (HL)

Hodgkin Lymphoma (HL)	
Etiology	Clonal B-cell population proliferating as RS cells.
Presentation	Supradiaphragmatic lymphadenopathy (typically seen in the neck and axilla), numerous constitutional symptoms, chest pain, intermittent fever, and pruritus. . Hepatosplenomegaly is typically evident on physical exam.
Diagnosis	ESR and LDH are elevated. CBC typically indicates an anemia of chronic disease. CT scans are used to identify the extent of disease, and flow cytometry is the key for diagnosis.
Treatment	Radiation therapy and chemotherapy. MOPP or ABVD regimen is often used. BMT is sometimes also used. PET scans are used to assess the success of the therapy.

NON-HODGKIN LYMPHOMA

ETIOLOGY AND PATHOPHYSIOLOGY

Non-Hodgkin lymphoma (NHL) is a lymphoid tumor with several distinct presentations. It may be due to malignant expansion of **B cells, T cells, natural killer (NK) cells, or macrophages**, but the majority are due to B cell expansion. NHL leads to over 25,000 deaths a year with over 50,000 new cases annually. Patients tend to be middle-aged adults at the time of diagnosis. Causes of NHL include a chromosomal translocation that predisposes to the patient to the lymphoma, history of infection by EBV, human T-cell leukemia virus (HTLV), HCV, and herpesvirus 8 (HHV 8), exposure to certain environmental toxins or chemotherapeutic agents, various congenital causes (severe combined immunodeficiency disease [SCID]), a state of chronic inflammation, and *H. pylori* infection.

PRESENTATION AND DIAGNOSIS

NHL presents as a painless peripheral adenopathy, extension to the **bone marrow** and subsequent pancytopenia, multiple constitutional symptoms, and extranodal manifestations. Bowel obstruction may occur, along with significant growth of the lymphoma leading to cranial nerve impingement. Hepatosplenomegaly is common, and more advanced disease may also present with testicular enlargement, skin lesions, and a mediastinal mass. Workup includes a CBC to detect the extent of the pancytopenia and lymphocytosis, elevation of LDH (which is tied to prognosis), and screen for involvement of other organs through various enzyme function tests. Imaging studies help to identify the extent of the tumor. Stage IV disease is confirmed by bone marrow biopsy. **Laparotomy is not indicated for staging for NHL**; CT scan is sufficient.

TREATMENT

Early stage NHL is treated with radiation therapy, but chemotherapy is sometimes used in high-risk patients. More advanced stages have a combination of radiotherapy and chemotherapy with the CHOP regimen (trade names for cyclophosphamide, hydroxydaunomycin, vincristine, and prednisone) or CVP (cyclophosphamide, vincristine, and prednisone). Monoclonal antibodies such as rituximab have been used with success. More aggressive tumors are treated with high dose chemotherapy, radiotherapy, followed by BMT. NHL is not an indication for laparotomy.

Table 92 Non-Hodgkin Lymphoma (NHL)

Non-Hodgkin Lymphoma (NHL)	
Etiology	Due to malignant expansion of B cells, T cells, NK cells, or macrophages. Majority due to B cells.
Presentation	Painless peripheral adenopathy, extension to bone marrow and pancytopenia, multiple constitutional symptoms, and extranodal manifestations. Bowel obstruction may occur, along with significant growth of the lymphoma leading to cranial nerve impingement. Hepatosplenomegaly is common, and more advanced disease may also present with testicular enlargement, skin lesions, and a mediastinal mass.
Diagnosis	CBC, elevation of LDH, and screen for involvement of other organs through various enzyme function tests. Imaging studies help to identify the extent of the tumor.
Treatment	Radiation therapy, chemotherapy (CHOP regimen or CVP) is used in high-risk patients. Monoclonal antibodies. Aggressive tumor is treated with high dose chemotherapy, radiotherapy, followed by BMT.

PLEURAL CAVITY

CONGENITAL AND STRUCTURAL

THORACIC OUTLET SYNDROME

Thoracic outlet syndrome has a T8-C1 distribution. Anterior scale muscle release leads to resolution of ulnar nerve symptoms and relieves supraclavicular pain. The most common intervention is excision of the first rib. The most common presentation of thoracic outlet syndrome is neurologic, typically presenting as compression of the ulnar nerve. Symptoms are worsened with abduction of the arm. A combination of thoracic outlet syndrome with vein thrombosis is initially treated with thrombolysis, anticoagulation, then excision of the first rib. This disorder is known as Paget-Schroetter disease.

TOS: Resect first rib. Ulnar nerve distribution pattern.

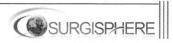

METABOLIC AND DEGENERATIVE

ATELECTASIS

ASSESSMENT

Collapse of a portion of the lung is one of the most common causes of postoperative fever due to activation of **alveolar macrophages** and secretion of **IL1**. Poor inspiratory effort in this period, lack of sufficient coughing and lung expansion, and failure to use devices that aid in inspiration and expiration have all been implicated in the development of lung collapse. Atelectasis presents with fever, tachycardia, dyspnea, tachypnea, and hypoxemia. Deviations of the trachea or elevations of the diaphragm may be present on CXR, while more significant atelectasis may have mediastinal shifts.

MANAGEMENT

Treatment of atelectasis involves incentive spirometry, inducing cough, and deep breathing in an attempt to reperfuse the affected lung regions with air. Treating any concomitant pulmonary disorders is also necessary, along with removing any obstructions or foreign bodies via bronchoscopy. Early ambulation following surgery reduces the risk. Fever is induced by alveolar macrophages. Aspiration pneumonia leading to atelectasis may be treated with nasotracheal suctioning, possible bronchoscopy, and **positive end expiration pressure ventilation**.

Table 93 Atelectasis

Atelectasis	
Causes	Poor inspiratory effort, lack of sufficient coughing and lung expansion, and failure to use devices that aid in inspiration and expiration.
Presentation	Fever, tachycardia, dyspnea, tachypnea, and hypoxemia. Deviations of the trachea or elevations of the diaphragm may be present on CXR, while more significant atelectasis may have mediastinal shifts.
Treatment	Incentive spirometry, inducing cough, and deep breathing. Treating any concomitant pulmonary disorders is also necessary, along with removing any obstructions or foreign bodies via bronchoscopy.

CHRONIC OBSTRUCTIVE PULMONARY DISEASE

ETIOLOGY AND PATHOPHYSIOLOGY

Chronic obstructive pulmonary disease (COPD) includes emphysema and chronic bronchitis. A long-standing expiratory obstruction is present with decreases in FEV1. COPD is an irreversible airway obstruction and presents with significant anatomical and functional changes. Chronic bronchitis presents with a chronic productive cough for at least three months within a two year period. Emphysema presents with airway enlargement distal to the terminal bronchioles. COPD is more common in men and carries a greater mortality in Caucasians. The most common cause of COPD is smoking, followed by air pollution, infection, allergy, and alpha-1-antitrypsin deficiency. Up to 90% of patients with COPD are smokers. Alpha-1-antitrypsin deficiency is an autosomal recessive (AR) disorder that is more common in patients of Mediterranean descent. Liver abnormalities are commonly present in this disorder. The underlying pathophysiology of COPD is increased airway resistance in bronchitis, and decreased lung recoil in emphysema. Patients with chronic bronchitis are typically known as blue bloaters and present with RHF, Polycythemia, and high PCO2 with low O2 on ABG. Patients with emphysema are typically known as pink puffers with a barrel chest, anorexic appearance, and a low PCO2 with normal PO2 on ABG. Congenital lobar emphysema is due to compression of normal alveoli.

PRESENTATION AND DIAGNOSIS

COPD diagnosis is made after physical exam, CXR, and PFTs. Chronic bronchitis presents with ronchi and wheezes upon auscultation; emphysema presents with distant breath sounds. CXR indicates pulmonary markings with chronic bronchitis. Emphysematous changes on CXR include lung hyperinflation, flattening of the diaphragm, small heart size, and increased retrosternal space. PFTs indicate an increased TLC and RV, but a reduction in FEV_1: FVC and FEF. D_{LCO} is decreased in emphysema. As COPD is irreversible, there is typically little change in FEV_1: FVC after administration of bronchodilators. PFT is the diagnostic method of choice for COPD.

TREATMENT

COPD is primarily treated with oxygenation via home oxygen support and nighttime oxygen support. The goal is to maintain PaO2 over 60 and hemoglobin saturated at over 90%. Vaccinations against influenza and *Streptococcus pneumoniae* are mandatory, and antibiotic treatment is given prophylactically against *Haemophilus influenzae* and *Streptococcus pneumoniae* to reduce hospitalization and acute symptoms. Beta agonists are used along with ipratropium bromide, and steroids are used with significantly poor FEV1. The first line treatment is composed of steroids, especially in acute exacerbations. Surgical options are limited, but include lung reduction to improve FEV_1. Regardless of what treatment is used, smoking cessation is mandatory to slow the progression.

PROGNOSIS

Survival in COPD is best predicted by FEV1, with a rapid decline indicative of increased morbidity and mortality. Dyspnea often occurs with exercise (DOE) when FEV1 drops below 50%. FEV1 below 25% often portends dyspnea at rest.

Table 94 Chronic Obstructive Pulmonary Disease (COPD)

Chronic Obstructive Pulmonary Disease (COPD)	
Diagnosis	Physical exam, CXR, and PFTs.
Presentation of bronchitis	Ronchi and wheezes upon auscultation, CXR indicates pulmonary markings.
Presentation of emphysema	Distant breath sounds, lung hyperinflation, flattening of diaphragm, small heart, and increased retrosternal space. PFTs indicate an increased TLC and RV, but a reduction in FEV_1: FVC and FEF. DL_{CO} is decreased, PFTs indicate an increased TLC and RV, but a reduction in FEV_1: FVC and FEF. DL_{CO}.
Diagnosis	PFT, CXR
Treatment	Oxygenation with home oxygen support and nighttime oxygen support. Vaccinations against influenza and *Streptococcus pneumoniae*, and antibiotic treatment given prophylactically against *Haemophilus influenzae* and *Streptococcus pneumoniae*. Beta agonists along with ipratropium bromide, and steroids with poor FEV1. The first line treatment is composed of steroids, especially in acute exacerbations. Surgical options include lung reduction to improve FEV_1. Smoking cessation is mandatory.

ACUTE RESPIRATORY DISTRESS SYNDROME

ETIOLOGY AND PATHOPHYSIOLOGY

Adult respiratory distress syndrome is a severe diffuse alveolar injury that leads to pulmonary infiltrates, hypoxemia, and failure of normal lung function. **Increased permeability of the alveoli** leads to **fluid infiltration** into the alveoli and

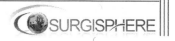

subsequent damage to their sensitive epithelia. Damage occurs primarily to the vascular endothelium or alveolar epithelium, depending on the nature of the infiltrate. **Pulmonary edema occurs with damage mostly to type I cells.** Longstanding damage leads to hypoxemia, pulmonary HTN, and in more severe cases, fibrosis with permanent and progressive pulmonary damage. Limited acute injury typically resolves. It is commonly due to sepsis and leads to significant V/Q mismatches.

PRESENTATION AND DIAGNOSIS

ARDS presents with acute onset of dyspnea and hypoxemia following an identifiable cause (i.e. drug overdose, **sepsis**, acute **pancreatitis**, aspiration). Physical findings include tachypnea, tachycardia, DOE, oxygen supplementation, signs of hypoxia, and signs of the underlying etiology. ARDS often occurs with sepsis and shock. Diagnosis is made by ABG that indicates **respiratory alkalosis or metabolic acidosis,** if ARDS occurs due to sepsis; and CXR that indicates **pulmonary infiltrates bilaterally with alveolar filling.** ARDS is primarily a clinical diagnosis that is confirmed with various diagnostic tests. The **PaO2 / FiO2 is less than 200.**

 ARDS: From sepsis, pancreatitis. Leads to bilateral pulmonary infiltrates and PaO2 / FiO2 < 200. Treat underlying etiology.

TREATMENT

Treatment of ARDS involves treating the underlying etiology. Respiratory support may be necessary. Fluid management is important for certain patients. **Permissive hypercapnia** should be allowed.

Table 95 Adult Respiratory Distress Syndrome (ARDS)

Adult Respiratory Distress Syndrome (ARDS)	
Etiology	Severe diffuse alveolar injury that leads to pulmonary infiltrates, hypoxemia, and failure of lung function.
Presentation	Dyspnea and hypoxemia following an identifiable cause. Tachypnea, tachycardia, DOE, oxygen supplementation, hypoxia, and signs of the underlying etiology. ARDS often occurs with sepsis and shock.
Diagnosis	ABG that indicates respiratory alkalosis or metabolic acidosis if ARDS occurs due to sepsis; and CXR that indicates pulmonary infiltrates bilaterally with alveolar filling.
Treatment	Treating the underlying etiology. Respiratory support. Fluid management is important for certain patients.

INFLAMMATORY AND INFECTIOUS

PNEUMONIA

ETIOLOGY AND PATHOPHYSIOLOGY

Pneumonia is commonly the result of infection by community-acquired sources such as *Streptococcus pneumoniae* or *Haemophilus influenzae*, or hospital acquired sources such as *Pseudomonas aeruginosa, Staphylococcus aureus,* or enteric organisms. Atypical sources of pneumonia include *Chlamydia pneumoniae, Legionella pneumoniae,* and *Mycoplasma pneumoniae*. A common cause of pneumonia in alcoholics, the elderly, and with blood products includes *Klebsiella*, especially if currant jelly sputum is present. Patients with chronic bronchitis are likely to be infected by *Haemophilus influenzae.* Immunocompromised (IC) patients are likely to be infected by *Pneumocystis carinii* pneumonia (PCP). *Streptococcus pneumoniae* presents with rust-colored sputum. It is also the likely cause of a complicated pneumonia arising after influenza.

ETIOLOGY IN IMMUNOCOMPROMISED STATES

HIV patients and others with significant immunocompromise are likely to be infected by a number of atypical sources. With CD4 counts above 200, *Mycobacterium tuberculosis* should be suspected. CD4 counts dropping below 200 should begin a search for, and prophylactic treatment against *Pneumocystis carinii*, *Histoplasma capsulatum*, and *Cryptococcus neoformans*. If the CD4 count continues to drop below 50, cytomegalovirus and MAC should be suspected. Neutropenic hosts should be suspected of having *Pseudomonas aeruginosa* or enteric bacteria. Those with splenectomy may be infected with encapsulated bacteria. Patients who abuse steroids may be infected by *Mycobacterium tuberculosis* or *Nocardia*. Alcoholics, in addition to being infected with *Klebsiella*, may also have *Streptococcus pneumoniae* or *Haemophilus influenzae*.

PRESENTATION AND DIAGNOSIS

Pneumonia generally presents with fever, productive cough, and pleuritic chest pain. Pneumonia is equally likely to present with atypical symptoms, such as dry cough, constitutional symptoms, and generalized GI symptoms. On physical exam, rales and tactile fremitus are typically present. Pectoriloquy is also present with egophony. Diagnosis is made by telltale CXR signs including a lobular or segmental infiltrate (upper lobe if TB or *Klebsiella*), cavities (small in TB, large in many others), and bilateral infiltrates (in PCP and TB). Gram stains are done on sputum samples. Encapsulated organisms may be detected, including *Streptococcus pneumoniae*, *Haemophilus influenzae*, *Klebsiella*, and *Neisseria meningitidis*. An idiopathic eosinophilic pneumonia can occasionally occur, known as Loeffler pneumonia. Elevated LDH is indicative of PCP. No bacteria on smear may be indicative of *Legionella* and *Mycoplasma* spp.

TREATMENT

Inpatient treatment is necessary for patients at extremes of age, residents of nursing homes (NHs), those with chronic conditions, any change in mental status, hypotension, tachypnea, tachycardia, a PaO2 < 60, and those with pleural effusions. Treatment consists of penicillins, cephalosporins, and quinolones. Atypical pneumonias get coverage with erythromycin; hospital-acquired pneumonias are covered for *P. aeruginosa*; and pneumonia in IC patients gets PCP coverage. Aspiration pneumonia is treated with nasotracheal suction and PEEP.

Table 96 Pneumonia

Pneumonia	
Etiology	Commonly the result *Streptococcus pneumoniae* or *Haemophilus influenzae*, or hospital acquired sources.
Presentation	Fever, productive cough, and pleuritic chest pain. It is equally likely to present with dry cough, constitutional symptoms, and generalized GI symptoms.
Diagnosis	CXR signs including a lobular or segmental infiltrate, cavities, and bilateral infiltrates. Gram stains are done on sputum samples.
Treatment	Penicillins, cephalosporins, and quinolones. Atypical pneumonias get coverage with erythromycin.

PNEUMOCYSTIS CARINII

P. carinii infection is a serious concern in HIV patients with a CD4 T-cell count below 200 / mm^3. Prophylaxis should be started in these and otherwise symptomatic patients with bactrim. Aerosolized pentamidine can also be given, although this has been associated with spontaneous pneumothorax and extrapulmonary pneumocystosis. Dapsone has also been shown to be effective in therapy.

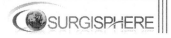

LUNG ABSCESS

ASSESSMENT

A lung abscess is the formation of an infectious cavity with subsequent pulmonary damage. Infectious sources such as *Staphylococcus, Streptococcus, Klebsiella*, HIB, *Actinomyces, Nocardia*, and other sources. Morbidity drastically increases with rupture or developing in high-risk patients, such as those who are immunocompromised. Lung abscess presents with fever, productive cough, night sweats, and weight loss with foul smelling sputum. Hemoptysis is sometimes present. Blood culture and sputum culture are often collected, and a bronchoscopy may be done. Plain films and CT are also done to precisely identify the location of the defect.

MANAGEMENT

Treatment involves clindamycin and specific coverage against identified agents. Hamartomas of the lung present as popcorn lesions on chest X-ray.

Table 97 Lung Abscess

Lung Abscess	
Etiology	Formation of an infectious cavity with subsequent pulmonary damage. Sources include *Staphylococcus, Streptococcus, Klebsiella*, HIB, *Actinomyces, Nocardia*.
Presentation	Fever, productive cough, night sweats, and weight loss with a foul smelling sputum. Hemoptysis is sometimes present.
Diagnosis	Blood culture, sputum culture and bronchoscopy may be done. Plain films and CT are also done to precisely identify the location of the defect.
Treatment	Clindamycin and specific coverage against identified agents.

PLEURAL EFFUSION

ETIOLOGY AND PATHOPHYSIOLOGY

Pleural effusions are transudative or exudative fluid collections within the pleural cavity. Common causes of a transudative effusion are from increased hydrostatic pressure or decreased oncotic pressure, which occurs in CHF, cirrhosis, and nephrotic syndrome. Transudative effusions are likely to be due to systemic causes and are bilateral in nature. Pulmonary embolism is another cause of transudative effusion. Exudative transfusions contain cells and are due to local processes such as cancer, infection, and trauma. Exudative effusions tend to be unilateral. **Pleural fluid has a turnover of 1-2 liters per day**.

PRESENTATION AND DIAGNOSIS

Pleural effusions are diagnosed by thoracentesis and the LDH and protein titers are measured. A LDH greater than 200, a ratio of LDH between the effusion and serum greater than 0.6, and a protein effusion to serum ratio more than 0.5 are indicative of an exudative effusion. Any positive value is indicative of exudative effusion. Transudative effusions have all three numbers below their cut-off values and relative ratios. A parapneumonic effusion is considered if the leukocyte count is greater than 10,000 with a high PMN number; these are always exudative effusions due to the high cellular content. Blood in the effusion brings the differential to trauma, infection, aortic dissection, and malignancy. Low glucose in the effusion leads to the consideration of tuberculosis, empyema, rheumatoid arthritis, and malignancy. Finally, elevated amylase titers require ruling out pancreatitis, renal failure, esophageal rupture, and tumors.

TREATMENT

Transudative and exudative effusions should be treated by treating the underlying cause(s).

Table 98 Pleural Effusion

Pleural Effusion	
Etiology	**Transudative effusion**: increased hydrostatic pressure or decreased oncotic pressure, which often occurs in CHF, cirrhosis, nephrotic syndrome, and pulmonary embolism **Exudative effusions:** Cancer, infection, and trauma, tend to be unilateral.
Diagnosis	Thoracentesis and the LDH and protein titers are measured as well as a leukocyte count. Check for blood, low glucose, and elevated amylase titers. Elevated amylase titers require ruling out pancreatitis, renal failure, esophageal rupture, and tumors.
Treatment	Transudative effusion and exudative effusions should be dealt with by treating the underlying cause(s).

VASCULAR

PULMONARY EMBOLISM

ETIOLOGY

Pulmonary embolism is a challenging diagnosis that must be made to avoid a potentially lethal outcome. PE is commonly due to **venous stasis, intimal injury, and hypercoagulability** (Virchow's triad), and often occurs in deep veins of the lower extremities. Motion of the deep vein thrombus (DVT) leads to travel through the inferior vena cava and eventually into the right atrium, followed by the right ventricle, then through the pulmonary artery into the pulmonary circulation. Large emboli may become lodged at the bifurcation of the pulmonary artery or major branches thereof, leading to a saddle embolus that leads to significant ischemia throughout that region of the lung and concomitant respiratory failure. Other causes of PE include use of oral contraceptives, cancer, thrombophilias (including factor V Leiden, antithrombin III (ATIII) deficiency), **protein C (PrC) deficiency**, protein S (PrS) deficiency, and antiphospholipid antibody (APA).

PATHOPHYSIOLOGY

Respiratory effects of PE include alveolar necrosis, hypoxemia, and hyperventilation. Pulmonary infarction often occurs with untreated PE, and surfactant loss in the affected lung region often occurs, leading to a loss of lung integrity. **Arterial hypoxemia** is a common finding due to ventilation-perfusion (V/Q) mismatch, formation of shunts, decreased cardiac output from increased pulmonary circulation pressure, and patency of a foramen ovale (PFO). Infarction of the lung is rare due to collateral circulation from the bronchial arteries. Increased pulmonary vascular resistance leads to increased RV afterload with subsequent RVH. Sudden increases in load can lead to sudden cardiac death from excessive RV load. Hemodynamic collapse is the effect of large PEs.

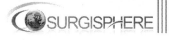

PRESENTATION

A large PE presents with circulatory collapse and death, and is a common cause of death in hospitalized postoperative patients, especially in the elderly. Smaller PEs can present with pulmonary infarction with pleuritic chest pain and hemoptysis. SOB, DOE, pallor, hypotension, and numerous atypical symptoms such as seizures, syncope, abdominal pain, wheezing, CNS changes, atrial fibrillation, and other signs and symptoms complicate the picture. The most common signs and symptoms include tachypnea, rales, tachycardia, S4 gallop, and accentuated P2 heart sound. A sudden decrease in end tidal CO_2 during surgical procedures likely indicates a pulmonary embolism. Most DVTs arise from the iliofemoral circulation.

DIAGNOSIS

PE diagnosis involves a host of exams and imaging studies with variable sensitivity and specificity. The diagnostic testing begins after a thorough history and physical exam are completed. **ABGs** are drawn, and may indicate hypoxemia, hypocapnia, and alkalosis with a decreased A-a gradient. D-dimer is a nonspecific test that indicates fibrin breakdown; it should not be used alone for diagnosis but raises the clinical suspicion if positive. CXR is normal in the acute phase, but later shows dilation of pulmonary vessels, atelectasis, pleural effusions, and an elevated diaphragm (Westermark sign). **V/Q scanning** provides a meaningful diagnosis in many cases; segmental perfusion defects are highly indicative of PE but many patients fall in the intermediate probability category. Additional testing is warranted, and includes ultrasound to detect a DVT, helical **CT with contrast** to identify a significant pulmonary embolus (smaller ones are not detected), and **pulmonary angiography** (the gold standard). MRI and echocardiography have been used with mixed results. Signs of a PE on EKG include ST-T wave changes, right-axis deviation, S waves in lead 1, Q waves in lead 3, and inverted T waves in lead 3 (**S1-Q3-T3**).

TREATMENT

Any patient with a high or medium clinical suspicion with a high-probability V/Q scan, or those with confirmed results should be treated for PE. Anticoagulation therapy starting with heparin followed by warfarin is used; treatment is typically continued for at least six months. **LMWH can also be substituted, especially in pregnant patients**. Thrombolytic therapy is often used in hemodynamically unstable patients and must be given shortly after the event to achieve maximal effectiveness. **An inferior vena cava filter is placed in patients with contraindications to anticoagulation, fragile patients who cannot tolerate another PE, and those with risk of recurrence.** The first occurrence of a DVT is treated with six months of warfarin. The second occurrence of a DVT is treated with one year of warfarin. A repeat occurrence requires lifetime warfarin therapy.

Table 99 Pulmonary Embolism (PE)

Pulmonary Embolism (PE)	
Etiology	Commonly due to venous stasis, intimal injury, and hypercoagulability, and often occurs in deep veins of the lower extremities. Use of oral contraceptives, cancer, thrombophilias, ATIII deficiency, PrC deficiency, PrS deficiency, and APA.
Presentation	A large PE presents with circulatory collapse and death. Smaller PEs can present with pulmonary infarction with pleuritic chest pain and hemoptysis. SOB, DOE, pallor, and hypotension. Common signs and symptoms include tachypnea, rales, tachycardia, S4 gallop, and accentuated P2 heart sound.
Diagnosis	ABG, D-dimer test, CXR , V/Q scanning, segmental perfusion defects, ultrasound, helical CT, pulmonary angiography, EKG.
Treatment	Anticoagulation therapy for at least six months. Thrombolytic therapy must be given shortly after the event to achieve maximal effectiveness. An IVC filter is placed in patients with contraindications to anticoagulation.

Table 100 Indications for IVC Filter

Indications for IVC Filter
DVT or PE in the presence of anticoagulation therapy
DVT or PE with contraindications to anticoagulation therapy (i.e. trauma, head bleeds, GI bleeding)
Persistent DVT or PE with maximum anticoagulation therapy
s/p Pulmonary embolectomy

TRAUMA

SPONTANEOUS PNEUMOTHORAX

ETIOLOGY AND PATHOPHYSIOLOGY

Spontaneous pneumothorax is a potentially devastating disorder that leads to air in the pleural cavity from a sudden rupture of a pleural **bleb**. It is most likely to occur in **tall and thin** people, or in those who **smoke**. Other causes include **COPD, cystic fibrosis**, pneumonia, cancer, and illicit drug abuse. Emphysema with increased airway pressures is due to pneumothorax.

PRESENTATION AND DIAGNOSIS

Spontaneous pneumothorax presents with **pleuritic chest pain and decreased breath sounds**. Hyperresonance due to increased conduction through the air is present on the affected side. The trachea may deviate towards the side of the pneumothorax. Diagnosis includes upright expiratory CXR, where a collapsed lung may be found. EKG changes are sometimes present in the form of ST changes. Volume-control mode on ventilation will increase airway pressures in the event of a pneumothorax.

TREATMENT

Treatment includes oxygen and observation. If the pneumothorax is significant, air may need to be removed via tube thoracostomy. Pleurodesis may be necessary to seal the hole.

Table 101 Spontaneous Pneumothorax

Spontaneous Pneumothorax	
Etiology	COPD, cystic fibrosis, pneumonia, cancer, and illicit drug abuse.
Presentation	Pleuritic chest pain and decreased breath sounds.
Treatment	Oxygen and observation. If the pneumothorax is significant, air may need to be removed via tube thoracostomy. Pleurodesis may be necessary to seal the hole.

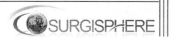

TENSION PNEUMOTHORAX

ETIOLOGY AND PATHOPHYSIOLOGY

Tension pneumothorax occurs with air under pressure within the pleural space, leading to impingement upon the airway and compromise in both ventilation and perfusion of the affected lung region. Tension pneumothorax can occur during general anesthesia due to traumatic intubation (pharyngeal or pyriform sinus perforation) or from injury during central line placement (subclavian > internal jugular). Trauma to the region may also lead to the presence of blood; tension pneumothorax must be excluded in patients with rib fractures or contusions to the chest. High peak inspiratory pressures can also lead to tension pneumothorax through barotrauma.

PRESENTATION AND DIAGNOSIS

It presents similarly to spontaneous pneumothorax, with the addition **of tracheal deviation away** from the side of the pneumothorax, hypotension, and tachycardia. **Diagnosis is made by clinical presentation, not by CXR.** Beware of tension pneumothorax following central line placement. **A tension pneumothorax exerts its physiologic compromise through vena cava compression, leading to decreased venous return. This leads to hypoxia, hypercapnia, hypotension, and sudden death.**

A tension pneumothorax will eventually lead to kinking of the great veins and occlusion of blood flow. A sign of tension pneumothorax while on a mechanical ventilator includes increasing inspiratory pressures. Caudal displacement of the diaphragm is sometimes seen intraoperatively or on a CXR.

Tension pneumothorax: Tracheal deviation away from PTX. Diagnose clinically. Needle decompression followed by chest tube.

TREATMENT

Tension pneumothorax requires emergency management and is treated with decompression by needle followed by tube thoracostomy. **An 18 gauge needle is inserted into the second intercostal space at the mid-clavicular line.** Trauma patients with a pneumothorax should be intubated first (preserve the airway first).

Table 102 Tension Pneumothorax

Tension Pneumothorax	
Presentation	Similar to spontaneous pneumothorax, with the addition of tracheal deviation away from the side of the pneumothorax, hypotension, and tachycardia. Trauma to the region may also lead to the presence of blood.
Treatment	Decompression by needle followed by tube thoracostomy.

PENETRATING PARASTERNAL INJURIES

ASSESSMENT

A parasternal stab wound may present with hypotension and shortness of breath. Diagnosis is made by CXR and EKG. Wounds that are anterior and below the fifth intercostal space also require a FAST and DPL to rule out abdominal injuries.

MANAGEMENT

Treatment includes chest tube placement. **If immediate chest tube output is greater than 1.5L or over 250cc/hr over 4 hours, a thoracotomy is required.** Other indications for thoracotomy include pericardial tamponade and hypovolemic shock, and a left anterolateral exposure is preferred. "Trap door" incisions can be made to expose a large length of the left subclavian or carotid artery. The presence of a widened mediastinum, hypotension, and the lack of hemothorax deserve evaluation for an aortic injury.

 Chest tube output > 1.5L or 250cc/hr over 4 hours = thoracotomy.

BLUNT PARASTERNAL INJURIES

ASSESSMENT

Deceleration injuries following a fall or motor vehicle accident may lead to shear injuries causing damage to important vascular structures in the chest. This primarily includes the **ligamentum arteriosum**, which is torn distal to the left subclavian. The majority of these injuries result in death prior to arrival in the ER.

CANCER

OVERVIEW

EPIDEMIOLOGY

The leading cause of cancer-related death is due to lung cancer, and is the number one killer in both men and women. Over 160,000 people die annually in the United States, surpassing the total number of deaths from breast cancer, prostate cancer, and colorectal cancer. Lung cancer has very high morbidity and mortality with only a fraction of patients surviving after five years. By the time tumors are found, malignant metastasis has already occurred in most people with rapid spread through lymph nodes and blood to the liver, adrenal glands, bones, and brain. The vast majority of lung cancer can be traced back to a longstanding history of smoking, and a history of smoking invariably worsens the prognosis of lung cancer. About 95% of all lung cancers are either small cell lung cancer (SCLC) or non-small cell lung cancer (NSCLC). Rarer varieties include carcinoid, lymphoma, metastatic cancers to the lung, and others. Of the NSCLCs, adenocarcinoma (adenoCA) and squamous cell carcinoma (SCC) are the most common, each making up 30% of all lung cancers. SCLC makes up another 30%. Overall, adenocarcinoma makes up 45% of all lung cancers, followed by squamous cell cancer at 30%, small cell cancer at 20%, and large cell cancer at 10%.

ETIOLOGY

Without question, the most significant positive predictor of lung cancer risk is a history of smoking. Further, the number of cigarettes smoked, the number of years of smoking, and the age that smoking started are specific positive predictors of risk. Other causes make up about 15% of all lung cancers, and include secondhand smoke, air pollution, asbestosis, chronic lung disease (including TB and COPD), radon exposure, exposure to heavy metals, and a prior history of lung cancer. One affected **oncogene** is **K-ras**, which is transformed through **point mutation**.

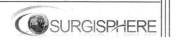

PRESENTATION

Lung cancer presents without symptoms in up to a quarter of patients at the time of diagnosis. The remainder develops a new, progressive cough that is sometimes blood-tinged, pleuritic chest pain, SOB, wheezing, hoarseness, recurrent URIs, and systemic effects based on metastasis. Paraneoplastic syndromes can also occur with production of gastrin, ACTH, ADH, calcitonin, ANF, and PTHrP. The result can be clubbing, metastatic ossification, anemia, weakness, constitution symptoms, neural degeneration, anorexia, and hyponatremia. **Squamous cell cancers tend to occur centrally, while adenocarcinomas tend to occur peripherally.**

DIAGNOSIS

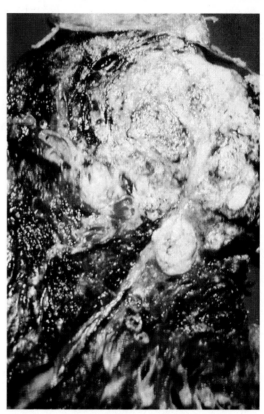

Lung cancer is diagnosed by a number of exams. A careful smoking history and complete physical exam are necessary. CXR is typically the first test, but abnormalities may include only small nodules in early cases – they may even be entirely negative due to the low sensitivity of this exam. **CT and MRI** are more sensitive and can detect smaller nodules, and are also useful for staging; a CT of the chest and abdomen is typically completed, along with the head as indicated. Biopsy, sputum testing, and bronchoscopy are other methods of obtaining cells and tissue for additional analysis. Collection of fluid via thoracentesis, or open procedures such as thoracotomy is necessary to collect an adequate tissue sample. **Local spread is often gauged by a mediastinoscopy. Definitive diagnosis is made by a thoracoscopic wedge resection.** Approximately half of all lung cancers are metastatic at the time of diagnosis. **A PFT with FEV1 > 0.8 is required prior to lung surgery. An FEV1 > 2L is required prior to pneumonectomy, over 1L for a lobectomy, and 0.6L for a wedge resection.** PCO2 > 60 and poor DLCO ratios are all prohibitive risks for lung resection due to the elevated chance for permanent ventilation.

FEATURES AND TREATMENT OF SCLC

The treatment of SCLC differs compared to NSCLC. SCLC tends to be more aggressive and rapidly growing. Histology often indicates dark nuclei with little cytoplasm. **SCLC produces gastrin, ACTH, ADH, ANF, and calcitonin**, which can lead to a number of secondary effects. The result can be clubbing, metastatic ossification, anemia, weakness, constitution symptoms, neural degeneration, anorexia, and hyponatremia. Treatment of SCLC involves **radiotherapy** and **chemotherapy**, as the majority of these tumors respond well to this modality. **Surgical resection is typically not possible.** SCLC has a low 5 year survival.

FEATURES AND TREATMENT OF NSCLC

SCLC = gastrin, ACTH, ADH, ANF, calcitonin
NSCLC = **PTHrP**

NSCLC features cells with pleomorphic nuclei and large amounts of cytoplasm. **NSCLC (i.e. squamous cell carcinoma) produces PTHrP.** This type of tumor is less responsive to radiotherapy, and barely responsive to chemotherapy. However, **surgical resection is an option** in cases with limited spread. Five year survival is better for NSCLC than it is for SCLC.

PROGNOSIS

Palliative care is often the final outcome of therapy when dealing with lung cancer. This is due to the high rate of recurrence, in which many lung cancers are present again within 2 years. Pain management with hospice care involves the use of high dose opioids and NSAIDs as indicated. Oxygen administration is often the key to patient comfort. The primary method of avoiding the lethal pitfalls of lung cancer is avoidance – smoking cessation is the first and most important step to reducing the risk of lung cancer. Survival with stage I NSCLC have a 70% 5 year survival; stage II offers a 30% survival, stage III offers a 20% survival, and higher stages offer only a 9 month survival period. SCLC that is treated with chemotherapy has a 10% 5 year survival; advanced SCLC has a 6 month survival period.

SCREENING

Some institutions offer CT scans as a screening test in high risk patients; early data appears to indicate that CT scans can detect lung cancer earlier, and in some patients, this may lead to earlier treatments and potential surgical resection before significant metastasis occurs. Whether this translates into less morbidity and mortality over a 5 year period remains to be determined.

COMPLICATIONS

Lung cancer is associated with numerous syndromes, including **superior vena cava syndrome**, **Horner syndrome**, **Pancoast tumor**, **SIADH**, **Eaton-Lambert syndrome**, and **Trousseau syndrome**. Superior vena cava syndrome occurs due to compression of the SVC with swelling of the upper extremity, head, and neck. Cough, headache, epistaxis, and syncope are commonly associated symptoms. SVC syndrome is most likely due to lung cancer (90%). It is treated with radiotherapy. Horner syndrome presents with paralysis of the sympathetic nerve due to damage to the ganglion; it presents with ptosis, enophthalmos, miosis, and anhidrosis. Pancoast tumor presents with damage to the 8th cervical nerve, 1st and 2nd thoracic nerve, and damage to the ribs that leads to pain that radiates to the ipsilateral arm. Pancoast tumor can lead to Horner syndrome, vessel or nerve compression, and injury to underlying structures. SIADH presents with hyposmolality and hyponatremia. Eaton-Lambert syndrome occurs with an autoimmune reaction to nerve terminals leading to decreased release of acetylcholine (ACh). Trousseau syndrome is a hypercoagulable state that leads to venous thrombosis. Right upper lobectomies require the use of a rigid 90 degree bronchoscope.

STAGING

Table 103 Lung Cancer Staging

Lung Cancer Staging	
Stage I	N0 with no direct invasion and greater than 2cm from the carina
Stage II	N+ with ipsilateral hilar nodes, no metastasis
Stage III	Invasion of chest wall, diaphragm, pericardium, or the presence of positive mediastinal lymph nodes
Stage IV	Metastatic cancer

MEDIASTINAL MASSES

- Anterior Mediastinum: Thymoma, thyroid enlargement, T-cell lymphoma
- Middle Mediastinum: Vascular lesion, enlarged lymph nodes
- Posterior Mediastinum: Neurogenic tumor

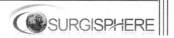

PRACTICE QUESTIONS

 A 28 year old male involved in a knife fight presents to the ER with several penetrating stab wounds to his right chest. Two chest tubes are inserted and his tension pneumothorax resolves. Over the next 4 hours, the patient has a chest tube output of 300 cc / hr. What is the next step in management?

A.   Chest CT
B.   Exploratory laparotomy
C.   Observation
D.   Pulmonary resection
E.   Thoracotomy

The best answer is <u>Thoracotomy</u>. This patient will go to the operating room for an immediate thoracotomy. Indications following placement of a chest tube include a spontaneous output of over 1500 cc upon placement, or an output rate of 200cc / hr over 4 hours. Any loss of vital signs or tamponade on FAST will lead to an ER thoracotomy. Left thoracoabdominal penetrating injuries require laparoscopy to exclude damage to abdominal organs. The best step in management of any questionable patient is immediate exploratory laparotomy of the abdominal cavity in hypotensive patients without other obvious primary causes.

 A 47 year old male who has had some difficulty with ventilation has an increase in his PEEP to 15. A transient decrease in urine output is noticed. Which of the following is the next step in management?

A.   Aggressive fluid boluses
B.   Decrease PEEP as tolerated
C.   FENA
D.   Observation
E.   Renal ultrasound

The best answer is <u>Decrease PEEP as tolerated</u>. This patient has an increase in thoracic pressure from the increase in PEEP, leading to release of renin and oliguria. Treatment is to decrease PEEP as tolerated. Fluid boluses are not necessary, and observation is not the initial best step in management. PEEP serves to avoid collapse of functional alveoli, thereby increasing recruitment and FRC / VC. PaO2 thereby increases. PEEP should be avoided in COPD due to the risk of puncture. Of the alveoli, type I cells are squamous and type II are glandular. The right upper lobe has the highest oxygen concentration, and so is also the site of most bacterial abscesses.

A 28 year old male presents to clinic with a small, firm, but mobile anterior neck mass. What is the next best step in management?

A. Excisional biopsy
B. Fine needle aspiration
C. Lymph node dissection
D. Observation
E. Open lymph node biopsy

 The best answer is <u>Fine needle aspiration</u>. All anterior neck masses initially undergo a fine needle aspiration as part of their workup. An excisional biopsy can be completed if additional testing is required. An open biopsy is not recommended due to the need to preserve lymph node architecture for possible future interventions. A fine needle aspiration is upwards of 90% sensitive for tumors – the most common being squamous cell carcinoma and lung cancer. Of note, a thyroglossal duct cyst is completely excised along with the hyoid bone. It presents as a mobile midline mass that is attached to the tongue. The presence of a buccal squamous cell carcinoma receives a wide resection with a selective neck dissection.

 A 32 year old female presents with her third complication due to a pulmonary embolism. She has a long history of deep vein thromboses. She initially started subcutaneous heparin therapy to avoid these thromboembolic phenomenon, but has apparently failed it. What is the next step in management?

A. Coumadin and thrombectomy
B. IVC filter
C. IVC filter and coumadin
D. IVC filter and heparin
E. Lifelong coumadin

 The best answer is <u>IVC filter</u>. Intracaval filters are the therapy of choice for recurrent pulmonary embolisms due to deep vein thrombosis within the lower extremities. Multisystem trauma, hemorrhagic cerebrovascular accidents, and failed anticoagulation therapy are also indications. The standard therapy otherwise is a heparin bridge to coumadin with a target INR of 2-2.5. This particular patient would receive an IVC filter only. There are some indications in the literature that the use of an IVC filter with coumadin or heparin may be even more beneficial.

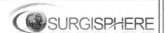

An 18 year old male has a difficult time with sports due to signs and symptoms of thoracic outlet obstruction. Hypertrophy of the anterior scalene muscle is deemed to be the culprit and a resection is completed. Which of the following describes the anatomy around this muscle?

A.   Lies anterior to the subclavian artery and brachial plexus, and anterior to the subclavian vein
B.   Lies anterior to the subclavian artery and brachial plexus, and posterior to the subclavian vein
C.   Lies lateral to the subclavian artery and brachial plexus, and medial to the subclavian vein
D.   Lies posterior to the subclavian artery and brachial plexus, and posterior to the subclavian vein
E.   Lies posterior to the subclavian artery and brachial plexus, and anterior to the subclavian vein

The best answer is <u>Lies anterior to the subclavian artery and brachial plexus, and posterior to the subclavian vein</u>. The anterior scalene muscle, also known as the scalenus anticus, lies deeply at the side of the neck, behind the sternocleidomastoideus. It arises from the anterior tubercles of the transverse processes of the third, fourth, fifth, and sixth cervical vertebra, and descending, almost vertically, is inserted by a narrow, flat tendon into the scalene tubercle on the inner border of the first rib, and into the ridge on the upper surface of the rib in front of the subclavian groove. It lies anterior to the subclavian artery and brachial plexus, posterior to the subclavian vein, and may lead to thoracic outlet obstruction through compression of the brachial plexus between the anterior and middle scalene muscles when it hypertrophies.

CARDIAC SURGERY

CHAPTER CONTENTS

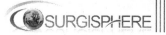

GENERAL CONCEPTS

ANATOMY

HEART

The heart is made of four chambers, including two atria and two ventricles. The flow that occurs throughout the pulmonary vasculature and systemic vasculature is due to the action of the muscular ventricles, while the atria serve primarily to store blood during diastole. One atrium works in conjunction with a ventricle, and the two systems are separated by a septum. The atrioventricular valves control flow of blood from the atria to the ventricles. The right atrium and ventricle are separated by the tricuspid valve, and the left atrium and ventricle are separated by the bicuspid (mitral) valve. **The SA node is located at the junction of the right atrium and superior vena cava.**

VASCULATURE

The internal mammary artery is the first branch off the subclavian artery. **The left internal mammary artery has the best patency for a CABG. The subclavian artery is located between the anterior and middle scalene muscles**

CORONARY ARTERIES

The blood supply to the heart consists of the coronary arteries. The left coronary artery (LCA) supplies the left side of the heart, and the left anterior descending (LAD) branch of the LCA supplies the anterior wall of the left ventricle and anterior 2/3's of the interventricular septum of the heart. The left circumflex (LCX) branch supplies the lateral wall of the left ventricle and posterior portions of the heart. The LCA arises distal to the posterior aortic sinus of Valsalva. The right coronary artery (RCA) supplies the inferior wall of the left ventricle and the SA and AV nodes of the heart. The RCA also gives off the marginal artery, which supplies the right atrium and right ventricle. The RCA arises directly from the aorta immediately distal to the anterior aortic sinus of Valsalva.

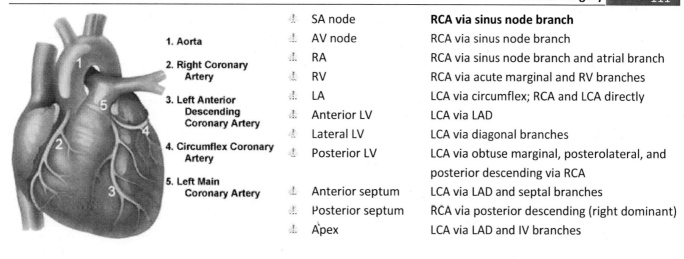

	SA node	**RCA via sinus node branch**
	AV node	RCA via sinus node branch
	RA	RCA via sinus node branch and atrial branch
	RV	RCA via acute marginal and RV branches
	LA	LCA via circumflex; RCA and LCA directly
	Anterior LV	LCA via LAD
	Lateral LV	LCA via diagonal branches
	Posterior LV	LCA via obtuse marginal, posterolateral, and posterior descending via RCA
	Anterior septum	LCA via LAD and septal branches
	Posterior septum	RCA via posterior descending (right dominant)
	Apex	LCA via LAD and IV branches

1. Aorta
2. Right Coronary Artery
3. Left Anterior Descending Coronary Artery
4. Circumflex Coronary Artery
5. Left Main Coronary Artery

THORACIC DUCT

The thoracic duct terminates at the junction of the left subclavian vein and the left internal jugular vein.

PHYSIOLOGY

HEMODYNAMICS

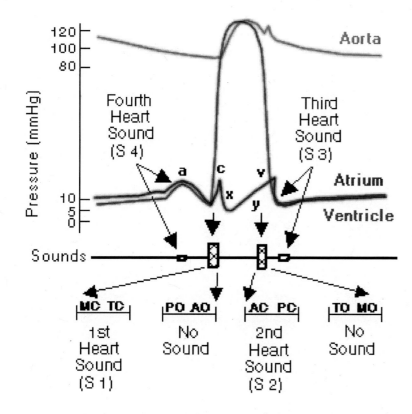

$$EF = \frac{(EDV - ESV)}{EDV} = \frac{SV}{EDV}$$

$$CO = HR \times SV$$

The compensatory reaction for mild, normovolemic anemia is via increased cardiac output.

Mean arterial pressure is 2/3s of the diastolic pressure plus 1/3 of the systolic pressure. MAPs should be kept above 60.

Components of MAP are cardiac output and peripheral vascular resistance.

Oxygen delivery is affected by cardiac output, hemoglobin, and oxygen saturation.

Per Starling's rule, cardiac output increases with left ventricular end diastolic volume.

Left heart valve disorders lead to distortions in pulmonary capillary wedge pressure.

A significant discordance in PCWP and central venous pressure indicate right heart failure.

Myocardial oxygen consumption is proportional to ventricular wall tension.

PULMONARY ARTERY CATHETER

A pulmonary artery catheter (PAC, also known as a Swan-Ganz catheter) is an excellent method for measuring pulmonary vascular resistance. Indications include hypovolemia with significant fluid management issues, and low urine output following an operation. A fixed reading on the pulmonary artery catheter with loss of respiratory variation is an indication for malposition.

INTRA-AORTIC BALLOON PUMP

An intra-aortic balloon pump (IABP) **decreases afterload** without increasing work on the heart. An IABP is indicated with significant ischemic damage to the heart that cannot be alleviated with afterload reducers. IABPs inflate 40ms before the T-wave and deflate with a P wave. Therefore, inflation occurs during diastole and augmentation of diastolic blood flow occurs.

 IABP decreases afterload and reduces myocardial oxygen consumption

Afterload reduction is the only method to prevent additional ischemic damage. Indications for the use of an IABP include acute MI leading to cardiogenic shock and the presence of acute mitral insufficiency. IABPs can be placed at the bedside.

PHARMACOLOGY

ADRENERGIC AGONISTS – CATECHOLAMINES

Table 104 Adrenergic Agonists - Catecholamines

DRUG	INDICATIONS	MECHANISM OF ACTION	COMPLICATIONS	NOTES
Dopamine	Shock with renal protection CHF	D1, D2 β1	Nausea, HTN, arrhythmia.	Given IV due to significant first pass effects
Norepinephrine	Shock	α1, α2, β1, β2		Given IV due to significant first pass effects
Epinephrine	Acute asthma Shock Increase local anesthetic duration	α1, α2, β1, β2 Increases aqueous humor outflow	Mydriasis	Given IV due to significant first pass effects
Dobutamine	CHF	β1	Avoid with atrial fibrillation.	Given IV due to significant first pass effects
Phenylephrine	Shock	α1		
Milrinone	Increase cardiac contractility	Phosphodieserase inhibitor		Increased mortality
Isoproterenol	Bradycardia	β1, β2	Arrhythmia, ischemia w/ CAD	Increased CO, HR & SP, decreased DP, & MAP, and SVR

ALPHA ADRENERGIC ANTAGONISTS

Table 105 Alpha-Adrenergic Antagonists

DRUG	INDICATIONS	MECHANISM OF ACTION	COMPLICATIONS	CONTRAINDICATIONS	NOTES
Terazosin	HTN, BPH	α1	Orthostatic hypotension on first dose, dizziness, syncope, and HA		Dilates arterioles and venules

BETA ADRENERGIC ANTAGONISTS

Table 106 Beta-Adrenergic Antagonists

DRUG	INDICATIONS		MECHANISM OF ACTION	COMPLICATIONS	CONTRAINDICATIONS	NOTES
Propranolol	HTN Angina pectoris MI	Akathisia, HTN, angina, migraine, IHSS	β1, β2	Sedation, hyperlipidemia	Impotence, asthma, CV disease, CNS disease, diabetes (relative)	Also used for performance anxiety and thyrotoxicosis
Metoprolol	SVT CHF Glaucoma	HTN	β1	Sedation, hyperlipidemia	Impotence, asthma, CV disease, CNS disease, diabetes (relative)	

- Cardioprotective when used preoperatively and following an MI. Also used to control the ventricular response to atrial fibrillation and atrial flutter (i.e. rate control).

SEROTONINERGIC AGENTS

Table 107 Serotoninergic Agents

DRUG	INDICATIONS	MECHANISM OF ACTION	COMPLICATIONS	CONTRAINDICATIONS	NOTES
Sumatriptan	Migraines Cluster headaches	5-HT$_{1D}$ agonist leading to acute vasoconstriction.	Distal paresthesia, ACS	CAD, variant (Prinzmetal) angina	Short half-life.
Ondansetron	Treatment of N/V in chemotherapy	5-HT$_3$ receptor antagonist to reduce vagus nerve activity and reduce serotonin receptor activity in CTZ	Dizziness, generally rare	Hepatic disease (P-450)	

CARDIAC GLYCOSIDES

Table 108 Cardiac Glycosides

DRUG	INDICATIONS	MECHANISM OF ACTION	COMPLICATIONS	CONTRAINDICATIONS	NOTES
Digoxin	CHF	Increases contractility through Na/K ATPase inhibition with inhibition of the Na/Ca antiport. An increase in intracellular calcium is the effect	N/V/D. Yellow vision. Hypokalemia leading to arrhythmia.	Avoid in patients with renal disease, hypokalemia, quinidine use, and propensity towards arrhythmias.	Positive inotrope. No change in mortality, but reduces hospital admissions.

- High bioavailability with long half-life. Treat arrhythmias induced by the cardiac glycosides with K+ normalization, lidocaine, and anti-digoxin Fab.

CLASS IA ANTIARRHYTHMICS

Table 109 Class IA Antiarrhythmics

DRUG	INDICATIONS	MECHANISM OF ACTION	COMPLICATIONS	CONTRAINDICATIONS	NOTES
Amiodarone	Suppress ectopic rhythms from abnormal pacemaker cells Phase 3 and 4 effects	↓ phase 4 depolarization and ↑ firing threshold State-dependent effects target abnormal pacemaker cells	AV block, ventricular arrhythmia	Use with care.	Sodium channel blocker
Procainamide					

- Antiarrhythmics are often used in an emergent setting for initial control of a dysrhythmia until a more permanent solution can be implemented.

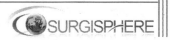

CLASS IB ANTIARRHYTHMICS

Table 110 Class IB Antiarrhythmics

DRUG	INDICATIONS	MECHANISM OF ACTION	COMPLICATIONS	CONTRAINDICATIONS	NOTES
Lidocaine	Ventricular arrhythmia Phase 3 and 4 effects	↓ AP duration	Local anesthesia CNS changes ↓CV, Proarrhythmic	Use with care.	Also used in digitalis toxicity Targets ischemic and depolarized tissue

CLASS IC ANTIARRHYTHMICS

Table 111 Class IC Antiarrhythmics

DRUG	INDICATIONS	MECHANISM OF ACTION	COMPLICATIONS	CONTRAINDICATIONS	NOTES
Flecainide	VT and VF	↑ threshold of firing and ↓ phase 4 depolarization	Proarrhythmic	Use with care.	No change in AP duration

CLASS II ANTIARRHYTHMICS

Table 112 Class II Antiarrhythmics

DRUG	INDICATIONS	MECHANISM OF ACTION	COMPLICATIONS	CONTRAINDICATIONS	NOTES
Metoprolol	Suppress ectopic focus, HTN	↓cAMP with ↓Ca2+ current ↓phase 4 in AV node with ↑PR	Proarrhythmic, impotence, asthma, CV and CNS effects, masks hypoglycemia	Use with care.	B-blocker

CLASS III ANTIARRHYTHMICS

Table 113 Class III Antiarrhythmics

DRUG	INDICATIONS	MECHANISM OF ACTION	COMPLICATIONS	CONTRAINDICATIONS	NOTES
Amiodarone !	Last line for arrhythmia	↑AP, ↑ERP, ↑QT, ↓I_K	Pulmonary fibrosis, hepatotoxicity, smurf skin, photodermatitis, CNS and CV effects, change in thyroid function	Use with care.	Long half-life, very toxic

CLASS IV ANTIARRHYTHMICS

Table 114 Class IV Antiarrhythmics

DRUG	INDICATIONS	MECHANISM OF ACTION	COMPLICATIONS	CONTRAINDICATIONS	NOTES
Diltiazem !	SVT	↓conduction velocity to ↑ERP and ↑PR from calcium-channel blockade	Flushing, constipation, CV effects	Do not use in VT due to progression to VF	Targets AV node

- Class IA and IC decrease phase 0 depolarization to slow conduction, class IB decrease phase 3 repolarization to slow conduction, class II suppresses phase 4 depolarization, class III prolongs phase 3 repolarization, and class IV shortens the action potential to make reaching threshold more difficult

ATYPICAL ANTIARRHYTHMICS

Table 115 Atypical Antiarrhythmics

DRUG	INDICATIONS	MECHANISM OF ACTION	COMPLICATIONS	CONTRAINDICATIONS	NOTES
Adenosine	SVT	Decreases cAMP	Arrhythmia		
Potassium	Ectopic focus Digoxin toxicity	Normalizes potassium and repolarization	Arrhythmia	Hyperkalemia	Insulin can be given as a temporary antidote in hyperkalemia
Magnesium	Torsade de pointes Digoxin toxicity	Substitutes for calcium effects without depolarization	Arrhythmia		

ACE-INHIBITORS

Table 116 ACE-Inhibitors

DRUG	INDICATIONS	MECHANISM OF ACTION	COMPLICATIONS	CONTRAINDICATIONS	NOTES
Enalapril	HTN CHF	Prevents conversion of ATI to ATII through inhibition of ACE	Cough, angioedema, hypotension	Do not use in pregnancy due to fetal renal damage Avoid in renal artery stenosis	Mediates cough and angioedema through bradykinin

ANGIOTENSIN RECEPTOR BLOCKERS

Table 117 Angiotensin Receptor Blockers

DRUG	INDICATIONS	MECHANISM OF ACTION	COMPLICATIONS	CONTRAINDICATIONS	NOTES
Losartan	HTN CHF	Prevents binding of ATII to receptor	Few	Avoid in pregnancy and renal artery stenosis	Does not affect bradykinin or upregulate renin like ACE-inhibitors

CARBONIC ANHYDRASE INHIBITORS

Table 118 Carbonic Anhydrase Inhibitors

DRUG	INDICATIONS	MECHANISM OF ACTION	COMPLICATIONS	CONTRAINDICATIONS	NOTES
Acetazolamide	Metabolic alkalosis Alkalinize urine	Causes diuresis of sodium bicarbonate in PCT	Hyperchloremic metabolic acidosis, ammonium build-up causing CNS effects	Avoid in patients with allergies to sulfa compounds	

LOOP DIURETICS

Table 119 Loop Diuretics

DRUG	INDICATIONS	MECHANISM OF ACTION	COMPLICATIONS	CONTRAINDICATIONS	NOTES
Furosemide	CHF HTN Hypercalcemia	Inhibits $Na^+/K^+/Cl^-$ cotransporter in ascending loop of Henle to decrease urine concentration.	Ototoxicity, hypokalemia, dehydration, interstitial nephritis, hyperglycemia.	Gout, sulfa allergy.	

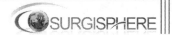

THIAZIDE DIURETICS

Table 120 Thiazide Diuretics

DRUG	INDICATIONS	MECHANISM OF ACTION	COMPLICATIONS	CONTRAINDICATIONS	NOTES
Hydrochlorothiazide	HTN CHF DI Hypercalciuria	Prevents absorption of Na in distal tubule leading to increased water and salt excretion from the kidney. This destroys the Na / Ca gradient leading to increased calcium secretion.	Hypokalemia, hyponatremia, metabolic alkalosis.	Avoid in people with sulfa allergies.	

- These drugs are secreted by the proximal tubule and compete with urea secretion in the kidney. The net effect may lead to hyperuricemia.

POTASSIUM-SPARING DIURETICS

Table 121 Potassium-Sparing Diuretics

DRUG	INDICATIONS	MECHANISM OF ACTION	COMPLICATIONS	CONTRAINDICATIONS	NOTES
Spironolactone	CHF Hyperaldosteronism	Competitive antagonist against aldosterone	Hyperkalemia Gynecomastia	Avoid in arrhythmia	Also used as an antiandrogen to decrease hirsutism

- These drugs require an intact RAA axis. As a result, they cannot be used to diagnose Addison disease.
- Weak diuretics with little water and sodium loss and significant potassium retention
- Typically combined with thiazide diuretics. Consider given insulin as a temporary measure to decrease potassium excess.

ADH AGONISTS

Table 122 ADH Agonists

DRUG	INDICATIONS	MECHANISM OF ACTION	COMPLICATIONS	CONTRAINDICATIONS	NOTES
Vasopressin	DI, control hemorrhage in esophagus and colon	Antidiuretic & vasopressor	Water intoxication, hyponatremia	Caution in pediatric and geriatric cases. Monitor fluid intake	

METABOLIC AND DEGENERATIVE

HYPERTENSION

Table 123 Hypertension

Hypertension	
Etiology	Increased SVR with a normal CO. This results in an increase in work by the heart in order to have the same SV with every heartbeat. Risk factors for HTN include a high salt diet, obesity, smoking, diabetes, family history, African American race, and males.
Presentation	Presents with few, if any symptoms unless severe. Severe symptoms may include epistaxis, hematuria, blurred vision, chest pain, light-headedness, headache, and CHF.
Diagnosis	Testing the BP in both arms and finding symmetrically abnormal readings of at least stage 1 HTN. Ophthalmoscope exam positive for papilledema, AV nicking, & punctate hemorrhages.
Risk factors	High salt diet, obesity, smoking, diabetes, family history, African American race, and male gender.
Treatment	Reduction in fatty-acid, weight loss and exercise, use of beta-receptor blockers and thiazide diuretics. The use of ACE inhibitors is especially effective in Caucasians and diabetics. African American patients benefit more from calcium-channel blockers.

CORONARY ARTERY DISEASE

INTRODUCTION

Coronary heart disease (CHD), also known as coronary artery disease (CAD), is a serious public health problem that affects nearly 14 million Americans. CHD is the result of years of fatty acid deposition, calcification, and subsequent plaque formation within the coronary arteries. Narrowing of the artery lumen by the plaque leads to decreased blood to the myocardium, followed by symptoms of angina and chest pain. Sudden complete blockage of the lumen, as can occur with the rupturing of the plaques, leads to signs and symptoms of an MI.

RISK FACTORS FOR CHD

There are a number of risk factors for the development and progression of CHD. Atherosclerosis is the most significant cause, and this disease may be exacerbated by a positive family history, smoking, elevated titers of low-density lipoprotein (LDL), decreased titers of high-density lipoprotein (HDL), hypertension (HTN), central obesity, diabetes mellitus (DM), elevated C-reactive protein (CRP), elevated homocysteine levels, and increase in the circulation of fibrinogen. Lack of regular exercise, poor diet, high levels of emotional stress, and a typical type A personality also contribute to the development of CHD. Anemia and carbon monoxide poisoning can significantly decrease the oxygen-carrying capacity of the blood and exacerbate CHD. A family history for CHD is considered positive if relatives have experienced a MI prior to the age of 45 in men, and 55 in women. The major causes of CHD are discussed below. CHD that presents with decreased blood supply and oxygen to the heart is often referred to as ischemic heart disease (IHD).

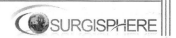

Table 124 Coronary Heart Disease

Coronary Heart Disease	
Etiology	The result of years of fatty acid deposition, calcification, and plaque formation within the coronary arteries. Narrowing of the artery lumen by the plaque leads to decreased blood to the myocardium, causing symptoms of angina and chest pain.
Risk factors	Atherosclerosis, a positive family history, smoking, elevated titers of LDL, decreased titers HDL, HTN, central obesity, DM, elevated CRP, elevated homocysteine levels, increase in circulation of fibrinogen. Lack of regular exercise, poor diet, high levels of emotional stress, and type A personality.

DYSLIPIDEMIA

Table 125 Dyslipidemia

Dyslipidemia	
Presentation	Presents with obvious signs and symptoms only in very severe disease. Severe hypercholesterolemia may present with xanthelasmas, xanthomas.
Diagnosis	Fasting lipid profile.
Treatment	Changes to dietary intake and increased exercise. Medication, if diet & exercise fail.
Medications	Statins, cholestyramine and colestipol, niacin, fish oils.

ANGINA

ETIOLOGY AND PATHOPHYSIOLOGY

Angina is chest pain associated with decreased oxygen flow to the myocardium leading to temporary, reversible ischemia. There are three major types of angina – stable angina, unstable angina, and Prinzmetal angina.

PRESENTATION

Angina presents with retrosternal pain that radiates to the left shoulder, arm, or jaw. The pain is typically a heavy pressure sensation, sometimes described as a squeezing or tightening inside the chest. Angina typically does not last more than 15 minutes – if it does, the clinician should seriously consider angina evolving into an MI. Angina is precipitated by factors that affect cardiovascular stability or increase cardiac work; these factors typically include vasoconstriction due to cold or exertion, psychoactive factors such as anxiety, and eating large meals. Angina also presents with shortness of breath, nausea and vomiting, diaphoresis, and palpitations. Angina is relieved by nitroglycerin within a few minutes; resting also ameliorates the symptoms of angina. Physical signs of angina include tachycardia with or without an S4 gallop.

STABLE ANGINA

Stable angina is due to **ischemia of the myocardium** leading to episodic pain. Stable angina is **chronic** in nature and does not progress over time. Stable angina occurs with predictive changes to myocardial oxygen consumption, such as with strenuous exercise. Stable angina is relieved with rest. This disease may evolve into unstable angina.

UNSTABLE ANGINA

Unstable angina is any **new-onset angina** that **progresses over time** with respect to location, frequency, or severity. Unstable angina can occur at rest, and typically requires increasing amounts of medication to have relief from symptoms. Unstable angina requires treatment to avoid **evolution into an MI**.

DIAGNOSIS

Diagnosing angina proceeds by ruling out other causes of chest pain by carefully obtaining a history, completing a physical exam, and running an EKG. EKG changes may be normal, or present with ST changes (depression or elevation), and T wave inversions. An exercise stress test (treadmill stress echocardiogram) is done to determine the type of angina that occurs and its severity. A TSE with thallium is done in patients with valvular defects, arrhythmia, young women, and those with acute ischemic changes. Other examinations available to diagnose and determine the prognosis of angina include dobutamine stress echocardiogram (DSE), persantine echocardiogram, and thallium imaging. Stress tests should not be performed on individuals with unstable angina due to the risk of evolution to MI. Patients with aortic stenosis (AS), hypertrophic subaortic stenosis, chronic obstructive pulmonary disease (COPD), congestive heart failure, aortic dissection, ischemic changes on EKG, uncontrolled HTN, and those with general contraindications to exercise should also not receive a stress echocardiogram.

TREATMENT

Angina is initially treated by lifestyle and dietary modifications. Patients with stable angina should receive sublingual nitroglycerin (SLN) during exacerbations, percutaneous transluminal coronary angioplasty (PCTA) or a coronary artery bypass graft (CABG), beta blockade to reduce oxygen demand by the myocardium, and aspirin (ASA) to decrease the risk of evolution to MI. Those with unstable angina should also receive SLN, PCTA and CABG as indicated, and should also be monitored in a cardiac care unit (CCU) due to the risk of MI. Heparin or low molecular weight heparin (LMWH) should be used in conjunction with ASA to decrease the risk of thrombosis. Finally, those patients with Prinzmetal angina should receive calcium channel blockers and nitrates to reduce coronary artery spasms; beta-blockers are contraindicated in this population.

Table 126 Angina

Angina	
Etiology	Severe BP increases that result in end-organ damage.
Presentation	Retrosternal pain that radiates to the left shoulder, arm, or jaw. Lasts a few minutes and is intermittent. The pain is typically a heavy pressure sensation. Angina also presents SOB, N+V, diaphoresis, and palpitations. Physical signs of angina include tachycardia with or without an S4 gallop.
Types	**Stable angina:** due to ischemia of the myocardium leading to episodic pain. Chronic in nature and does not progress over time. Occurs with predictive changes to myocardial oxygen consumption, is relieved with rest. **Unstable angina:** new-onset angina that progresses over time with respect to location, frequency, or severity. Can occur at rest, and requires increasing amounts of medication to have relief from symptoms. **Prinzmetal angina:** rare variant of angina that is due to vasospasms of coronary arteries. Chronic, intermittent chest pain unrelated to exertion, tends to occur at predictable times in the morning. Pain awakens patient at night. Presents with ischemic changes and STe during exacerbation.
Treatment	**Stable angina:** SLN during exacerbations, PCTA or a coronary artery CABG, beta blockade, and ASA. **Unstable angina:** SLN, PCTA and CABG as indicated, and should also be monitored CCU. Heparin or low LMWH should be used in conjunction with ASA. **Prinzmetal angina:** calcium channel blockers and nitrates.

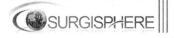

MYOCARDIAL INFARCTION

ETIOLOGY AND EPIDEMIOLOGY

MI is the development of myocardial necrosis following prolonged ischemia. MI is typically attributed to sudden rupture of a plaque leading to coronary artery blockade, an embolism from a secondary source, shock leading to impaired cardiac perfusion, and coronary vasospasm. Hypercoagulable states such as thrombocytosis and polycythemia vera can contribute to embolism, and direct embolisms can occur from atrial myxoma and coronary thrombi. Spasms of the coronary arteries are common in cocaine abuse and in Prinzmetal angina. Finally, inflammation of the vasculature can lead to MI, as in systemic lupus erythematosus (SLE), polyarteritis nodosa (PAN), Takayasu arteritis, and Kawasaki disease. Risk factors for MI include males over 55 years of age, postmenopausal women, smokers, HTN, hyperlipidemia, DM, and atherosclerosis.

PATHOPHYSIOLOGY

The typical MI is a progressive process that leads to significantly greater damage to the myocardium with the passage of time. If therapy is not immediately started after coronary vasocculsion, permanent damage to the myocytes sets in within 20 minutes. Coagulation necrosis begins within about 6 hours with the influx of PMNs. Total coagulative necrosis sets in after a day or two, and granulation tissue starts to form around 3-7 days. It is during this time that the destroyed myocytes are being cleared and fibrotic tissue is being formed. Rupture through the heart wall can occur, leading to cardiac tamponade and significant morbidity and mortality. Acute MI (AMI) can occur as a transmural lesion, which is typically accompanied with Q waves. A subendocardial infarct is confined to the innermost portion of the ventricular wall and does not present with Q waves; regardless of the cause of the MI, the subendocardial tissue of the left ventricle is the most susceptible to damage due to the tenuous oxygen supply from lack of direct arterial flow.

Table 127 Pathophysiology of an MI

Pathophysiology of an MI	
After 20 minutes	Permanent damage to myocytes.
After 6 hours	**Coagulation necrosis with influx of PMNs.**
After 1-2 days	**Total coagulation necrosis.**
After 3-7 days	**Granulation tissue starts to form**.

PRESENTATION

The typical MI presents with symptoms of severe, retrosternal chest pain for more than 20 minutes. This severe crushing pressure or squeezing sensation leads to nausea and vomiting, diaphoresis, weakness, and anxiety. Shortness of breath develops with failure of heart function. In order to compensate for the ischemic changes taking place, tachycardia ensues with an S4 gallop. Cardiogenic shock with hypotension, jugular venous distention (JVD), and S3 gallop, and rales may develop if more than half of the myocardium has been compromised. Depending on the severity of the damage, arrhythmias and septal rupture may occur. Inferior MIs may present with bradycardia. Typically, an MI will present as pain that radiates to the left arm or shoulder, or the jaw. It is most likely to occur in the early waking hours as this is when the blood pressure can be the highest. MI may be entirely silent in diabetics, the elderly, patients with HTN, and in postsurgical patients. Psychological symptoms include a feeling of impending doom.

DIAGNOSIS WITH EKG

The initial test in diagnosing an MI is the use of an EKG. In inferior wall MI, there will be an STe in leads II, III, and aVF. Anteroseptal MI has STe in leads V1-V3. Lateral wall MI has STe in V4-V6, and posterior wall MI has STd in V1 and V2. New onset of Q waves is indicative of a transmural MI, and is the most common EKG finding after an ST elevation MI (STEMI). Flattening of the ST segment typically does not progress to Q waves, and this is known as a non-ST elevation MI (NSTEMI). A new LBBB is also diagnostic of MI. Echocardiograms in order to demonstrate hypokinesia of the ventricular wall are used in patients with nondiscernable EKGs but who otherwise fit the clinical picture of MI. The EKG changes that occur immediately upon onset of MI include sharp, peaked T waves and STe, followed by Q waves, then T wave inversions (Twi) after several hours. The Q waves may remain as an indicator of prior MI, and the Twi may remain for several years.

Table 128 EKG Findings

EKG Findings	
Inferior wall MI	STe in leads II, III, and aVF
Anteroseptal MI	STe in leads V1-V3
Lateral wall MI	STe in V4-V6
Posterior wall MI	STd in V1 and V2
Transmural MI	Q waves after an ST elevation MI (STEMI)

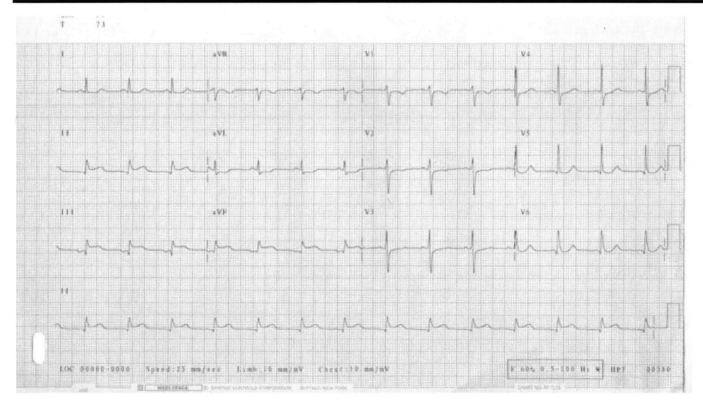

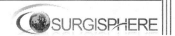

DIAGNOSIS WITH CARDIAC ENZYMES

The progression of an MI leads to a predictable rise in cardiac markers of myocardial damage. Some of these markers are specific, others sensitive, and some useful only as early markers of disease. Myoglobin is typically one of the earliest markers to become serologically positive with elevations within one hour of experiencing an MI; however, myoglobin is found in numerous tissues and so is not very specific. Rises in CPK occur within 6 hours, but this marker is similar to myoglobin in that it is not specific. Troponin T (TnT) and troponin I (TnI) rise within 3-4 hours, remain elevated for up to a week, and are highly sensitive markers for even minimal myocardial damage (so called microinfarcts). Creatine kinase, MB fraction (CK-MB) is a highly specific and sensitive

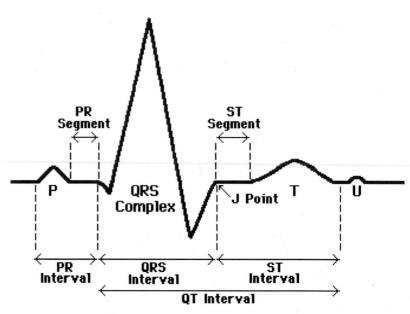

marker for cardiac damage that is positive within 4-6 hours and remains so for at least one or two days. The CK-MB fraction rises only with myocardial necrosis, but CK itself may rise with general cardiac trauma or manipulation with resuscitation procedures. Lactate dehydrogenase (LDH) is rarely used as a marker for cardiac damage due to its lack of specificity and sensitivity, but it tends to be positive after 12 hours and remains elevated for up to two weeks. Most centers in the United States now measure serial cardiac enzymes in patients suspected of MI (especially in ruling out MI). Cardiac enzymes including CK-MB, TnT, and CPK are typically collected every 6 hours three consecutive times along with EKG tracings. A patient typically rules out for MI with lack of EKG signs and no increases in cardiac enzymes.

Table 129 Diagnosis with Cardiac Enzymes

Diagnosis with Cardiac Enzymes	
Myoglobin	One of the **earliest markers** within one hour of experiencing an MI; Not very specific.
CPK	Occurs within 6 hours. Not specific.
TnT, TnI	Rise within 3-4 hours, remain elevated for up to a week, and are highly sensitive markers.
CK-MB	**Highly specific** and **sensitive** marker for cardiac damage that is positive within 4-6 hours and remains so for at least 1 or 2 days. The CK-MB fraction rises only with myocardial necrosis, but CK itself may rise with general cardiac trauma or manipulation with resuscitation procedures.

TREATMENT

Aspirin, or its alternative, clopidogrel, are administered immediately given evidence that aspirin can reduce mortality from MI by over 25% through decreased clot formation. Beta-blockers have also been shown to decrease mortality by limiting the extent of damage; metoprolol is typically given three times every 5 minutes and stopped if the heart rate falls below 60. If given in the first few hours after an MI, thrombolytic therapy has also been shown to decrease mortality by breaking up clots; agents include streptokinase and alteplase. Heparin is given to prevent the further development of clots. Oxygen is given to increase oxygen saturation and for patient comfort. Nitroglycerin is also given to relieve symptoms by dilating coronary arteries and reducing cardiac oxygen demand through decreased preload. Morphine is given to reduce pain and anxiety, and thereby further decrease oxygen demand by the damaged myocardium. PTCA can be done on an emergent basis and within an hour or two of MI onset to restore the patency of the coronary arteries, especially if there is multiple vessel disease.

Angioplasty is preferred in patients with contraindications to normal thrombolytic therapy, have CHF or poor EF, risk of dangerous arrhythmia development, and patients who fail thrombolytic therapy. Cardiac pacing may be required if arrhythmias develop as a result of damage to the heart. Patients should also be counseled with regard to dietary changes and exercise as discussed above for dyslipidemia and HTN. **Indications for a CABG** include moderate to severe **angina** that is refractory to medical therapy, **greater than 50% blockage** in the **left main** coronary artery or **triple vessel disease**, and **greater than 70% blockage** in the **LAD and one other** vessel. The **internal mammary artery has the best patency**; it is the first branch from the subclavian artery. CABG has a 1% mortality risk. There is greater than 95% patency at 20 years. Vein grafts have 80% patency at 5 years. Angioplasty has a 20% restenosis rate at 1 year.

Table 130 Myocardial Infarction (MI)

Myocardial Infarction (MI)	
Etiology	Development of myocardial necrosis following prolonged ischemia. Sudden rupture of a plaque, an embolism from a secondary source, shock, and coronary vasospasm.
Risk factors	Males over 55 years of age, postmenopausal women, smokers, HTN, hyperlipidemia, DM, and atherosclerosis.
Presentation	Severe, retrosternal chest pain for more than 20 minutes. Leads to nausea and vomiting, diaphoresis, weakness, and anxiety. SOB, tachycardia. Cardiogenic shock with hypotension, JVD. Arrhythmias and septal rupture may occur. Inferior MIs may present with bradycardia. Typically, an MI will present as pain that radiates to the left arm or shoulder, or the jaw. It is most likely to occur in the early waking hours. MI may be entirely silent in diabetics, the elderly, patients with HTN, in postsurgical patients, and in those following heart transplantation. Psychological symptoms include a feeling of impending doom.
Diagnosis	EKG, myoglobin, CPK, TnT, TnI, CK, CK-MB, LDH.
Treatment	Aspirin or clopidogrel, Beta-blockers, metoprolol, streptokinase and alteplase, heparin oxygen, nitroglycerin, morphine, PTCA , angioplasty, patient counseling, pacemaker.

STAGING

MI is broken down into four classes with specific clinical findings and objective signs that are indicative of mortality. Class I MI presents with no pulmonary symptoms, indicating reasonable cardiac function without heart failure. The cardiac index (CI) is greater than 2.2, and the pulmonary capillary wedge pressure (PCWP) less than 15. The hospital mortality is less than 1%. Class II MI presents with pulmonary congestion, CI greater than 2.2, and PCWP more than 15. There is a 10% hospital mortality. Class III MI has systemic hypoperfusion with CI less than 2.2, PCWP less than 15, and a hospital mortality of about 20%. Class IV MI has pulmonary congestion with systemic hypoperfusion, CI less than 2.2, PCWP more than 15, and a hospital mortality exceeding 50%.

Table 131 Staging of MI

Staging of MI	
Class I	Presents with no pulmonary symptoms, CI is greater than 2.2, and the PCWP less than 15.
Class II	Presents with pulmonary congestion, CI greater than 2.2, and PCWP more than 15.
Class III	Systemic hypoperfusion with CI less than 2.2, PCWP less than 15.
Class IV	Pulmonary congestion with systemic hypoperfusion, CI less than 2.2, PCWP more than 15.

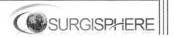

COMPLICATIONS

ARRHYTHMIA

Complications arising from MI include those leading to arrhythmias, dysfunction leading to pump failure, ischemic changes, pericarditis, and sudden cardiac death. Arrhythmias that develop following an MI include bradycardia that may require the use of atropine to prevent ectopic foci from developing and the use of a pacemaker, if the bradycardia is severe enough. Premature atrial contractions (PACs) or premature ventricular contractions (PVCs) can develop, although these tend to be benign, if isolated. Supraventricular tachycardia (SVT) can occur with the development of atrial fibrillation, atrial flutter, or a junctional focus. Ventricular tachycardias (VT) can also occur, which heralds a more dismal prognosis, especially with ventricular fibrillation. Hemiblocks and bundle branch blocks can also occur, in addition to first, second, and third order atrioventricular (AV) blocks.

HEART FAILURE

Heart failure is an all too common occurrence following a significant heart attack, and can present with either mechanical disruption due to anatomic failure, or with contractile dysfunction due to failure of normal expansion and contraction from direct muscle damage. In addition, the conduction system of the heart can become dissociated from the targets it innervates.

ISCHEMIA

Ischemia can continue and even progress following an MI. Extension of the infarct site can also occur, and is especially common if there is a sustained increase in myocardial oxygen demand but without the concomitant increase in supply. Thrombolytics should be used along with measures to ensure vessel patency prior to discharge.

PERICARDITIS

Dressler syndrome is the development of a pericarditis following an MI. **Dressler syndrome** may occur between a few days to a few months following an MI, and is due to an **inflammatory process** that runs rampant and leads to damage to otherwise healthy cells. Dressler syndrome may also complicate other heart disorders, especially those that require open surgical management. It is a rare complication of MI, affecting fewer than one in a hundred patients. Dressler syndrome is treated with **NSAIDs and steroids.**

PRO-THROMBOTIC STATE

MI can lend to a pro-thrombotic state due to relative stasis of blood residing in a now dysfunctional portion of the heart. This meets one of the three requirements of Virchow's triad for vascular thrombosis (the other two being endothelial damage and a hypercoagulable state). These clots can go on to cause pulmonary dysfunction in a right-sided MI, or systemic complications such as stroke and renal destruction in a left-sided MI. Immobilization immediately after an MI can also predispose an individual to deep vein thrombosis (DVT) and subsequent PE.

PAPILLARY MUSCLE RUPTURE

Greatest risk of ventricular septal rupture occurs 3-5 days post MI from macrophage-effect. Presents as loud holosystolic murmur.

Rupture of the papillary muscles can lead to **mitral regurgitation and sudden cardiac decompensation** following a posteroinferior MI. It tends to occur approximately 3-5 days after an MI and presents with a **loud holosystolic murmur.** Echocardiography demonstrates a valve leaflet moving around with the flow and regurgitation.

VENTRICULAR SEPTAL RUPTURE

Septal rupture is more likely in anterior MI and occurs **3-5 days** afterwards. It presents with a **loud holosystolic** murmur that radiates to many locations, and also tends to have a palpable thrill. TTE is used for diagnosis. Ventricular septal rupture is **more common** than a papillary muscle rupture.

SUDDEN CARDIAC DEATH

Sudden cardiac death is occasionally a result of a fatal arrhythmia that develops following an MI, such as ventricular tachycardia and ventricular fibrillation. Repeated myocardial ischemia is the largest positive predictor of risk for arrhythmias leading to sudden cardiac death.

BYPASS

Cardiopulmonary bypass has constant flow to the brain, lung, muscle, and liver. The lack of pulsatile flow may lead to "pump-organ." Though the cause is controversial, most investigators believe that this occurs due to microinfarction. The presence of dark blood after coming off cardiopulmonary bypass should lead to the reintroduction of pulmonary ventilation. Post-operative bypass pump failure presents as a cool patient with increased PCWP, decreased CO, and increased SVR. It is treated with dobutamine.

Table 132 Complications of MI

Complications of MI	
Arrhythmia	Bradycardia, PACs, PVCs, SVT, atrial fibrillation, atrial flutter, or a junctional focus. VT Hemiblocks & BBB can also occur, in addition to first, second, and third order AV blocks.
Heart failure	Mechanical or contractile dysfunction. Conduction system of heart can become dissociated from the targets it innervates.
Ischemia	Ischemia can continue and progress following an MI. Extension of the infarct site can also occur.
Pericarditis	Dressler syndrome.
Prothrombotic state	Relative stasis of blood residing in a dysfunctional portion of the heart. Clots can go on to cause pulmonary dysfunction.
Papillary muscle rupture	Leads to mitral regurgitation and sudden cardiac decompensation following a posteroinferior MI.
Ventricular septal rupture	More likely in anterior MI.
Sudden cardiac death	Occasionally a result of a fatal arrhythmia that develops following an MI.

POSTINFARCT MANAGEMENT

Patients who have had an MI should receive a stress echocardiogram prior to discharge to ensure reasonable cardiac function. Left ventricular function may be assessed using a multigated acquisition (MUGA) scan. Patients should be advised to continue ASA and beta-blockers, and patients with poor EF should be started on ACE-inhibitors. Close management of existing risk factors such as HTN, DM, hyperlipidemia, and poor lifestyle habits should be done to minimize these contributing causes and

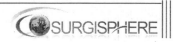

avoid a repeated MI. Patients at particular risk of continued cardiac dysfunction should be evaluated for PTCA and CABG. Post-MI patients should achieve at least 70% of their ideal target rate on a stress test.

Table 133 Postinfarct Management

Postinfarct Management
Stress echocardiogram, MUGA, ASA, beta-blockers, ACE inhibitors, PTCA, CABG, lifestyle change.

CONGESTIVE HEART FAILURE

ETIOLOGY

Congestive heart failure is the loss in the heart's ability to properly replenish the systemic or pulmonary blood volume. Right-sided CHF (RHF) leads to overflow in the systemic circulation leading to systemic venous congestion. Left-sided CHF (LHF) leads to pulmonary symptoms due to pulmonary venous congestion. The most common cause of CHF is following MI and the resultant ischemic changes. Abnormalities in myocardial cells also contributes to CHF; for example, cardiomyopathy arising from substance abuse, diseases such as sarcoidosis or hemochromatosis, and intrinsic cardiopulmonary diseases such as pulmonary HTN or aortic regurgitation can all lead to symptoms of CHF. Structural abnormalities such as valvular heart disease, congenital heart disease, CAD, constrictive pericarditis, restrictive cardiomyopathy (RCM), and high-output failure (such as wet beriberi) can exacerbate CHF. CHF can also be worsened with a high salt diet, arrhythmias that compromise the proper dynamics of heart function, infection (such as systemic infections or pneumonia), renal failure, high fluid loads, anemia, thyrotoxicosis, PE, and excessive exercise. The most common cause of right-sided CHF is left-sided CHF.

PATHOPHYSIOLOGY

DIASTOLIC DYSFUNCTION

CHF can present with either a diastolic dysfunction or a systolic dysfunction. Diastolic dysfunction leads to decreased cardiac output (CO) due to elevated systolic pressure (SBP) with normal EF. EF is allowed to remain approximately normal as both SV and EDV decrease proportionately. Recall the formula for EF:

$$EF = \frac{(EDV - ESV)}{EDV} = \frac{SV}{EDV}$$

The decrease in EF due to decreased SV leads to a decrease in CO in the absence of any change in HR. Recall the formula for CO to understand how diastolic dysfunction occurs:

$$CO = HR \times SV$$

The EF in diastolic dysfunction can be measured with echocardiography.

SYSTOLIC DYSFUNCTION

In systolic dysfunction, there is decreased contractility leading to decreased EF. The decrease in EF is proportional to changes in SV and inversely proportional to changes in EDV. As a result, decreased EF leads to decreased SV, which in the absence of changes to HR, leads to decreased CO. In both diastolic and systolic dysfunction, congestion in either the pulmonary or systemic circulation is the end result.

CARDIOVASCULAR COMPENSATION

As indicated by the formula for CO, the output per beat is directly **proportional to HR and SV**. With decreases in SV as found in CHF, the first compensatory mechanism is to increase the HR in order to return CO to baseline. The heart can also function along its Frank-Starling curve by increasing stretch, leading to ventricular dilation and thereby increasing EDV. While the heart is along its Frank-Starling curve, it is able to compensate for the increased EDV by increasing its contractility, leading to a return of SV to baseline but at higher pressures. Myocardial hypertrophy results from the increased pressures, and after some time, the heart decompensates, falls off the Frank-Starling curve, and any further dilation only leads to worsening CHF. A systemic compensation can also occur by way of decreased activation of stretch receptors in the heart and carotid artery, leading to increased systemic vascular resistance, increased afterload, and decreased SV. In other words, the systemic compensation is hardly helpful to restoring normal cardiac function.

RENAL COMPENSATION

The kidneys also attempt to compensate for the decreased renal perfusion pressures. The renin-angiotensin-aldosterone (RAA) system is activated, leading to vasoconstriction and the retention of sodium chloride and water. This increased volume load leads to an increase in preload, which worsens the congestion as the heart is unable to compensate for the increased stretch by increasing its contractility — the reason is that by the time the kidneys attempt to compensate for the failing heart, the heart has already fallen off its Frank-Starling curve and can no longer adequately compensate for changes in EDV. Stretch within the atria releases BNP, which also stimulates the RAA.

PRESENTATION

RHF

CHF presents differently depending on whether it is right-sided CHF or left-sided CHF. Right-sided CHF presents with hepatic congestion due to backing up of fluid from the right heart to the vena cava. The resultant hepatomegaly can lead to RUQ pain, distention of the jugular veins (JVD), ascites, peripheral edema, cyanosis, and a hepatojugular reflex (HJR). The HJR is increased distention of the jugular veins with gentle upward abdominal pressure due to a fluid wave that travels superiorly.

LHF

Left-sided CHF presents with signs and symptoms of dyspnea on exertion (DOE), paroxysmal nocturnal dyspnea (PND), orthopnea, rales, nocturia, diaphoresis, an S3 gallop, and tachycardia. Both RHF and LHF can present with ankle edema, white sputum with flecks of blood, and cardiomegaly. Dyspnea is also a complaint in CHF, and cardiac dyspnea can present with sudden complaints of SOB, no change in sputum production with no risk factors or objective signs of pulmonary disease, and a restrictive lung defect (RLD) demonstrable by pulmonary function tests (PFTs).

DIAGNOSIS

Diagnosis of CHF is made by plain films of the chest demonstrating cardiomegaly, congestion of the pulmonary vasculature, Kerley B lines, and pulmonary effusion. Echocardiography can be used to demonstrate abnormalities in ventricular wall motion and diminished EF. EF can also be evaluated using a MUGA scan. A urinalysis (UA) will demonstrate oliguria (from activation of the RAA axis), increased specific gravity (SG), hyaline casts, and proteinuria. Diastolic dysfunction will present with normal EF and decreased CO; systolic dysfunction will present with decreased EF and decreased CO. SBP is often increased in diastolic dysfunction.

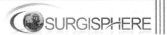

Table 134 Congestive Heart Failure (CHF)

	Congestive Heart Failure (CHF)
Etiology	Most common cause of CHF is following MI and the resultant ischemic changes. Cardiomyopathy, sarcoidosis or hemochromatosis, pulmonary HTN or aortic regurgitation. Structural abnormalities, congenital heart disease, CAD, constrictive pericarditis, RCM,
Diastolic dysfunction	Decreased CO due to elevated SBP with normal EF. Decrease in EF due to decreased SV leads to a decrease in CO in the absence of any change in HR
Systolic dysfunction	Decreased contractility leading to decreased EF. Decreased EF leads to decreased SV, which in the absence of changes to HR, leads to decreased CO.
Pericarditis	Dressler syndrome.
Cardiovascular compensation	Decreases in SV causes increase in the HR. The heart increases stretch, leading to ventricular dilation and thereby increasing EDV. Myocardial hypertrophy results from the increased pressures, and after some time, the heart decompensates, and any further dilation only leads to worsening CHF. A systemic compensation can also occur by way of decreased activation of stretch receptors in the heart and carotid artery, leading to increased systemic vascular resistance, increased afterload, and decreased SV.
Renal compensation	RAA system is activated, leading to vasoconstriction & retention of sodium chloride & water. Increased volume load leads to an increase in preload, which worsens the congestion as the heart is unable to compensate for the increased stretch by increasing its contractility.
Presentation	**RHF--** hepatic congestion, hepatomegaly, RUQ pain, JVD, ascites, peripheral edema, cyanosis, HJR. **LHF--** DOE, PND, orthopnea, rales, nocturia, diaphoresis, an S3 gallop, and tachycardia **Both RHF & LHF--**ankle edema, white sputum with flecks of blood, & cardiomegaly. Dyspnea, sudden complaints of SOB.
Diagnosis	CXR demonstrating cardiomegaly, congestion of pulmonary vasculature, Kerley B lines, pulmonary effusion. Echocardiography, EF can also be evaluated using a MUGA scan. A UA will demonstrate oliguria, increased SG, hyaline casts, and proteinuria. Diastolic dysfunction will present with normal EF and decreased CO; systolic dysfunction will present with decreased EF and decreased CO. SBP is often increased in diastolic dysfunction.

TREATMENT OF DIASTOLIC DYSFUNCTION

Diastolic dysfunction is typically treated with surgical options as medical options such as diuretics and negative inotropes have limited utility. Diuretics are recommended in situations of volume overload, while beta-blockers and calcium-channel blockers are used decrease the inotropic activity of the heart. Digoxin and vasodilators are not used. The main treatment for CHF is to decrease preload through sodium restriction, furosemide diuresis, and venodilation with nitrates. Afterload reduction is typically accomplished with ACE inhibitors. The Caucasian population responds best to ACE inhibitors and beta blockers, while African Americans respond best to calcium-channel blockers. The elderly respond better to thiazides, and diabetics respond better to ACE inhibitors.

TREATMENT OF SYSTOLIC DYSFUNCTION

The cornerstones of treatment involve decreased cardiac oxygen demand, improving cardiac function, and reducing vascular load. Systolic dysfunction is primarily treated by reversing dietary trends such as excessive salt intake, and decreasing major stressors (physical and mental) for the patient. Medical treatment is essential, and is composed of diuretics and vasodilators such as ACE-inhibitors and hydralazine or nitrates. Beta-blockers such as carvedilol or metoprolol are used. Other agents that are often added to manage systolic dysfunction include spironolactone (which reduces mortality), digoxin, dobutamine, and amrinone (which decrease symptoms but have no effect on mortality), and ARBs. Surgery and heart transplant are the final options when all other recourses are exhausted.

Table 135 Treatment of Dysfunctions

Treatment of Dysfunctions	
Diastolic	Surgery, diuretics, beta-blockers and calcium-channel blockers, decrease preload through sodium restriction, furosemide diuresis, and venodilation with nitrates, ACE inhibitors.
Systolic	Decreased cardiac oxygen demand, improving cardiac function, and reducing vascular load. Decrease salt intake, and decreasing major stressors. Diuretics and vasodilators, beta-blockers. Spironolactone, digoxin, dobutamine, and amrinone, and ARBs. Surgery and heart transplant are the final options.

COMPLICATIONS

PULMONARY EDEMA

Acute pulmonary edema is the result of cardiac decompensation leading to fluid collection in the perivascular, peribronchial, and alveolar spaces. It is commonly the result of CHF, arrhythmia, MI, severe HTN, PE, adult respiratory distress syndrome (ARDS), uremia, shock, anaphylaxis, and drug reactions. APE presents with tachypnea, pink sputum discharged with cough, cyanosis, dyspnea, rales, ronchi, wheezing, and crackles. CXR indicates Kerley B lines, pulmonary effusion, Cardiomegaly, and prominent, congested pulmonary vessels. Early ABGs indicate respiratory alkalosis, and later evolve into respiratory acidosis. Treatment of pulmonary edema involves nitroglycerin for preload reduction, oxygen with positive end expiratory pressure (PEEP), morphine, aspirin, and diuretics to further reduce preload. Amrinone may be used to increase inotropy and cause vasodilation, dobutamine can be used to further increase inotropy, and dopamine to cause an inotropic action with vasoconstriction.

Table 136 Pulmonary Edema (APE)

Pulmonary Edema (APE)	
Etiology	Commonly the result of CHF, arrhythmia, MI, severe HTN, PE, ARDS, uremia, shock, anaphylaxis, and drug reactions.
Presentation	Tachypnea, pink sputum discharged with cough, cyanosis, dyspnea, rales, ronchi, wheezing, and crackles.
Diagnosis	CXR indicating Kerley B lines, pulmonary effusion, cardiomegaly. ABG.
Treatment	Nitroglycerin, PEEP, morphine, aspirin, diuretics, amrinone, dobutamine, dopamine.

PAROXYSMAL NOCTURNAL DYSPNEA

PND is the development of difficulty in breathing that awakens a person. During night, the volume of blood that was redistributed to the dependent extremities begins to flow superiorly to the head and chest. This increased fluid load is initially handled by the heart as it stays on the Frank-Starling curve, but the heart in CHF is already at its limits in terms of how much more it can increase contractility in response to increased EDV. The heart falls off the Frank-Starling curve, contractility ceases to keep pace with EDV, and the volume backs up into the lungs. Over a few hours, increasing pulmonary congestion occurs leading to pulmonary edema and impaired oxygen exchange. Hypoxia and dyspnea are the result. PND is treated by having the patient stand up, walk a few paces, and attempt to sleep sitting up. Standard CHF therapies are also used such as vasodilators and volume reducers.

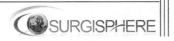

Table 137 Paroxysmal Nocturnal Dyspnea (PND)

Paroxysmal Nocturnal Dyspnea (PND)	
Etiology	At night, blood begins to flow superiorly to the head and chest. Contractility ceases to keep pace with EDV, and the blood backs up into the lungs.
Presentation	Hypoxia, dyspnea wakens patient.
Treatment	Stand up, walk, sleep sitting up, vasodilators, volume reducers.

VALVULAR HEART DISEASE

MITRAL STENOSIS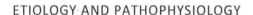

ETIOLOGY AND PATHOPHYSIOLOGY

Mitral stenosis is the development of a narrowing between the left atrium and left ventricle. Abnormalities of the valvular leaflets are the typical cause, and most cases are secondary to RF and subsequent RHD. The majority of patients are female, and congenital causes of MS are rare. Deficits in the valve leaflets and narrowing of the outflow tract lead to impaired LV function (LVF). There is increased pressure in the LA as a result of outflow tract failure, and this causes pulmonary edema and finally RHF.

PRESENTATION

MS presents over a period of time with onset of cough, DOE, hemoptysis, RHF with ventricular failure, hoarseness from laryngeal nerve impingement by the expanding LA, and thromboembolic phenomenon in the systemic vasculature due to hemostasis in the LA. Orthopnea, PND, fatigue, hepatomegaly, ascites, and peripheral edema are other symptoms and are especially likely in the later stages of MS. On physical exam, a significant precordial thrust can be palpated with a sternal lift, atrial fibrillation may be present on EKG, and auscultation may yield a loud S1 with an opening snap. Decreased pulse pressure and a typical apical diastolic rumble may also be present.

DIAGNOSIS

An **apical diastolic murmur with an S1 that has an opening snap** is indicative of MS. A CXR may indicate a straight left edge of the heart due to LAH, and Kerley B lines may be present as a result of the pulmonary congestion; a large pulmonary artery and pulmonary HTN may also be indicated on CXR. EKG typically indicates RVH, atrial fibrillation, and LAH. Echocardiography demonstrates thickened mitral valve leaflets and LAH.

TREATMENT

Treatment of MS starts with **prophylaxis for endocarditis** by beginning regimens typically used for CHF, controlling any arrhythmia that is present, beginning anticoagulation therapy (especially in the presence of atrial fibrillation), and considering balloon valvuloplasty or open surgical repair with significantly narrowed outflow tracts. Balloon valvuloplasty is more successful in MS than in AS. Specific medications include digitalis, diuretics, and warfarin.

Table 138 Mitral Stenosis (MS)

Mitral Stenosis (MS)	
Etiology	Development of a narrowing between LA and LV. Abnormalities of the valvular leaflets are the typical cause, and most cases are secondary to RF and subsequent RHD.
Presentation	Onset of cough, DOE, hemoptysis, RHF with ventricular failure, hoarseness, and thromboembolic phenomenon in the systemic vasculature. Orthopnea, PND, fatigue, hepatomegaly, ascites, and peripheral edema are other symptoms and are especially likely in the later stages.
Diagnosis	Apical diastolic murmur. CXR, a large pulmonary artery and pulmonary HTN. EKG typically indicates RVH, atrial fibrillation, and LAH. Echocardiography demonstrates thickened mitral valve leaflets and LAH.
Treatment	Prophylaxis for endocarditis, controlling any arrhythmia that is present, beginning anticoagulation therapy, and considering balloon valvuloplasty or open surgical repair.

MITRAL REGURGITATION

ETIOLOGY

MR is the result of ischemic changes leading to dysfunction of the papillary muscles, sudden rupture of the chordae tendineae, damage secondary to RHD, progressive changes from MVP, endocarditis, HCM, congenital defects, and severe LV dilation. MR leads to the return of blood during systole from the LV to the LA. MR is more common in men.

PATHOPHYSIOLOGY

MR leads to a compromise of systolic function by causing the left ventricle to exert more energy than necessary against a greater volume load in order to pump blood throughout the systemic circulation. Due to a relative patency in the mitral valve, part of the SV pumped during systole is transmitted into the LA instead of into the systemic circulation. Preload increases, and with the increase in EDV, there is an increase in myocardial contractility, abnormally high EF to compensate for part of the volume going to the LA, and eventual damage to the myocardium from the abnormally high work load as the MR continues to worsen.

PRESENTATION

MR presents with the development of thromboemboli from the relative stasis in the LA, dyspnea, fatigue and weakness, orthopnea, PND, and RHF with pulmonary HTN. A displaced point of maximal impulse (PMI) with a palpable thrill and diminished carotid upstroke, a **holosystolic apical murmur** that radiates to the axilla, an **S3** from rapid LV filling with a split S2 that worsens with inspiration, and JVD.

DIAGNOSIS

Diagnosis of MR includes the presence of the physical symptoms, LAH on CXR and EKG, and valvular dysfunction on echocardiogram. LA overload is obvious on catheterization.

TREATMENT

Medical treatment is typically of low utility, but is the only option available until surgical correction can be achieved. The goal of treatment is to maintain LV function, which heralds a good prognosis. To this extent, diuretics are used to decrease

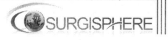

preload, anticoagulation is used to minimize thromboembolic phenomenon, vasodilators such as ACE inhibitors are used to decrease afterload and attempt to shunt the blood away from the bicuspid valve, and digitalis is occasionally used as an inotropic agent. **Replacement of the valve** is done as soon as possible. Criteria for surgery include symptomatic heart failure due to severe MR.

Table 139 Mitral Regurgitation (MR)

Mitral Regurgitation (MR)	
Etiology	Ischemic changes leading to dysfunction of the papillary muscles, sudden rupture of the chordae tendineae, damage secondary to RHD, progressive changes from MVP, endocarditis, HCM, congenital defects, and severe LV dilation.
Presentation	Development of thromboemboli, dyspnea, fatigue & weakness, orthopnea, PND, and RHF with pulmonary HTN.
Diagnosis	Presence of physical symptoms, LAH on CXR and EKG, and valvular dysfunction on echocardiogram. LA overload is obvious on catheterization.
Treatment	Medical treatment is the only option available until surgical correction can be achieved. Diuretics, anticoagulation, vasodilators, and replacement of the valve.

MITRAL VALVE PROLAPSE

Table 140 Mitral Valve Prolapse (MVP)

Mitral Valve Prolapse (MVP)	
Etiology	Most commonly seen in Marfan disease and other connective tissue diseases. RHD, IHD, and ASD. MVP is a congenital valve defect that leads to mild regurgitation.
Presentation	Typically asymptomatic, but may present with atypical chest pain, a mid-systolic click, lightheadedness, syncope, palpitations, fatigue, SOB, and the development of arrhythmias.
Diagnosis	Echocardiography demonstrates displacement of the bicuspid valve leaflets and subsequent meeting at some point distal to the valve opening.
Treatment	Chest pain and arrhythmias are controlled with beta-blockers, and prophylaxis for endocarditis is started in all individuals. Close observation is required to avoid complications.

AORTIC STENOSIS

ETIOLOGY

AS is the result of a congenital disorder, abnormal calcification of the valve leaflets in an otherwise normal adult, presence of a bicuspid valve that predisposes to fibrosis and calcification, or secondary to RHD.

PATHOPHYSIOLOGY

AS leads to increased afterload due to difficulty with transmitted blood through the aortic orifice. In order to avoid the decrease in SV that occurs as a result of the afterload elevation, there is increased contractility of the ventricle in order to maintain CO. Hypertrophic cardiomyopathy (HCM) occurs. Until cardiac decompensation takes place, SV is maintained and CO remains normal. Unfortunately, the hypertrophy that occurs in the ventricle leads to increased oxygen demand, but this is confounded by the elevated pressures within the ventricle that decrease oxygen supply. AS can therefore lead to angina through ischemia. Subsequent failure of the LV can lead to backflow congestion into the lungs and cause pulmonary edema.

PRESENTATION

The high pressures generated within the LV lead to an S4 gallop. **Syncope, angina, and DOE** are all symptoms of AS. Angina and syncope are particularly noted for being worse with exertion. This triad eventually leads to CHF. None of these symptoms occur until late in the course of AS – the early presentation is asymptomatic. Survival after development of angina is typically about five years; after syncope it is about 3 years; and after heart failure, it is typically about one year.

DIFFERENTIAL DIAGNOSIS

The differential diagnosis of AS includes HCM, MR, and pulmonary stenosis (PS). HCM presents with Q waves on EKG, has a bifid carotid upstroke, and has a murmur that decreases with squatting and increases with the Valsalva maneuver. MR presents as a holosystolic murmur that radiates to the axilla. PS presents as a murmur that worsens with inspiration and is loudest along the left upper sternal border (LUSB). Echocardiography is the definitive procedure to distinguish all of these causes. With regard to maneuvers, the Valsalva maneuver decreases the murmur of AS but increases that of HCM; squatting increases the murmur of AS but decreases that of HCM.

AS presents with syncope, angina, and dyspnea on exertion. Triad leads to CHF → 1 year survival.

DIAGNOSIS

Diagnosis of AS is made with physical signs of an aortic ejection click, harsh systolic ejection murmur (SEM) leading to a palpable thrill, especially at the PMI, and S4 gallop, split S2, narrow pulse pressure, and a carotid thrill. The SEM may radiate to the carotids. On echocardiography, a pulsus tardus et parvus may be present – a specific waveform of blood flow velocity that occurs distal to the AS and has a prolonged early systolic acceleration and flattening of the systolic peak (a late pulse that is wider than normal). EKG changes indicate LV stain, and echocardiography demonstrates the damaged aortic valve. CXR can detect calcification of the aortic valve, along with cardiomegaly and pulmonary HTN.

TREATMENT

AS requires endocarditis prophylaxis. The standard therapy, as defined by the American Heart Association, for dental procedures, esophageal procedures, and pulmonary procedures is to administer amoxicillin one hour prior to the procedure. Patients who cannot take oral medications are given ampicillin. Those who are allergic to penicillins are given clindamycin, cephalosporins, or azithromycin. Prior to gastrointestinal or genitourinary (GU) procedures, ampicillin and gentamicin should be given; if the patient is allergic to penicillins, vancomycin plus gentamycin should be administered. Surgery via balloon valvuloplasty to correct the aortic valve defect is done with severe symptoms, but the rate of restenosis is very high and may eventually require replacement of the entire valve. Patients should be advised to avoid exercise.

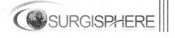

Table 141 Aortic Stenosis (AS)

	Aortic Stenosis (AS)
Etiology	A congenital disorder. Abnormal calcification of the valve leaflets in an otherwise normal adult, presence of a bicuspid valve that predisposes to fibrosis and calcification, or secondary to RHD.
Presentation	S4 gallop. Syncope& angina (worse with exertion), and DOE, CHF. Symptoms occur late in the course of AS
Diagnosis	Physical signs of an aortic ejection click, harsh SEM leading to a palpable thrill, narrow pulse pressure, and a carotid thrill. On echocardiography, a pulsus tardus et parvus. EKG changes indicate LV stain, and echocardiography demonstrates the damaged aortic valve. CXR can detect calcification of the aortic valve, along with cardiomegaly and pulmonary HTN.
Treatment	Endocarditis prophylaxis. Prior to GI or GU procedures, ampicillin and gentamicin should be given Surgery via balloon valvuloplasty to correct the aortic valve defect is done with severe symptoms, but the rate of restenosis is very high and may eventually require replacement of the entire valve. Patients should be advised to avoid exercise.

AORTIC REGURGITATION

ETIOLOGY

AR is commonly the result of RHD, but may also occur in infective endocarditis, in dilations of the aortic root due to HTN, collagen vascular disease (CVD), or Marfan syndrome, in proximal dissections of the aortic root (as in cystic medial necrosis), syphilis, pregnancy, Turner syndrome, in conditions that affect the ascending aorta (such as aortic dissection), ankylosing spondylitis, and trauma.

PATHOPHYSIOLOGY

AR leads to its effects through **volume overload of the LV**. The increased fluid load leads to increased EDV, which in turn increases preload and causes increased myocardial contractility in order to meet the same EF. This attempt to maintain SV and CO leads to overstretching of the myofibrils, and eventually, decompensation by the LV, as it can no longer stretch enough to have a sufficiently forceful contraction. Acute presentations of AR present with very high LV EDP due to lack of sufficient compensation by the ventricle to generate the necessary contractile force. Sudden AR can even lead to unexpected cardiac death by total heart decompensation and cessation of contractions due to fatal EDP. Acute AR leads to decreased CO and a narrow aortic pulse pressure (PP).

PRESENTATION

AR presents with **dyspnea, orthopnea, and PND**. Angina is common from decreased circulation and increased oxygen demand in the myocardium. There is typically a wide pulse pressure, a bounding pulse known as Corrigan pulse, a bisferiens pulse with a dicrotic pulse (two fluid waves), and a rapid femoral pulse (referred to as a pistol-shot pulse). Compression of the femoral artery leads to a bruit, known as Duroziez sign; the Hill sign is SBP that is higher in the lower extremities (LE) than the upper extremities (UE); Quincke sign is fingernail color that changes with the heartbeat; and De Musset sign is bobbing of the head in synchrony with the HR. Other manifestations include a diastolic decrescendo murmur, a systolic flow murmur, and S3, and an Austin-Flint murmur (in which blood enters the LV simultaneously from the aorta due to AR), and from the mitral valve (normal flow).

DIAGNOSIS

Diagnosis of AR is made by physical exam (in which a **blowing diastolic murmur** is worsened by leaning the patient forward). A2 is accentuated, the PMI is displaced laterally and inferiorly, EKG demonstrates LVH with narrow Q waves in the left precordial leads, and echocardiography demonstrates regurgitation. CXR demonstrates LVH and aortic dilation.

TREATMENT

Treatment of AS involves prophylaxis against endocarditis, treating LV failure with preload and afterload reduction, digitalis for positive inotropy, and valve replacement with cardiac decompensation.

Table 142 Aortic Regurgitation (AR)

Aortic Regurgitation (AR)	
Etiology	Commonly the result of RHD, also occurs in infective endocarditis, in dilations of the aortic root due to HTN, CVD, or Marfan syndrome, in proximal dissections of the aortic root , syphilis, HTN, CVD, pregnancy, and Turner syndrome, and in conditions that affect the ascending aorta, ankylosing spondylitis, and trauma.
Presentation	Dyspnea, orthopnea, and PND, angina, a wide pulse pressure, bounding, bisferiens, and rapid femoral pulses. Duroziez sign; Hill sign; Quincke; De Musset sign.
Diagnosis	Physical exam in which a blowing diastolic murmur is worsened by leaning the patient forward. EKG demonstrates LVH. Echocardiography demonstrates regurgitation. CXR demonstrates LVH and aortic dilation.
Treatment	Prophylaxis against endocarditis, treating LV failure with preload and afterload reduction, digitalis for positive inotropy, and valve replacement with cardiac decompensation.

TRICUSPID STENOSIS

Table 143 Tricuspid Stenosis (TS)

Tricuspid Stenosis (TS)	
Etiology	Commonly secondary to RHD, carcinoid, and congenital malformations. It presents with JVD, peripheral edema, and signs of hepatic congestion leading to hepatomegaly, ascites, and jaundice.
Diagnosis	Low-pitched, rumbling, diastolic murmur. A thrill is palpable at the LLSB, and there is a RV thrust present. TS is distinguished from MS in that TS worsens with inspiration.
Treatment	Treatment requires surgical repair.

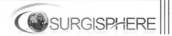

TRICUSPID REGURGITATION

Table 144 Tricuspid Regurgitation

Tricuspid Regurgitation	
Etiology	The result of LHF or mitral valve deficits leading to increased pressure from the pulmonary artery. Stretching of the RV. Presents with signs and symptoms of liver congestion, JVD, & RHF.
Diagnosis	Holosystolic, blowing murmur loudest along the LLSB. Worsens with inspiration. EKG signs indicate RVH, and atrial fibrillation.
Treatment	Treat as LHF. Preload reduction, surgery, endocarditis prophylaxis.

Table 145 Summary Diagnoses of Murmurs

Summary Diagnoses of Murmurs				
Diagnosis	Murmur	S1	S2	Clinical Findings
Mitral stenosis	Apical diastolic rumble	Loud with opening snap	Normal	Murmur worsens with exercise
Mitral regurgitation	Holosystolic murmur	Soft	Split S2	S3 with strong carotid upstroke
Mitral valve prolapse	Mid systolic murmur with click	Normal	Normal	Murmur worsens when standing
Aortic stenosis	Mid systolic murmur, soft when severe	Normal	Paradoxical split	S3, S4, and diminished carotid upstrokes
Aortic regurgitation	Blowing diastolic murmur	Soft	Normal	Wide pulse pressure, SBP elevated
Pulmonary stenosis	Systolic		Single	Prominent "a" wave in the JVP, right ventricular lift, ejection click.
Pulmonary regurgitation	Inaudible in the absence of pulmonary HTN		Widened splitting	Usually related to the underlying disease process.
Tricuspid stenosis	Murmur upon inspiration	Louder at lower left sternal border		Large jugular "a" wave with a slow Y descent. Often occurs with RHD.
Tricuspid regurgitation	Systolic			Atrial enlargement, ventricular hypertrophy, echocardiography is descriptive.

ARRHYTHMIA

INTRODUCTION

Normal electrical conduction within the heart begins with the sinoatrial (SA) node, located in the RA. This natural pacemaker of the heart receives innervation from both the parasympathetic nervous system (PNS) and sympathetic nervous system

(SNS), and responds to the body's need for heart rate modulation as in exercise or in combating illnesses. The impulses leave the SA node and travel to the AV node, where they are briefly delayed to permit atrial contraction and ventricular filling. Once the impulses are transmitted from the AV node, they travel via the bundle of His and the Purkinje fibers to reach the ventricles and cause ventricular depolarization and contraction. The intact conduction system is referred to as normal sinus rhythm (NSR). Abnormal heartbeats due to electrical abnormalities are known as arrhythmia. Arrhythmias are classified by where they begin.

PREMATURE CONTRACTIONS

Premature atrial contractions (PACs) and premature ventricular complexes (PVCs) are early electrical impulses that cause a premature contraction of the heart. They are typically benign and disappear on their own.

SINUS BRADYCARDIA

ETIOLOGY

Sinus bradycardia is a regular heart beat with normal P waves and regular PR intervals but with a rate less than 60 beats per minute (BPM). It is caused by excessive vagal tone, which in turn may be due to vasovagal syncope, MI, carotid sinus pressure, vomiting, parasympathetic agonists such as edrophonium, cardiac glycosides, and Valsalva maneuvers. Overmedication with beta-blockers and calcium-channel blockers also contribute. Increased intracranial pressure (ICP), hypothyroidism, and hypothermia are other causes. Sinus bradycardia may be an entirely normal finding, especially in athletes. It is typically asymptomatic.

TREATMENT

Symptomatic patients are typically treated with atropine. Continuing bradycardia with symptoms requires the use of a pacemaker. A dopamine drip may also be used in an emergent situation.

Table 146 Sinus Bradycardia

Sinus Bradycardia	
Etiology & presentation	It is caused by excessive vagal tone, which in turn may be due to vasovagal syncope, MI, carotid sinus pressure, vomiting, parasympathetic agonists, cardiac glycosides, and Valsalva maneuvers. Overmedication with beta-blockers and calcium-channel blockers also contribute. Increased ICP, hypothyroidism, and hypothermia are other causes. It is typically asymptomatic.
Treatment	Symptomatic patients are typically treated with atropine. Continuing bradycardia with symptoms requires the use of a pacemaker. A dopamine drip may also be used in an emergent situation.

SINUS TACHYCARDIA

ETIOLOGY AND TREATMENT

Sinus tachycardia is a sustained HR over 100 BPM, commonly due to fever, low BP, stress, medications, and hyperthyroidism. It may also occur for a short period of time following the cessation of beta-blocker therapy. Treatment often involves carotid sinus massage and otherwise increasing vagal tone.

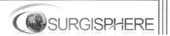

Table 147 Sinus Tachycardia

Sinus Tachycardia	
Etiology	Commonly due to fever, low BP, stress, medications, and hyperthyroidism. May occur for a short period of time following cessation of beta-blockers.
Treatment	Carotid sinus massage and increasing vagal tone.

PAROXYSMAL ATRIAL TACHYCARDIA (PAT)

ETIOLOGY AND TREATMENT

Paroxysmal atrial tachycardia (PAT) is the result of a premature supraventricular beat leading to an AV nodal re-entry rhythm with a rate greater than 130 BPM. It is typically treated by increasing vagal tone, using calcium-channel blockers or adenosine, beta-blockers, and cardioversion.

Table 148 Paroxysmal Atrial Tachycardia

Paroxysmal Atrial Tachycardia	
Etiology	Premature supraventricular beat leading to an AV nodal re-entry rhythm with a rate greater than 130 BPM.
Treatment	Increase vagal tone, calcium-channel blockers or adenosine, beta-blockers, and cardioversion.

ATRIAL FLUTTER

ETIOLOGY AND TREATMENT

Atrial flutter is a regular atrial rhythm of about 300 BPM and a **2:1 block** through the AV node leading to a ventricular rhythm of 150 BPM. It is commonly the result of COPD, PE, MVP, ETOH, and **thyrotoxicosis**. Treatment involves cardioversion, calcium-channel blockers, and digoxin. Atrial flutter is distinguished from atrial fibrillation by its regular rate and rhythm.

Table 149 Atrial Flutter

Atrial Flutter	
Etiology	It is commonly the result of COPD, PE, MVP, ETOH, and thyrotoxicosis.
Treatment	**Cardioversion, calcium-channel blockers, and digoxin.**

ATRIAL FIBRILLATION

ETIOLOGY

Atrial fibrillation is the development of impotent atrial contractions as a result of chaotic electrical activity through the conduction system. It is commonly found in patients with dilated atria, CHF, valvular heart disease, elderly patients, CAD, cardiomyopathy, ETOH abuse, sepsis, RHD, and **thyrotoxicosis**.

PRESENTATION AND DIAGNOSIS

Atrial fibrillation presents with palpitations, missed heart beats, fatigue, chest pain, and TIAs due to thromboembolic phenomenon likely in this condition. Atrial fibrillation is diagnosed as an irregularly irregular pulse, and nondistinct P waves on EKG. Atrial fibrillation has been described as having a "bag of worms" appearance.

TREATMENT

Atrial fibrillation is treated with thromboembolism prophylaxis using warfarin. Patients with a HR greater than 100 BPM may receive IV **beta-blockers** or **calcium-channel blockers**, **digoxin**, and **cardioversion**. Unstable patients receive cardioversion followed by maintenance therapy. Quinidine or **procainamide** may also be used with variable effect.

Table 150 Atrial Fibrillation

Atrial Fibrillation	
Etiology	Result of chaotic electrical activity through the conduction system. Commonly in patients with dilated atria, CHF, valvular heart disease, elderly patients, CAD, cardiomyopathy, ETOH abuse, sepsis, RHD, and thyrotoxicosis.
Diagnosis	Presents with palpitations, missed heart beats, fatigue, chest pain, and TIAs, irregularly irregular pulse, and nondistinct P waves on EKG.
Treatment	Warfarin. Patients with a HR greater than 100 BPM may receive IV beta-blockers or calcium-channel blockers, digoxin, and cardioversion. Unstable patients receive cardioversion followed by maintenance therapy.

ATRIOVENTRICULAR (AV) BLOCK

ETIOLOGY AND PATHOPHYSIOLOGY

Atrioventricular (AV) block can be divided into three distinct classes: first-degree heart block, second-degree heart block, and third-degree heart block. **First-degree heart block is a PR interval greater than 0.20s** at a normal resting HR. It is commonly due to AV conduction system degeneration with aging, excessive vagal tone, inflammation, ischemia, and digoxin toxicity. Second-degree heart block is divided into Mobitz I and Mobitz II. **Mobitz I** second-degree heart block, also known as Wenckebach rhythm, is a **progressive increase in the PR interval** with shortening of the RR interval until a ventricular beat is dropped. It is typically due to AV nodal block in conduction, and this may occur due to poor perfusion. **Mobitz II** second-degree heart block is a **prolonged but stable PR interval with regularly dropped beats**. The site of blockage is usually infranodal. **Third-degree AV block** arises from discontinuity between the atria and ventricles, and leads to independent activity in the atria compared to the ventricles. Third-degree heart block is also known as **complete heart block**, and the source of ventricular rhythm is an ectopic focus distal to the point of conduction blockade. Complete heart block is typically attributed to Lenegre disease, which is age-related degeneration in the conduction system. Other causes include inferior or posterior MI, infection, inflammation, digoxin toxicity, and ankylosing spondylitis. HLA-B27 is linked with the development of complete heart block.

PRESENTATION

First-degree and second-degree heart blocks are typically asymptomatic. Third-degree heart block may present with intermittent CHF, transient ventricular arrhythmias leading to circulatory failure (known as Adams-Stoke attacks), and bradycardia which can worsen CHF.

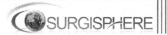

DIAGNOSIS

First-degree heart block is diagnosed by EKG with the characteristic prolonged PR interval. Mobitz I second-degree heart block is diagnosed by progressive PR prolongation with intermittent dropped QRS complexes. Mobitz I may worsen with increased vagal tone, while atropine may ameliorate this condition. Mobitz II second-degree heart block has a stable and prolonged PR interval with predictable dropped beats. Atropine has no effect. Third-degree heart block is diagnosed by independent activity of the atria and ventricles.

TREATMENT

First-degree heart block is typically asymptomatic and not treated. Mobitz I is treated with atropine and pacing. Mobitz II typically requires a pacemaker. Complete heart block requires epinephrine or isoproterenol to establish a sustainable ventricular rate, then maintenance with a pacemaker.

Table 151 Atrioventricular Block

Atrioventricular Block	
Etiology	**First-degree heart block**: Commonly due to AV conduction system degeneration with aging, excessive vagal tone, inflammation, ischemia, and digoxin toxicity. **Second-degree:** is divided into Mobitz I and Mobitz II. *Mobitz I* is typically due to AV nodal block in conduction, and this may occur due to poor perfusion. *Mobitz II* site is usually infranodal. **Third-degree**: Typically attributed to Lenegre disease. Other causes include inferior or posterior MI, infection, inflammation, digoxin toxicity, and ankylosing spondylitis. HLA-B27 is linked with the development of complete heart block.
Presentation	**First-degree** and **second-degree** heart blocks are typically asymptomatic. **Third-degree** heart block may present with intermittent CHF, transient ventricular arrhythmias leading to circulatory failure, and bradycardia which can worsen CHF.
Treatment	**First-degree** heart block is typically not treated. **Mobitz I** is treated with atropine and pacing. **Mobitz II** typically requires a pacemaker. **Complete heart block** requires epinephrine or isoproterenol, then maintenance with a pacemaker.

VENTRICULAR ARRHYTHMIAS

ETIOLOGY

Ventricular arrhythmias are composed of ventricular tachycardia (VT), ventricular fibrillation (VF), WPW, and Torsade de Pointes (the latter two are discussed separately below). VT is a serious condition due to its degeneration into VF. VF is incompatible with life and patients with VF lasting more than a few seconds will lose consciousness. VT is an organized depolarization of the ventricles from a focus of ventricular origin that leads to more than 120 BPM. VT is characterized as having bizarre QRS complexes, and typically has some level of AV dissociation. VT is common in patients with MI, cardiomyopathy, metabolic changes, and digoxin toxicity. WPW and antiarrhythmic agents can also lead to VT. VF is the end result of a chaotic electrical activity within the ventricles leading to haphazard depolarization of the ventricles and an impotent contraction.

PRESENTATION

VT presents with hypotension, CHF, syncope, and cardiac failure. SBP varies over time, and extra heart sounds may be present. Cannon waves may be present in the JVP due to simultaneous contraction of the chambers of the heart. There is also wide splitting of S1 and S2. VF presents with syncope and leads to death if no emergent interventions are taken.

TREATMENT

Increasing voltage cardioversion is used to restore normal heart rhythm, followed by epinephrine, and repeated cardioversion. Amiodarone, lidocaine, magnesium, and procainamide are given with cardioversion repeated between each medication administration. If successful, maintenance therapy includes pacemaker implantation, an implanted cardioverter and defibrillator (ICD), and ablation of any bypass tracts.

Table 152 Ventricular Arrhythmias

Ventricular Arrhythmias	
Etiology	VT, VF, WPW, and Torsade de Pointes. VT is common in patients with MI, cardiomyopathy, metabolic changes, and digoxin toxicity. WPW and antiarrhythmic agents can also lead to VT. VF is the end result of a chaotic electrical activity within the ventricles.
Presentation	Hypotension, CHF, syncope, and cardiac failure. SBP varies over time, and extra heart sounds may be present. Cannon waves may be present in the JVP. There is also wide splitting of S1 and S2. VF presents with syncope and leads to death if no emergent interventions are taken.
Treatment	Increasing voltage cardioversion, followed by epinephrine, and repeated cardioversion. Amiodarone, lidocaine, magnesium, and procainamide are given with cardioversion repeated between each medication administration. If successful, maintenance therapy includes pacemaker implantation, an ICD, and ablation of any bypass tracts.

WOLFF-PARKINSON-WHITE SYNDROME (WPW)

Table 153 Wolf-Parkinson-White Syndrome (WPW)

Wolf-Parkinson-White Syndrome (WPW)	
Etiology	Premature activation of parts of the ventricle. WPW is especially common in congenital heart defects such as Ebstein anomaly, ToV. It can also occur in CHF, HCM, SVT, PAT, and atrial fibrillation.
Diagnosis	EKG typically shows a wide QRS wave with a delta wave indicating early depolarization of the ventricle by the bypass tract. The bypass is identified through electrophysiological tests and cardiac catheterization.
Treatment	Cardioversion may be required and with destructive arrhythmias. Maintenance therapy may be instituted until radioablation can take place; the medications used include amiodarone, flecainide, procainamide, or sotalol.

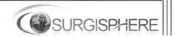

TORSADE DE POINTES

Table 154 Torsade de Pointes

Torsade de Pointes	
Etiology	Caused by hypokalemia, hypomagnesemia, TCAs, procainamide, disopyramide, psychotropic agents, CVA, congenital QT syndrome, quinidine, bradycardia, complete heart block, & idiopathic causes.
Diagnosis/ treatment	Syncope which may worsen into ventricular fibrillation. It may also be initiated by sudden auditory stimuli. Long QT syndrome presents with recurrent lightheadedness and syncope.
Treatment	Treat the underlying etiology, use magnesium to stabilize the heart rhythm, and using beta-blockers for maintenance. Pacing may be necessary.

EISENMENGER SYNDROME

Eisenmenger syndrome occurs later in life with long-term RVH that eventually reverses a L→R shunt and makes it R→L. Occurs with PHTN and requires heart-lung transplant. Shunt reversal leads to cyanosis, hypoxia, clubbing, and polycythemia.

INFLAMMATORY AND INFECTIOUS

CARDIOMYOPATHY

DILATED CARDIOMYOPATHY

ETIOLOGY

DCM is the enlargement of the RV or LV with the loss of normal contractility. The end result is CHF, arrhythmia, and a predisposition towards thromboembolic phenomenon. It typically involves both ventricles, and is the most common cause of cardiac transplant. Causes of DCM include viral infections, alcohol abuse, cocaine abuse, heavy metal poisoning, doxorubicin poisoning, endocrine disease (such as hypothyroidism or hyperthyroidism), pheochromocytoma, CTD, glycogen storage disease (GSD), neuromuscular disease (DMD), pregnancy, metabolic disorders (such as hypocalcemia and hypophosphatemia), inherited disorders (such as Fabry disease or Gaucher disease), and genetic predilections.

PATHOPHYSIOLOGY

Dilation of the ventricles leads to regurgitation through failure of coaptation of the valve leaflets. The combination of poor cardiac contraction, decreased EF, increased preload, and poor valvular function leads to CHF. Relative stasis of blood predisposes individuals to developing thromboembolisms. Finally, the dilation may impinge upon the conduction system and lead to arrhythmia. DCM is distinguished with decreased CO due to decreased SV and EF, an increase in ventricular filling pressure, increase in ventricular volume, and decreased compliance.

PRESENTATION AND DIAGNOSIS

DCM presents as heart failure. Angina is typically present due to increased oxygen demand and poor supply. Diagnosis of DCM is by CXR that indicates cardiomegaly and pulmonary edema, EKG that indicates LVH with LBBB or RVH with RBBB, and confirmation with echocardiography that demonstrates a dilated ventricle, wall motion abnormalities, and valve regurgitation. Physical exam often yields an S3 and S4 murmur, rales, and regurgitation murmurs.

TREATMENT

DCM is symptomatically treated as CHF, with preload and afterload reduction and volume reduction through diuretics and vasodilators, and positive inotropic agents such as digoxin. Pacemaker implantation may be necessary with arrhythmia, especially if rhythm suppressants such as procainamide and quinidine fail. The definitive treatment is heart transplant. All patients require lifelong anticoagulation.

Table 155 Dilated Cardiomyopathy (DCM)

Dilated Cardiomyopathy (DCM)	
Etiology	Viral infections, alcohol abuse, cocaine abuse, heavy metal poisoning, doxorubicin poisoning, endocrine disease, pheochromocytoma, CTD, GSD, DMD, pregnancy, metabolic disorders, inherited disorders, and genetic predilections.
Diagnosis	Presents as heart failure & angina. Diagnosis: CXR that indicates cardiomegaly and pulmonary edema, EKG that indicates LVH with LBBB or RVH with RBBB, echocardiography that demonstrates a dilated ventricle, wall motion abnormalities, and valve regurgitation. Physical exam: often yields murmur, rales, and regurgitation murmurs.
Treatment	Preload, afterload, and volume reduction through diuretics, vasodilators, and positive inotropic agents. Pacemaker (with arrhythmia). **Heart transplant**. Lifelong anticoagulation therapy.

HYPERTROPHIC CARDIOMYOPATHY

ETIOLOGY

HCM is the thickening in the heart wall with narrowing of the intraventricular (IV) septum and sporadic obstruction of the outflow tract. Causes of HCM include generally idiopathic conditions (about half of all cases), and genetic causes (the remainder of all cases). The genetic defects are typically on chromosome 14 with the familial form, and autosomal dominant (AD) with variable penetrance. HCM is sometimes referred to as idiopathic hypertrophic subaortic stenosis (IHSS).

PATHOPHYSIOLOGY

HCM leads to decreased ventricular compliance but an increase in CO, as the heart function moves along the Frank-Starling curve due to volume changes. Diastolic dysfunction may occur as the heart is unable to relax. HCM is exacerbated with inotropic agents, tachycardia, preload reduction, and afterload reduction. HCM is improved with B-blockers, calcium-channel blockers, preload increases, afterload increases, and alpha-adrenergic stimulation. HCM is distinguished by normal CO due to increased SV and EF, an increase in EDP, and a decrease in chamber size. HCM has decreased compliance.

PRESENTATION

HCM presents with syncope and angina, but may proceed directly to sudden cardiac death. Syncope often occurs following exercise, arrhythmia, and CHF. Angina may occur at rest, is not responsive to nitrates, but may improve by lying down. Angina may be due to outflow obstruction, but the precise cause remains to be elucidated. It is the development of arrhythmia that leads to sudden death in HCM. Clinical findings may include palpitations, paradoxical S2 splitting, bifid carotid pulse, S4 gallop, SEM along the LLSB that decreases with squatting and increases with exercise, decreased LV EDV, and regurgitation murmurs.

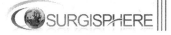

DIAGNOSIS

HCM diagnosis is by EKG (which indicates arrhythmia including PVCs), atrial fibrillation, Q waves, ST changes, and T wave changes. Echocardiography is definitive with septal hypertrophy, LVH, reduced LV EDV, and midsystolic aortic valve closure. A CXR indicates LVH with a dilated LA.

TREATMENT

HCM is treated with arrhythmia suppressants such as amiodarone, beta-blockers decrease HR and permit increased filling time, increasing ventricular space with septal myomectomy, replacement of the mitral valve to reduce obstruction, pacemaker or defibrillator implantation, and avoiding exercise. Heart transplantation is required in most cases. HCM with a resting obstruction is often medically treated with dipyramide, beta-blockers, and calcium-channel blockers; surgical interventions replace the mitral valve or do a ventriculomyotomy. HCM with latent obstruction is treated first with beta-blockers, then by calcium-channel blockers and disopyramide; mitral valve replacement is the surgical procedure of choice. HCM without obstruction is treated with calcium-channel blockers and beta-blockers, and surgery is usually not required. Dopamine will worsen outflow obstruction in HCM.

Table 156 Hypertrophic Cardiomyopathy (HCM)

Hypertrophic Cardiomyopathy (HCM)	
Etiology	Idiopathic conditions & genetic causes. The genetic defects are typically on chromosome 14, and AD with variable penetrance.
Presentation	Syncope & angina, but may proceed directly to sudden cardiac death.
Diagnosis	EKG indicates PVCs, atrial fibrillation, Q, ST, and T wave changes. Echocardiography is definitive with septal hypertrophy, LVH, reduced LV EDV, and midsystolic aortic valve closure. A CXR indicates LVH with dilated LA.
Treatment	Arrhythmia suppressants, beta-blockers, septal myomectomy, replacement of the mitral valve and avoiding exercise. **Heart transplantation** is required in most cases.

RESTRICTIVE CARDIOMYOPATHY

ETIOLOGY

RCM is the result of fibrosis and infiltrative changes to the myocardium, leading to decreased compliance and filling of the ventricles. Causes of RCM include fibroelastosis, hypereosinophilia, amyloidosis, sarcoidosis, hemochromatosis, carcinoid, and cancer. Primary endocardial fibroelastosis is most likely to affect infants and has a thickened aortic and mitral valve with cardiac dilation and hyperplasia. Endomyocardial fibrosis is more common in Africa. Löffler endocarditis typically follows inflammation of the arteries and has an eosinophilia associated with it. Scleroderma (and the CREST syndrome), radiation exposure, GSD, and Becker disease are other causes of RCM. Becker disease occurs mostly in southern Africa with fibrosis of the papillary muscle, concomitant necrosis of the endocardium, and dilation of the ventricles.

PATHOPHYSIOLOGY

RCM leads to scarring of the ventricles and thereby decreases compliance. The rigid myocardium retards filling and leads to abnormalities in diastole. While systolic function is also compromised to some extent, RCM is primarily a diastolic disorder. It must be differentiated from constrictive pericarditis (discussed below), and biopsy is usually done for confirmation of RCM.

DIAGNOSIS

Upon physical exam, an S3 and S4 gallop with mitral valve regurgitation are evident. Low voltage EKG with ST and T wave changes and conduction changes are present. Echocardiography reveals large atria and thickened ventricular walls; some regurgitation is also present. Biopsy clinches the diagnosis.

TREATMENT

RCM is treated with heart transplantation. Medical treatment is effective only in reversible causes such as hemochromatosis (treat with phlebotomy and deferoxamine).

Table 157 Restrictive Cardiomyopathy (RCM)

Restrictive Cardiomyopathy (RCM)	
Etiology	Fibroelastosis, hypereosinophilia, amyloidosis, sarcoidosis, hemochromatosis, carcinoid, & cancer. Scleroderma (and the CREST syndrome), radiation exposure, GSD, and Becker disease are other causes of RCM.
Diagnosis	Biopsy clinches the diagnosis. S3 and S4 gallop with mitral valve regurgitation. Low voltage EKG with ST and T wave changes and conduction changes are present. Echocardiography reveals large atria and thickened ventricular walls; some regurgitation is also present.
Treatment	**Heart transplant.**

PERICARDIAL DISEASE

INTRODUCTION

Nearly all forms of pericardial disease are accompanied by pericardial effusion. Analysis of the fluid helps distinguish the underlying cause of the disease. A transudative effusion has a low specific gravity and is primarily composed of fluid bereft of proteins and cells; transudative effusion is most common in CHF, excessive hydration, and hypoproteinemia. Exudative effusions are more common with direct injury to the pericardium. Serosanguineous effusions are indicative of TB and cancer, while bright red blood should immediately begin a search for aortic dissection and rupture. Other causes of blood within the pericardium include direct trauma, rupture of the heart several days after MI, and coagulopathies. Rapid accumulation of fluid may lead to pericardial tamponade.

Table 158 Pericardial Disease

Pericardial Disease	
Transudative effusion	Has a low specific gravity and is primarily composed of fluid bereft of proteins and cells. Most common in CHF, excessive hydration, and hypoproteinemia.
Exudative effusion	More common with direct injury to the pericardium
Serosanguineous effusions	Indicative of TB and cancer
Aortic dissection	Bright red blood

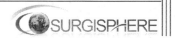

PERICARDITIS

ETIOLOGY

Pericarditis is the inflammation of the pericardium leading to chest pain and a friction rub. Pericarditis is commonly a result of various infectious causes, primary tumors from the breast or lung, a complication of MI, uremia, radiation, Gaucher disease, immunologic disorders, allergic reactions to drugs (such as hydralazine), INH, and procainamide, CVD, thyroid disturbances, trauma, and idiopathic in nature. Recent viral infections can grow into pericarditis; bacterial causes include tuberculosis, streptococci, and staphylococci.

PRESENTATION AND DIAGNOSIS

Pericarditis presents as substernal, pleuritic chest pain relieved by leaning forward. SLN has no effect on ameliorating the symptoms. Upon auscultation, a pericardial friction rub is commonly heard – it is highly specific to pericarditis, but not always present. EKG changes indicate STe; STe in children is most commonly due to pericarditis. CXR may indicate an enlarged cardiac silhouette due to pericardial effusion. Echocardiography may be used to confirm the effusion.

TREATMENT

Pericarditis is treated by symptomatic management, including the use of NSAIDs, and steroids for Dressler syndrome. The underlying etiology should be treated to control progression of pericarditis.

Table 159 Pericarditis

Pericarditis	
Etiology	Inflammation of the pericardium leading to chest pain & a friction rub. Result of various infectious causes, primary tumors from the breast or lung, a complication of MI, uremia, radiation, Gaucher disease, immunologic disorders, allergic reactions to drugs, INH, and procainamide, CVD, thyroid disturbances, trauma, and idiopathic in nature. Recent viral infections can grow into pericarditis.
Diagnosis	Substernal, pleuritic chest pain relieved by leaning forward. Upon auscultation, a pericardial friction rub is commonly heard – it is highly specific to pericarditis, but not always present. EKG changes indicate STe; CXR may indicate an enlarged cardiac silhouette. Echocardiography may be used to confirm the effusion.
Treatment	**NSAIDs and steroids**. The underlying etiology should be treated.

CONSTRICTIVE PERICARDITIS

ETIOLOGY

Constrictive pericarditis is the result of scarring and granulation tissue within the pericardium that limits CO. The subsequent diffuse thickening of the pericardium leads to abnormal diastole. Most causes are idiopathic, but open-heart procedures, radiation, and viral infections have all been attributed.

PRESENTATION

Constrictive pericarditis presents similar to pericardial tamponade but without the rapid circulatory collapse. Orthopnea and dyspnea are the most common signs. Kussmaul sign with continuing JVP during inspiration is a common sign. A pericardial knock manifesting similar to an S3 gallop is typically present, along with distant heart sounds.

DIFFERENTIAL DIAGNOSIS

Pericarditis must be distinguished from RCM (in which LV EF is likely to be decreased). CT can also be used to differentiate pericarditis from RCM.

DIAGNOSIS

Pericarditis is diagnosed through auscultation of distant heart sounds, calcification within the pericardium evident on CXR, low voltage EKG with inverted T waves in V1 and V2 and notched P waves, CT or MRI demonstrating a thickened pericardium, and confirmation of these findings with echocardiography.

TREATMENT

Treatment of pericarditis is to remove the pericardium. Sodium restriction and diuretics typically fail with more severe disease.

Table 160 Constrictive Pericarditis

Constrictive Pericarditis	
Etiology	Result of scarring and granulation tissue within the pericardium that limits CO. The subsequent diffuse thickening of the pericardium leads to abnormal diastole. Most causes are idiopathic, but open-heart procedures, radiation, and viral infections have all been attributed.
Presentation	Presents similar to pericardial tamponade but without the rapid circulatory collapse. Orthopnea and dyspnea. Kussmaul sign with continuing JVP during inspiration. A pericardial knock along with distant heart sounds.
Diagnosis	Pericardium evident on CXR, low voltage EKG with inverted T waves in V1 and V2 and notched P waves. CT or MRI demonstrating a thickened pericardium, and confirmation of these findings with echocardiography.
Treatment	Remove pericardium.

MYOCARDIAL DISEASE

MYOCARDITIS

ETIOLOGY

Myocarditis is the inflammation of the myocardium, commonly due to Coxsackie's B virus infection. Other viruses that can lead to myocarditis include Coxsackie's A, CMV, Epstein-Barr virus (EBV), hepatitis B virus (HBV), echovirus, HIV, and adenovirus. Bacterial causes include group A streptococcus (GAS) leading to RF, corynebacterium, meningococcus, *Borrelia burgdorferi*, and *Mycoplasma pneumoniae*. Parasitic infections include Chagas disease from *Trypanosoma cruzi*, *Toxoplasma*, *Trichinella*, and *Echinococcus*. Arteritis from Kawasaki disease, general inflammation, sarcoid, SLE, cocaine abuse, and drug allergies to penicillin and sulfonamides can also lead to myocarditis. Idiopathic causes are the most common.

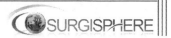

PATHOPHYSIOLOGY

Myocarditis is often associated with pericarditis due to the inflammatory changes taking place. Regurgitation and pericardial friction rubs can occur as a result of the infiltrate of PMNs and other mediators of inflammation and infection; this can also lead to conduction abnormalities. Myocarditis is a progressive disease that requires immediate hospitalization and treatment.

PRESENTATION AND DIAGNOSIS

Myocarditis presents with fever, fatigue, chest pain, and syncope. CHF may also be present due to diminished myocardial function. A history of URI may be present. Diagnosis of myocarditis is definitively made by biopsy. Serology raises the clinical suspicion with elevated ESR, WBC count, and cardiac enzyme elevations. Echocardiography indicates wall motion abnormalities, a generally dilated heart, and pericardial effusions. CXR is typically normal, and EKG changes sometimes find ST changes, arrhythmia, and may be low voltage. On physical exam, an S3 and S4 murmur is present along with regurgitation murmurs; a pericardial friction rub may also be heard. Presentation of symptoms prior to 30 years of age heralds a poor prognosis and increased risk of sudden death. Severity of symptoms is not correlated with increased risk of sudden death.

TREATMENT

Myocarditis is treated with supportive therapy, antibiotics and antivirals as indicated, and treatment of the heart failure and arrhythmia. The patient should be observed in the ICU. Immunosuppressive agents should not be used. Intravenous immunoglobulin (IVIG) may be beneficial.

Table 161 Myocarditis

Myocarditis	
Etiology	Idiopathic causes most common. **Viral:** Coxsackie's A & B, CMV, EBV, HBV, echovirus, HIV, and adenovirus. **Bacterial:** GAS, corynebacterium, meningococcus, *Borrelia burgdorferi*, and *Mycoplasma pneumoniae*. **Parasitic** infections include Chagas disease , *Trichinella*, and *Echinococcus*. **Other:** Arteritis from Kawasaki disease, general inflammation, sarcoid, SLE, cocaine abuse, and drug allergies.
Diagnosis	Diagnosis of myocarditis is definitively made by biopsy. Fever, fatigue, chest pain, and syncope. History of CHF or URI. Serology raises the clinical suspicion with elevated ESR, WBC count, and cardiac enzyme elevations. Echocardiography indicates wall motion abnormalities, a generally dilated heart, and pericardial effusions. CXR is typically normal.
Treatment	Supportive therapy, antibiotics and antivirals, and treatment of the heart failure and arrhythmia.

ENDOCARDIAL DISEASE

INTRODUCTION

Endocarditis is most commonly the result of infection by bacteria leading to infection of the endocardium and subsequent cardiac dysfunction and systemic phenomenon. It is especially likely in individuals with a pre-existing heart defect, those with a history of RHD, and in the elderly with a history of calcific AS. Non-infectious endocarditis is the result of iatrogenic damage to a heart valve followed by the development of infectious endocarditis. Rarer causes of endocarditis include complications of systemic lupus erythematosus (SLE) leading to Libman-Sacks endocarditis (LSE), and nonbacterial thrombotic endocarditis (which is typically a late-stage finding in numerous autoimmune disorders), chronic infections, and systemic illnesses.

INFECTIVE ENDOCARDITIS

ETIOLOGY

Endocarditis is typically the result of an infective process leading to vegetation on the leaflets. Both acute bacterial endocarditis (ABE) and subacute bacterial endocarditis (SBE) can occur. Infective endocarditis is rare, but is increasing in incidence in children with congenital heart defects, especially those with tetralogy of Fallot (TOF), VSD, and AS.

PATHOPHYSIOLOGY

The deposition of platelets and fibrin in regions of endothelial injury provide a region for bacteria to implant and multiply. Dental procedures, oral manipulation, esophageal procedures, respiratory procedures, GI procedures, and GU procedures all require prophylaxis as they may inadvertently allow bacteria to enter the blood (bacteremia), which may permit seeding of the damaged endocardium. About 80% of all cases are attributable to gram-positive bacteria such as *Streptococcus viridans* and *Staphylococcus aureus*. IV drug abusers and those with indwelling catheters are more likely to have fungal causes such as *Candida*. Patients with ABE are likely to have had normal, healthy valves and are typically infected with *S. aureus*. Death is likely within a month unless treatment is obtained. Patients with SBE have a history of heart damage, and are most likely to have *S. viridans*. The mitral valve is most likely to be affected in these patients. Infection by *S. bovis* should raise the suspicion for colon cancer. Most infection by *S. viridans*, group D streptococci, nonenterococcal group D streptococci, HACEK (*Haemophilus aphrophilus*, *Actinobacillus actinomycetemcomitans*, *Cardiobacterium hominis*, *Eikenella corrodens*, and *Kingella kinkae*) organisms, and fungi tend to cause subacute disease. Group B streptococcus, *Staphylococcus aureus*, and *Pseudomonas* tend to cause acute disease.

PRESENTATION

Infective endocarditis should be suspected in any patient with a fever of unknown origin (FUO). Common signs and symptoms include fever, anorexia, headache, arthralgia, and a new heart murmur (common finding that strongly raises the clinical suspicion). ABE in particular presents with acute onset of infection, a new murmur, and infections in other parts of the body from bacteremia leading to meningitis and pneumonia. SBE presents with gradual onset of infection and has splenomegaly. Patients with a right-sided endocarditis should be suspected of IV drug abuse, and septic PE may be the result from the tricuspid infestation. However, left-sided endocarditis is the most common type of endocarditis overall. Aortic valve endocarditis is an indication for replacement of the mitral valve.

DIAGNOSIS

Objective findings of infective endocarditis include multiple petechiae on the chest and mucous membranes, Osler nodes, Janeway lesions, splinter hemorrhages, Roth spots, and hemorrhage. Osler nodes are tender subcutaneous nodules on the distal extremities. Janeway lesions are hemorrhagic, nontender nodules on the distal extremities. Splinter hemorrhages are found in the nail bed, while Roth spots are points of retinal hemorrhage. Three positive blood cultures (BCx) are required for diagnosis. Vegetation on valve leaflets is pathognomonic and can be demonstrated best by TEE. Elevations in ESR, CRP, and WBCs are common, and the UA may have hematuria. CXR may indicate a water-bottle configuration.

TREATMENT

The primary treatment of infective endocarditis is prophylaxis, as discussed above with antibiotic treatment prior to major procedures. Following infection, treatment with ceftriaxone for one month is required for streptococcus infection and oxacillin for a month with staphylococcus infection. Vancomycin is used for resistant strains.

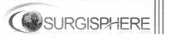

Table 162 Endocarditis

Endocarditis	
Etiology	Result of an infective process leading to vegetation on the leaflets. Both ABE and SBE can occur. Rare, but is increasing in incidence in children with congenital heart defects.
Presentation	Fever, anorexia, headache, arthralgia, and a new heart murmur. **ABE** in particular presents with acute onset of infection, a new murmur, and infections in other parts of the body from bacteremia leading to meningitis and pneumonia. SBE presents with gradual onset of infection and has splenomegaly. Patients with a right-sided endocarditis should be suspected of IV drug abuse, and septic PE may be from tricuspid infestation.
Diagnosis	Three positive BCx are required for diagnosis. Multiple petechiae on the chest and mucous membranes, Osler nodes, Janeway lesions, splinter hemorrhages, Roth spots, and hemorrhage. Vegetation on valve leaflets are pathognomonic, TEE. Elevations in ESR, CRP, and WBCs are common, and the UA may have hematuria. CXR may indicate a water-bottle configuration.
Treatment	Prophylactic antibiotic treatment prior to major procedures. Following infection, treatment with ceftriaxone for one month is required for streptococcus infection and oxacillin for a month with staphylococcus infection. Vancomycin is used for resistant strains.

NONBACTERIAL THROMBOTIC ENDOCARDITIS (NBTE)

Table 163 Nonbacterial Thrombotic Endocarditis (NBTE)

Nonbacterial Thrombotic Endocarditis (NBTE)	
Etiology	Deposition of fibrin is the general underlying cause. Late manifestation of numerous chronic infections, autoimmune disorders, and wasting diseases that lead to a degenerative series of endocardial lesions. NBTE appears to be related to DIC, and the underlying cause may be a variety of neoplasms and systemic infections.
Diagnosis	TEE provides the best chance of identifying this disease. There is no known treatment.

TRAUMA

PERICARDIAL TAMPONADE

ETIOLOGY

Tamponade is the result of a rapid pericardial effusion leading to fluid constriction around the heart and impeding normal cardiac function. It is typically the result of severe pericarditis, direct trauma, rupture of the heart wall following an MI, and dissection of the aorta with subsequent rupture. Cardiac filling is impaired, CO reduced, and systemic cardiovascular decompensation can lead to death. Numerous other causes also exist, such as uremia, radiation therapy to the chest, CVD and CTD, infection, and cancer. Traumatic injuries such as penetrating wounds to the chest or blunt trauma leading to myocardial rupture can all lead to pericardial tamponade.

PATHOPHYSIOLOGY

Pericardial tamponade leads to decreased ventricular volume due to increased external cardiac pressure from the pericardial effusion. **The decreased filling leads to decreased SV and CO, with a subsequent drop in SBP. The body attempts to** compensate for these changes by increased PVR, increasing HR, increased blood volume, and increasing contractility. However, as the effusion increases, the heart is not able to compensate for these changes and cardiac failure ensues with circulatory collapse. **Failure in tamponade occurs from impaired diastolic filling.**

PRESENTATION

Pericardial tamponade presents with **Beck's triad in 33% of patients, which includes JVD, muffled heart sounds, and hypotension.** Other common symptoms include dyspnea, tachycardia, narrow pulse pressure, fatigue, and orthopnea. Pulsus paradoxus is present with a drop in SBP with inspiration (this finding can also occur in other heart failure causes, asthma, and lung disease). Symptoms may develop over 2 hours.

DIAGNOSIS AND TREATMENT

Tamponade is diagnosed by auscultation, a low voltage EKG that shifts over time, CXR that shows enlargement of the cardiac shadow, and echocardiogram that demonstrates the effusion. Pericardiocentesis and surgical drainage are the treatments of choice, and must be done on an emergent basis.

Table 164 Pericardial Tamponade

Pericardial Tamponade	
Etiology	Typically the result of severe pericarditis, direct trauma, rupture of the heart wall following an MI, and dissection of the aorta with subsequent rupture. Numerous other causes also exist, such as uremia, radiation therapy to the chest, CVD and CTD, infection, and cancer.
Presentation	Beck's triad, dyspnea, tachycardia, narrow pulse pressure, fatigue, and orthopnea. Pulsus paradoxus, drop in SBP with inspiration.
Diagnosis	Auscultation, a low voltage EKG that shifts over time, CXR that shows enlargement of the cardiac shadow, and echocardiogram that demonstrates the effusion.
Treatment	Pericardiocentesis and surgical drainage.

AIR EMBOLISM

The initial treatment of an air embolus is placing the patient in Trendelenburg with the left side down. The purpose of this maneuver is to have the air embolism float in the right ventricle and slowly be dissolved by the passing blood.

CANCER

MYXOMA

Cardiac myxoma is the most common primary tumor of the heart in adults. Rhabdomyoma is the most common primary tumor of the heart in children. Cardiac myxoma presents as a left atrial ball-valve obstruction tumor that leads to episodic obstruction. **The presence of spindle cells elsewhere is an indication for an echocardiogram to search for a myxoma.**

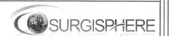

PRACTICE QUESTIONS

 Which of the following medications can be used in CABG patients to improve left ventricular function given high pulmonary artery pressure while avoiding tachycardia?

A. Dobutamine
B. Dopamine
C. Epinephrine
D. Milrinone
   E.   Norepinephrine

 The best answer is <u>Milrinone</u>. Milrinone is used in CABG patients to improve left ventricular function in patients with an elevation in pulmonary artery pressure without causing any tachycardia. Although long term studies debate the effects on morbidity and mortality, it's short term benefits are helpful.

 Which of the following best describes the function of amrinone, an inotrope used following cardiac surgery?

A. Activator of adenylate cyclase leading to inhibition of cAMP, vasodilation, and increased cardiac output
B. Activator of guanylate cyclase leading to vasodilation and increased cardiac output
C. Inhibitor of guanylate cyclase leading to vasodilation and increased cardiac output
D. Phosphodiesterase inhibitor that activates cAMP, leads to vasodilation, and increases cardiac output
E. Phosphodiesterase inhibitor that inhibits cAMP, leads to vasoconstriction, and increases cardiac output

 The best answer is <u>Phosphodiesterase inhibitor that activates cAMP, leads to vasodilation, and increases cardiac output</u>. Amrinone is a phosphodiesterase inhibitor that activates cAMP, leads to vasodilation, and increases cardiac output. It is one of the inotropes, along with milrinone, that leads to utilization of catecholamine stores. The end result is an increase in myocardial oxygen consumption (typically 60%), noted by the equation: oxygen extraction ratio = (arterial oxygen - venous oxygen) / arterial oxygen.

 An 84 year old male who has a myocardial infarction is transferred to the ICU. A Swan-Ganz catheter is floated and a significant elevation in PCWP is noted. What is the underlying cause?

A. Decreased CO
B. Increased EDV
C. Increased EDV and increased SVR
D. Increased EDV, increased SVR, and decreased CO
E. Increased SVR

The best answer is <u>Increased EDV, increased SVR, and decreased CO</u>. This patient has an increase in end diastolic volume due to cardiac hypocontractility, leading to an increase in systemic vascular resistance. The hypocontractility directly leads to a drop in cardiac output.

A 76 year old male who has a myocardial infarction is brought to the ICU in cardiogenic shock. Which of the following is the best initial course of therapy?

A. Dobutamine
B. Epinephrine
C. Milrinone
D. Norepinephrine
E. Vasopressin

 The best answer is <u>Dobutamine</u>. The best initial vasopressor is dobutamine due to its improvement in cardiac contractility without significantly increasing myocardial oxygen consumption. The result is a mitigation in ischemic damage due to failure to increase oxygenation. Hypertrophic subaortic stenosis should be treated with ACE inhibitors, beta blockers, and a possible balloon pump placement to decrease myocardial oxygen demand. Pressors that increase oxygen demand should be avoided in hypertrophic subaortic stenosis.

 Which of the following best describes the most common cause of late death in patients with heart transplantation?

A. Congestive heart failure
B. Graft failure
C. Papillary muscle rupture
D. Silent myocardial infarction
E. Ventricular septal rupture

 The best answer is <u>Silent myocardial infarction</u>. The most common cause of late death following heart transplantation is atherosclerosis leading to silent myocardial infarction. There are few initial warning signs due to denervation of the transplanted heart.

 A 53 year old male presents to the ER with crushing substernal chest pain. He is diagnosed with a myocardial infarction and treatment is started immediately. Four days later, he is seen in urgent care complaining of difficulty breathing and additional chest pain. A holosystolic murmur is auscultated. A transthoracic echocardiogram is most likely to reveal which of the following?

A. Aortic dissection
B. Atrial septal rupture
C. Dressler syndrome
D. Papillary muscle rupture
E. Ventricular septal rupture

 The best answer is <u>Ventricular septal rupture</u>. Septal rupture is more likely in anterior MI and occurs 3-5 days afterwards. It presents with a loud holosystolic murmur that radiates to many locations, and also tends to have a palpable thrill. Echocardiography is used for diagnosis. Rupture of the papillary muscles can lead to mitral regurgitation and sudden cardiac decompensation following a posteroinferior MI. It tends to occur approximately 3-5 days after an MI and presents with a loud holosystolic murmur. Echocardiography demonstrates a valve leaflet moving around with the flow and regurgitation. A ventricular septal rupture is the most common disruption, and occurs in up to 2% of patients who have a myocardial infarction.

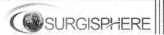

Which of the following is a major contributor to blood oxygen content leading to perfusion of peripheral tissues?

A. Heart rate
B. Hemoglobin concentration and %SO2
C. Hemoglobin concentration and PaO2
D. PaO2
E. PAO2

The best answer is <u>Hemoglobin concentration and %SO2</u>. The greatest contributor to oxygenation is hemoglobin concentration and percent of oxygen saturation within the blood. The initial treatment to improve peripheral oxygenation is to increase oxygen saturation to 100%. Further increases lead to an increase in dissolved oxygen within the blood, but this has a negligible effect at low oxygen flow levels. The next step is to give blood transfusions as clinically indicated in order to improve oxygenation. The relevant equation is 1.37 x oxygen saturation x hemoglobin concentration + 0.003 x PaO2.

A 38 year old male s/p CABGx4 is brought to the ICU in stable condition. Due to continued oozing from various surgical sites, the decision is made to reverse heparin with protamine. What is the most common complication of this maneuver?

A. Anaphylaxis
B. Fever
C. Hypotension
D. Thrombosis
E. Urticaria

The best answer is <u>Hypotension</u>. The most common complication with reversing heparinization with protamine is hypotension, and occurs in up to 10% of all patients. 1mg of protamine per 100 units of heparin should be given for adequate reversal. Serial PTT should be followed. LMWH can also be reversed with protamine to some extent.

Which of the following is not one of the changes that occur in cardiogenic shock?

A. Decreased CO
B. Increased CVP
C. Increased PCWP
D. Increased SVO2
E. Increased SVR

The best answer is <u>Increased SVO2</u>. Cardiogenic shock includes a drop in cardiac output, an increase in central venous pressure, an increase in systemic vascular resistance to maintain blood pressure, an increase in pulmonary capillary wedge pressure due to backflow, and a decrease in SVO2. In right heart failure, CVP is equal to PCWP due faulty right ventricular contraction.

A 32 year old male involved in a motorcycle accident presents to the ER with pulsus paradoxus and cardiovascular decompensation. He is found to have cardiac tamponade on an echocardiogram. What is the mechanism of his decompensation?

A. Collapse of right and left atria
B. Collapse of the thoracic aorta
C. Enlarged left ventricle
D. Hemorrhagic blood loss
E. Pulmonary collapse

The best answer is <u>Collapse of right and left atria</u>. This patient has tamponade, which leads to collapse of the right and left atria and impaired filling of the ventricles. During inspiration, the left ventricle collapses further while the right ventricle enlarges somewhat. Collapse of the great vessels is more likely to occur with tension pneumothorax. Blunt cardiac injuries should be monitored with telemetry. A widened mediastinum on CXR requires a CTA for diagnosis and management.

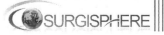

AV Fistula Formation

    ① must obtain flow > 300 mL/min

    ② native AV Fistula requires minimum 4-6 whs to heal ! mature
         (ideally 3-4 mo) !

    ③ Surgical indications
        1) CrCl ≤ 25 mL/min
        2) Cr ≥ 4
        3) likely needs dialysis w/in 1 year

Non-invasive Criteria for Access Procedures

VASCULAR SURGERY

CHAPTER CONTENTS

GENERAL CONCEPTS

CAROTID ANATOMY

Bulb = Baroreceptor

- Carotid bulb: Baroreceptor. Stimulation leads to bradycardia and vasodilation (parasympathetic reaction).

- Carotid sinus: Chemoreceptor. Stimulation leads to a sympathetic response and serves as a detector for CO2 and acidosis.
  (CO_2, H^+)

AV FISTULA FORMATION

The preferred site of AVF is **radial-cephalic** access. Second is brachial-cephalic, third is basilica vein transposition, and the fourth is a synthetic AV graft. Synthetic material is associated with a longer patency in the forearm.

1st option for AVF = radial-cephalic

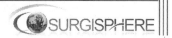

FORMATION OF PLAQUE

Plaque formation occurs in a three step process starting with deposit of lipid within the vessel wall. This leads to the **recruitment of macrophages** that attempt to resorb this lipid, leading to the formation of **foam cells**. **Intimal hyperplasia** sets in with smooth muscle cell proliferation. This is then followed by sudden **plaque rupture**, leading to thromboembolic phenomenon.

MEAN BLOOD PRESSURE

Mean blood pressure is calculated as: $MBP = DP + \frac{(SP-DP)}{3}$

ANKLE-BRACHIAL INDEX

The ankle-brachial index is calculated as the ratio of systolic blood pressure at the dorsalis pedis or posterior tibial artery to that of the brachial artery pressure. **Normal values range from 1.0 – 1.2. Ranges with claudication are 0.5-0.9. Rest pain tends to occur with values less than 0.4**. Patients taking part in an aggressive exercise regimen experience a **drop** in ABI in the presence of peripheral vascular disease.

 ABI < 0.4, rest pain, tissue loss, and failed conservative Rx = intervention, possible bypass

NITRIC OXIDE

Nitric oxide is also known as endothelium-derived relaxing factor, and is produced by **endothelial cells, macrophages, neutrophils, and smooth muscle cells**. It is produced by **L-arginine** and leads to an **increase in cGMP**. Nitric oxide functions as a **vasodilator** and **inhibits platelet aggregation**. Free radical formation is also suppressed. Nitric oxide may be given as a therapy for pulmonary hypertension.

REPERFUSION INJURY

Reperfusion injury occurs following removal of a thrombus and reperfusion to an affected area. Free radicals in the area lead to edema and cell membrane destruction and additional damage. This damage tends to occur in the penumbra region surrounding the necrotic focus. The resultant edema may lead to compartment syndrome, requiring a **four compartment fasciotomy**.

STRUCTURAL AND CONGENITAL

CAROTID ARTERY STENOSIS

Carotid artery stenosis is a serious problem that can lead to CVA and other concomitant head and neck problems. Asymptomatic disease with stenosis > 60%: CEA leads to a decrease in 5 year stroke rate from 10% to 5%. Symptomatic disease with stenosis > 70%: CEA leads to a decrease in 5 year stroke rate from 25% to 10%. Stenting of the carotid artery in high risk patients leads to a decrease in morbidity compared to CEA due to a reduced rate of MI. Amaurosis fugax is a unilateral loss of vision due to atheroembolism to the ophthalmic artery. The ophthalmic artery is the first branch of the ICA. The presence of retrograde ophthalmic artery flow indicates ICA stenosis. The presence of pseudoaneurysm typically occurs six months following repair. Diagnosis is made by duplex and treated by exclusion and bypass. The sequence in traditional CEA is common carotid, followed by the external and internal carotids. The **vagus nerve** is the most commonly injured nerve during a CEA and leads to unilateral vocal cord paralysis, presenting as **hoarseness**.

Table 165 Indications for Repair

Indications for Repair
>50% ICA stenosis and amaurosis fugax
Carotid pseudoaneurysm

SUBCLAVIAN STEAL SYNDROME

Subclavian steal syndrome presents as **subclavian stenosis** proximal to the vertebral artery and leads to a **reversal** of flow in the **vertebral artery** with concomitant lightheadedness and presyncope. Treatment is angioplasty with possible stenting or a carotid to subclavian bypass operation.

ARTERIOVENOUS FISTULAS

 Large arteriovenous fistulas lead to a **decrease in peripheral vascular resistance**.

FIBROMUSCULAR DYSPLASIA

Fibromuscular dysplasia predominantly occurs in **young women** and leads to eccentric arterial stenosis with interspersed dilation. The **right renal artery** is affected in the majority of renal cases. It is the most common cause of arterial stenosis in young females.

 Young woman with RAS / CAS → fibromuscular dysplasia

AORTA

THORACIC AORTIC ANEURYSM

Thoracic aortic aneurysms are separated into various categories. Crawford type I: Aneurysm distal to subclavian artery and terminating proximally to the renal vessels. Crawford type II: Aneurysm distal to subclavian artery and terminating at the aortic bifurcation. Crawford type III: Found more than 7cm distal to subclavian artery and terminating at the aortic bifurcation. Crawford type IV: Aneurysm below diaphragm and extending to aortic bifurcation. Repair is completed by a bypass procedure with intermittent short aorta segment clamping allowing for reimplantation. Repair is indicated for thoracic segments longer than 7.5cm, abdominal segments longer than 5.5 cm, rapidly enlarging size, or symptomatic disease.

ABDOMINAL AORTIC ANEURYSM

ETIOLOGY

An abdominal aorta aneurysm is a dilation of the abdominal aorta secondary to atherosclerosis. Other causes include cystic medial necrosis in CTD, syphilis, fungal infections, aortitis, and trauma. Expansion of the AAA over 5.5 cm heralds a significant risk of rupture, and thus a very high morbidity

 AAA surgery indications: Size > 5.5cm, enlargement > 0.5cm/yr, infection, symptomatic disease.

and mortality. A true aneurysm has a defect in all three layers of the aortic wall, while a pseudoaneurysm affects only the tunica intima and media. A decrease in TIMP1 and 2 occur followed by an increase in MMP1 and 9, IL1, and TNF-alpha; metalloproteases play a role in degradation of the tunica media and adventitia. Risk factors for rupture include **size**, **rapid enlargement** (> 0.5cm / year), **infection** (mycotic aneurysm), HTN, COPD, smoking, and females of gestational age.

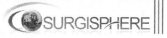

Table 166 Rates of Rupture of AAA

Rates of Rupture of AAA			
3-5.5cm	0.6% / year	5.6-5.9cm	10% / year
6-6.9cm	20% / year	7-7.9cm	30% / year
> 8.0cm	50% / year		

PRESENTATION AND DIAGNOSIS

AAA presents with abdominal pain or back pain and a palpable, pulsatile mass in the abdomen. Syncope is sometimes present, as well as hypotension. There is typically a history of CAD. Most patients are asymptomatic. Diagnosis of AAA is by US, but MRI with IV contrast is preferred to demonstrate the precise dimensions of the mass and whether a leak is present. Angiogram was previously the gold standard.

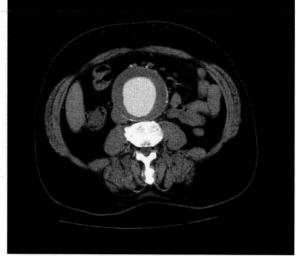

TREATMENT

After diagnosis, patients should have two large bore IV access points and a type and cross (TxC). Patients in whom rupture has occurred should receive emergent laparotomy and surgical correction. Unstable patients with a high clinical suspicion of AAA should be taken immediately to the operating room (OR). An endovascular repair (EVAR) is appropriate in older patients – it is still not the treatment of choice in younger patients as the long-term reliability of this repair remains unproven. Contraindications to EVAR include an infrarenal neck less than 15mm, angulation over 45 degrees, and an insufficient landing zone at the iliac arteries. Serial CT scans are required following EVAR to evaluate for leak.

 Bloody BM s/p AAA = bowel ischemia. Dx w/ colonoscopy.

COMPLICATIONS

The presence of bloody bowel movements following AAA repair requires colonoscopy to rule out ischemia. The presence of an aorto-enteric fistula is treated with an extra-anatomic bypass and exclusion of the graft. Bowel resection may be required.

Table 167 Abdominal Aortic Aneurysm (AAA)

Abdominal Aortic Aneurysm (AAA)	
Etiology	Dilation of the abdominal aorta secondary to atherosclerosis. Other causes include cystic medial necrosis in CTD, syphilis, fungal infections, aortitis, and trauma.
Presentation	Abdominal pain and a pulsatile mass in the abdomen. Syncope is sometimes present as well as HTN.
Diagnosis	US, but MRI with IV contrast is preferred.
Treatment	Patients in whom rupture has occurred should receive emergent laparotomy and surgical correction. Unstable patients with a high clinical suspicion of AAA should be taken immediately to the OR.
Complications	**Type I endoleak:** Perigraft flow into the aneurysm sac around either the proximal or distal attachment sites. **Type II endoleak:** Backbleeding due to collateral blood flow into the aneurysmal sac via patent lumbar arteries or IMA. **Type III endoleak:** Leakage of blood through structural defects in the graft. **Type IV endoleak:** Diffusion of blood through microscopic defects.

AORTIC DISSECTION

ETIOLOGY

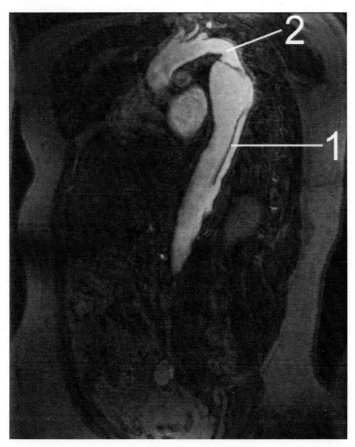

Aortic dissection is the result of a transverse tear through the intima and media of the aortic wall leading to extravasation of blood, potential compromise of flow to other arterial branches, and the possibility of rupture and hemorrhage. Aortic dissection is attributable to HTN, congenital heart defects, CTD, syphilis, pregnancy, coarctation of the aorta (as in Turner syndrome), abuse of cocaine, and trauma. The *Treponema pallidum* organisms of syphilis cause aortic dissection through infection of the vasa vasorum with subsequent irritation by the inflammatory and immune reaction. Aortic dissection is classified by the DeBakey system into three types: type I involves the ascending aorta and part of the distal aorta, and is the most common of the three types; type II involves only the ascending aorta; and type III involves only the descending aorta. The Stanford system classifies aortic dissections into the type A class if the ascending aorta is affected, and the type B class if the descending aorta is affected. **In simpler terms, ascending dissections require surgical management to avoid aortic root rupture. Descending dissections are treated with blood pressure control via beta-blockers and hydralazine.**

PRESENTATION AND DIAGNOSIS

Aortic dissection presents as a tearing sensation with severe chest pain that radiates to the back. HTN is typically present, discordant pulses between extremities can be measured, and AR is typically present. Diagnosis is made by CXR that indicates loss of the aortic knob and a widened mediastinum, CT with IV contrast or TEE that demonstrates an intimal flap with extravasation of blood, and angiogram as the gold standard. A CXR should be obtained in all patients suspected of MI, as the thrombolytic therapy used in MI is absolutely contraindicated in aortic dissection. **Indications for repair** include compromise of **blood flow**, **enlargement** rate over 0.5cm / year, and **pain** associated with dissection; these are all associated with an increase in risk of rupture.

TREATMENT

Aortic dissection is treated with BP control, **immediate surgical repair for type A / type II dissections**, and medical management for type B / type III dissections. Complications of treatment include the development of MI, stroke, and tamponade.

 Fix type A aortic dissections immediately.

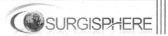

Table 168 Aortic Dissection

Aortic Dissection	
Etiology	Attributable to HTN, congenital heart defects, CTD, syphilis pregnancy, coarctation of the aorta, cocaine abuse, & trauma.
Classifications *DeBakey* *Stanford*	**Type I** involves the ascending aorta and part of the distal aorta **Type II** involves only the ascending aorta **Type III** involves only the descending aorta. **Type A** if the ascending aorta is affected **Type B** if the descending aorta is affected.
Presentation	A tearing sensation with severe chest pain that radiates to the back. HTN, discordant pulses, and AR.
Diagnosis	CXR indicates loss of the aortic knob & a widened mediastinum, CT with IV contrast or TEE that demonstrates an intimal flap with extravasation of blood, and angiogram.
Treatment	BP control, immediate surgical repair for type A / type II dissections, and medical management for type B / type III dissections.

MESENTERIC ARTERY ISCHEMIA

ETIOLOGY

Mesenteric ischemia is the compromise of GI blood flow. It is typically caused by CAD leading to celiac artery, superior mesenteric artery (SMA) or inferior mesenteric artery (IMA) obstruction. **Atrial fibrillation** leading to thromboembolic phenomenon, low flow states contributing to hemostasis, mesenteric thrombi, and hypercoagulable states also contribute to mesenteric ischemia.

PRESENTATION AND DIAGNOSIS

Mesenteric ischemia presents with severe abdominal pain that **worsens with ingestion**. Late signs include **metabolic lactic acidosis** with BRBPR. Diagnosis is confirmed by angiography, but a spiral CT with contrast can also be used.

TREATMENT

Mesenteric ischemia is treated supportively with tissue perfusion. Surgery is required.

Table 169 Mesenteric Ischemia

Mesenteric Ischemia	
Etiology	It is typically caused by CAD leading to celiac artery, SMA or IMA obstruction. Atrial fibrillation, low flow states, mesenteric thrombi, & hypercoagulable states also contribute to mesenteric ischemia.
Presentation	Severe abdominal pain that worsens with ingestion. Late signs include metabolic lactic acidosis with BRBPR.
Diagnosis	Angiography, but a spiral CT with contrast can also be used.
Treatment	Surgery is required. Supportively with tissue perfusion.

SPLENIC ARTERY

The **most common visceral aneurysm** is a splenic artery aneurysm. Repair is done in women of **childbearing age** or if it is larger than 2cm.

> **Splenic aneurysm**: fix if > 2cm or young woman
> **Popliteal aneurysm**: fix if > 2cm by exclusion and bypass due to distal embolization risk
> **Tibial aneurysm**: observe

FEMORAL ARTERY

A cold leg following an aortobifemoral bypass is an indication for return to the operating room for exploration of the groin. Doppler findings changing from biphasic to monophasic is the earliest sign of a thrombosed femoral-popliteal bypass. Reversed venous flow and swelling of the leg with negative Doppler signals indicate obstruction of lymphatic channels. **Treatment of early onset claudication is done with an aggressive exercise regimen and lifestyle changes including cessation of smoking**. Pletal (cilostazol) can be used for peripheral vasodilation and inhibit platelets. Failure of conservative therapy leads to angiography and possible bypass surgery. The best outcome following angioplasty is with the common iliac artery.

POPLITEAL ANEURYSM

Popliteal aneurysms are the most common peripheral aneurysm. Half of all patients have bilateral disease, and 75% have additional aneurysms elsewhere (i.e. AAA). The most common complication of a popliteal aneurysm is **distal embolization**. Popliteal aneurysms greater than 2cm require exclusion and bypass.

TIBIAL ANEURYSM

Indications for a bypass at the tibial artery include limb salvage procedures only. Claudication is not an indication for an infrapopliteal bypass surgery.

VEIN GRAFT FAILURE

Early failure of a vein-graft is likely due to technical error and presents as thrombosis. Late failure of a vein graft is due to fibrointimal hyperplasia and atherosclerosis. Superficial signs of arterial thrombosis include demarcation 10cm below the site of thrombosis. Common femoral artery or external iliac artery thrombosis presents with a midthigh demarcation. Popliteal artery occlusion presents with mid-calf demarcation.

METABOLIC AND DEGENERATIVE

WEGENER GRANULOMATOSIS

Table 170 Wegener Granulomatosis

Wegener Granulomatosis	
Etiology	Formation of necrotizing granulomas in the respiratory tract and renal parenchyma.
Presentation	Inflammation of the respiratory tract, vasculitis of smaller vessels, and focal glomerulonephritis. Septal perforation, otitis media, hearing loss, facial paralysis, oral ulcerations, subglottic stenosis, pulmonary symptoms such as cough, hemoptysis, and pleuritis, focal glomerulonephritis and ESRD, uveitis, myalgias, petechiae, and GI symptoms. **Triad of sinusitis, pulmonary infiltrates, and nephritis**.
Diagnosis	Clinical history, elevated C-ANCA, and confirmation by biopsy.
Treatment	Glucocorticoids. Cyclophosphamide and methotrexate serious disease. TMP-SMX to avoid relapse.

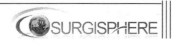

HENOCH-SCHONEIN PURPURA

Table 171 Henoch-Schönlein Purpura (HSP)

Henoch-Schönlein Purpura (HSP)	
Etiology	Aggregation of IgA and deposition of this immunoglobulin within vessel walls and the renal mesangium. An allergic reaction to foods, insects, cold exposure, and various medications have been implicated as being the basis for the faulty immune reaction and IgA release. Other causes include infections by EBV, VZV, parvovirus B19, GAS, HCV, and SBE, and vaccinations including those for typhoid, measles, cholera, and yellow fever.
Presentation	A symmetrical erythematous macular rash begins on the lower extremities followed by the development of purpura. Edema of the scalp and distal extremities occurs. Abdominal pain, bloody diarrhea, arthralgias, and acute renal damage occur. Eosinophilia is often present along with IgA.
Diagnosis	Ultrasound, plain films, and MRI are used to confirm the findings, and a renal biopsy often clinches the diagnosis. The distinguishing feature of HSP is the presence of arthralgias.
Treatment	Supportive management of renal failure and abdominal complications. Corticosteroids have been used with some benefit.

TAKAYASU ARTERITIS

ASSESSMENT

Takayasu arteritis is an autoimmune complex that affects medium and large-sized arteries. It is especially common in Asian women. Takayasu arteritis is also known as pulseless arteritis because it leads to a loss of a palpable pulse in the upper extremities and carotid vessels. Raynaud's phenomenon occurs as a result of this decreased flow, along with decreased perfusion of the brain and the resultant sequelae. Mesenteric ischemia leading to abdominal pain also occurs. Diagnosis of Takayasu arteritis is made by arteriography.

MANAGEMENT

Takayasu arteritis is treated with corticosteroids and methotrexate to induce remission. A related disorder, giant cell arteritis (temporal arteritis), is also treated with steroids.

Table 172 Takayasu Arteritis

Takayasu Arteritis	
Etiology	Autoimmune disorder of medium and large arteries.
Presentation	Loss of palpable pulse in upper extremities and carotids. Raynaud's, abdominal pain.
Diagnosis	Arteriography.
Treatment	Corticosteroids, methotrexate.

⚠ Buerger disease occurs in smokers and leads to medium and small artery vasculopathy.

THROMBOTIC THROMBOCYTOPENIC PURPURA

Table 173 Thrombotic Thrombocytopenic Purpura (TTP)

Thrombotic Thrombocytopenic Purpura (TTP)	
Etiology	Consequence of vascular injury from inflammatory or toxic damage.
Presentation	Widespread capillary thrombosis to kidney and brain. Evolves over a week with fever and purpura. Hematuria and hematochezia with hemorrhage in mucosal membranes and retina. Pancreatitis and arthralgia also evolve. HUS may be preceded by a viral or bacterial prodrome. HUS presents with abdominal pain, nausea and vomiting, diarrhea, GI bleeding, ARF, uremia, HTN, CNS changes, and high fever. A microangiopathic hemolytic anemia with hematuria and proteinuria occur in both TTP and HUS.
Diagnosis	Biopsy is typically required to detect the focal necrotizing arteritis.
Treatment	Plasmapheresis, FFP, and corticosteroids. Splenectomy. HUS requires blood transfusions in most patients. Dialysis is necessary in about half of all patients due to the severe ARF. Fluid and electrolyte management is required, and reduction of HTN is necessary. Anticoagulation, thrombolysis, plasmapheresis, and prostacyclin infusion are necessary in some cases. Mesenteric infarction leading to ischemia of the colon in HUS may necessitate bowel resection.

CHURG-STRAUSS DISEASE

Table 174 Churg-Strauss Disease

Churg-Strauss Disease	
Etiology	Systemic vasculitis of medium sized arteries.
Presentation	Systemic necrotizing vasculitis, bronchospasm, maculopapular rashes.
Diagnosis	Hypereosinophilia
Treatment	Corticosteroids, azathioprine, and cyclophosphamide.

AVASCULAR NECROSIS

ASSESSMENT

The blood supply to the **scaphoid** bone of the wrist and the **head of the femur** are particularly limited and therefore susceptible to distal ischemia, if the perfusion is disturbed. Wrist fractures in the anatomical snuff box and fractures of the head of the femur must therefore be managed quickly and efficiently to prevent avascular necrosis (AVN). Other conditions that can lead to avascular necrosis of the hip include use of steroids, radiation therapy, alcoholism, sickle cell anemia, and Gaucher disease. AVN of the hip presents as referred pain to the knee and is worsened with internal rotation of the hip. It is for this reason, and many other related conditions, that all knee pain elicits a full examination of the entire lower extremity, including the hip. Diagnosis of AVN of the hip or scaphoid is made by MRI or bone scans. Plain films are nonspecific early in the disease.

MANAGEMENT

If surgical repair cannot be done and the blood supply reestablished to the ischemic region, total replacement of the joint may become necessary.

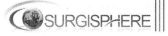

Table 175 Avascular Necrosis (AVN)

Avascular Necrosis (AVN)	
Etiology	Ischemia due to Wrist fractures in the anatomical snuff box and fractures of the head of the femur. Use of steroids, radiation therapy, alcoholism, sickle cell anemia, & Gaucher disease.
Presentation	AVN of the hip presents as referred pain to the knee and is worsened with internal rotation of the hip.
Diagnosis	MRI and bone scans.
Treatment	Surgery, replacement of joint.

LYMPHEDEMA

Lymphedema can be imaged using lymphoscintography. Lymphedema findings include thickening of the skin on MRI. The presence of pitting edema is typically treated with pressure stockings. Organs that do not have drainage of lymph include muscle and brain.

LYMPHADENITIS

Lymphadenitis presents as tender and enlarged lymph nodes typically secondary to a local infection. Suppurative lymphadenitis is the result of infection by gram positive cocci and presents with fever. Treatment involves a third generation cephalosporin and possible incision and drainage of the affected node if an abscess forms. In instances of chronic disease, complete excision and culture is necessary due to the risk of infection by TB or fungus. Necrotizing disease should raise the suspicion for cat-scratch disease; complete resection is required.

TRAUMA

UPPER GASTROINTESTINAL BLEEDING

PATHOPHYSIOLOGY

Upper gastrointestinal (GI) bleeds are arbitrarily defined as those located proximal to the ligament of Treitz, also known as the suspensory ligament of the duodenum. Upper GI bleeds can occur at any level between the oral mucosa and the proximal portion of the duodenum, and include causes such as epistaxis, esophageal varices, tears, or ruptures, gastric erosion, PUD, arteriovenous malformations (AVMs) and tumors.

PRESENTATION

Upper GI bleeds present with a variety of symptoms, depending on the severity of the blood loss. Minor bleeding is often asymptomatic, but may lead to nausea and subsequent hematemesis with the appearance of bright red blood or coffee grounds, if the blood has been exposed to stomach acid for a long time. More severe bleeding leads to melena with black, tar-like stools, hypotension, and tachycardia from the decrease in blood volume. Very brisk bleeds may lead to hypovolemic shock and bright red blood per rectum (BRBPR). Orthostatic hypotension indicates that more than 20% of the intravascular volume has been lost due to hemorrhage. Breakdown of blood by intestinal flora may lead to elevations in blood urea nitrogen (BUN), leading to false positive kidney function tests. Finally, chronic stomach bleeding may lead to iron deficiency anemia.

DIAGNOSIS

Diagnosis of upper GI bleeds is made by directly visualizing the blood via a nasogastric (NG) lavage. A rectal exam with hemoccult testing is always performed. Bleeding sites can often be directly assessed and sometimes immediately corrected via endoscopy. Active bleeding is often identified using tagged red blood cells (RBCs) or arteriography. Finally, laboratory tests include a complete blood count (CBC) to help determine the severity of the hemorrhage. Endoscopy is the standard of care in all upper GI bleeds.

TREATMENT

Treatment for upper GI bleeds is often carried out using an esophagogastroduodenoscopy (EGD), which permits the clinician to carry out a number of procedures to ameliorate the hemorrhage. EGD permits outpatient procedures such as electrocoagulation, sclerotherapy, ligation of ruptured varices, and tamponade if more severe. Severe bleeds also require intravenous (IV) fluids and replacement of lost blood as needed (PRN). Total bowel immobilization to minimize blood flow to the gastrointestinal system may be required through the use of somatostatin. Finally, the risk of recurrent bleeds due to PUD may be reduced through the use of proton pump inhibitors such as omeprazole.

Table 176 Upper Gastrointestinal Bleeding

Upper Gastrointestinal Bleeding	
Pathophysiology	Bleed proximal to the ligament of Treitz (epistaxis, esophageal varices, ruptures, PUD, gastric erosion, AVMs, tumors).
Presentation	Minor bleeding-asymptomatic, hematemesis (bright red or coffee ground); Severe bleeds (tar-like stools, hypotension, tachycardia, shock, BRBPR, elevated BUN.
Diagnosis	Visualized blood via NG lavage, rectal exam, FBOT, tagged RBCs, CBC, endoscopy.
Treatment	EGD with electrocoagulation, sclerotherapy, ligation of varices, tamponade, Ivs.

LOWER GASTROINTESTINAL BLEEDING

PATHOPHYSIOLOGY

Lower GI bleeds occur distal to the suspensory ligament of the duodenum, and may occur at any location between the duodenum and the anus. Although the most common cause of lower GI bleed in the elderly is due to diverticulosis, all GI bleeds in this population should be suspected as heralding gastrointestinal cancer until this etiology is ruled out. Younger patients are more likely to have lower GI bleeding from hemorrhoids, but this particular etiology is commonly managed by the patient and not seen in a clinical setting unless very severe or troublesome. Other causes of lower GI bleeds include inflammatory bowel disease, mesenteric ischemia, arteriovenous malformation (AVM) such as angiodysplasia, and infections. AVMs may present as part of a hereditary conditions that predispose to angiodysplasias, such as Osler-Rendu-Weber syndrome. **The most common cause in adults is from diverticulosis. The most common cause in children is from Meckel diverticulum.**

GI bleed mgmt: Tagged RBC scan if brisk bleed to identify source. Consider angiogram for coil embolization. Colonoscopy for lower GI bleed to ID source. If no source or failed embolization, then OR for bowel resection. Worst case is TAC w/ end ileostomy.

PRESENTATION

Lower GI bleeds present with BRBPR, and such bleeding should begin an immediate investigation of lower GI causes. However, not all incidents of BRBPR are due to lower GI bleeds – a particularly brisk upper GI bleed may also lead to fresh blood expressed from the rectum. Laboratory tests for

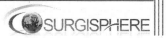

occult bleeding are positive, and other systemic symptoms such as tachycardia and hypovolemia may present in a manner similar to upper GI bleeds.

DIAGNOSIS

Diagnosis of lower GI bleeds is made after ruling out causes of upper GI bleed (through NG lavage). A digital rectal exam is mandatory to test for occult bleeding, followed by a colonoscopy in an attempt to directly visualize and potentially correct obvious sources of bleeding. As per upper GI bleeds, a tagged RBC scan and arteriography are often done. A CBC is done. The most common cause of a lower GI bleed is an upper GI bleed.

TREATMENT

Treatment for a lower GI bleed is similar to that for upper GI bleed. All patients with GI bleeds should receive two large bore IV lines in preparation for significant volume resuscitation. A type and cross should be ordered should emergent use of blood products become necessary. Severe cases of bleeding from the lower GI tract are sometimes treated with colectomy. Moderate bleeding can be isolated with a tagged red blood cell nuclear scan or angiography. Bleeding can sometimes be stopped with angiography and coil embolization. Failure to do so requires surgical intervention and segmental resection. If the bleed cannot be localized, a total abdominal colectomy is required.

Table 177 Lower Gastrointestinal Bleeding

Lower Gastrointestinal Bleeding	
Pathophysiology	Occur distal to the duodenal suspensory ligament. May be diverticulosis (elderly), hemorrhoids (young), cancer, inflammatory bowel disease, AVM, Meckel diverticulum.
Presentation	BRBPR.
Diagnosis	Rule out upper GI bleed. Digital rectal exam, colonoscopy, tagged RBCs, CBC.
Treatment	IVs, colectomy.

PRACTICE QUESTIONS

 Which of the following is an effect of an AV fistula graft formed in a diabetic patient on dialysis?

    A. Bradycardia
    B. Decreased SVO2
    C. Distal thrombosis
    D. Increased cardiac output
    E. Increased peripheral vascular resistance

 The best answer is <u>Increased cardiac output</u>. A patient who has an AV fistula has an increase in cardiac output, decreased peripheral vascular resistance, and tachycardia. The preferred choice for fistula formation is a radiocephalic fistula. The presence of high outflow occlusion should be treated with angioplasty through the venous limb.

A 65 year old female presents to surgery clinic with significant pain in her calf after walking 20 feet. She has dopplerable pulses in both extremities and ABIs of 0.5 and 0.6 (right and left). What is the next best step in management?

A. Anticoagulation

B. Arteriogram

C. Femoral-popliteal bypass graft

D. MRI

E. Smoking cessation and walking regimen

 The best answer is <u>Smoking cessation and walking regimen</u>. This patient has symptomatic claudication with lifestyle limitations. The initial therapy is smoking cessation with an aggressive walking regimen. Control of hyperlipidemia is also important.

 A patient presents with a 3cm popliteal aneurysm. What is the next step in management?

A. Anticoagulation

B. Femoral-popliteal bypass

C. Observation

D. Resection of the aneurysm

E. Stenting of the aneurysm

 The best answer is <u>Resection of the aneurysm</u>. This patient presents with a popliteal aneurysm over 2cm in size, which leads to a significant risk of thrombosis. The treatment is resection of the aneurysm with bypass. Dislocation of the knee can also lead to popliteal artery injury and thrombosis; therapy is with a saphenous vein graft following angiography.

 A 76 year old male is taken to the OR for a 6 cm AAA that has a small leak. Which of the following leads to the formation of an abdominal aortic aneurysm?

A. Decreased MMP activity

B. Destruction of the medial layer

C. Ischemic wall disease

D. Plaque rupture

E. Release of nitric oxide

 The best answer is <u>Destruction of the medial layer</u>. The formation of an AAA can be attributed to destruction of the medial layer of the vessel wall, secondary to an increase in matrix metalloprotease activity. AAA must be repaired when it is over 5 cm in size, becomes symptomatic or develops a leak, or grows by over ½ cm per year. Endovascular repair can be undertaken with infrarenal aneurysms and must have suitable distance between the renal artery and the beginning of the aneurysm. This is important for stent fixation. Symptomatic carotid disease must be repaired prior to AAA repair. Embolectomy is required if distal cyanosis is present at the end of the surgery. Bloody diarrhea following surgery is likely due to ischemic sigmoid disease and requires reimplantation of the IMA to prevent complications. Treatment once ischemia starts is a colonoscopy and sigmoidectomy if full thickness necrosis is present. Graft infections are most commonly attributed to S. aureus, S. epidermidis, and E. coli. Infection of a graft may present as GI bleeding.

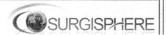

Which of the following is the most common intra-abdominal aneurysm second to a AAA?

A. GDA aneurysm
B. Hepatic artery aneurysm
C. Renal artery aneurysm
D. SMA aneurysm
E. Splenic artery aneurysm

The best answer is <u>Splenic artery aneurysm</u>. Splenic artery aneurysms require resection and bypass if they are over 2cm in size or if they occur in a gestational female. They are the second most common type of abdominal aneurysm.

A 54 patient is found to have 60% stenosis in his right carotid artery. Over the past several months, he has experienced occasional blurry vision and a brief limitation in function of his left hand. What is the next best step in management?

A. Anticoagulation
B. Bilateral CEA
C. CABGx4
D. Observation
E. Right CEA

The best answer is <u>Right CEA</u>. This patient has symptomatic carotid disease with over 50% stenosis, which is treated by carotid endarterectomy. The right side should be corrected first as it is the symptomatic side. Asymptomatic disease with over 70% blockage should be surgically corrected. Simultaneous CABG and CEA can be conducted if there is critical stenosis of the coronary vessels. Angioplasty is the treatment of choice if a younger patient presents with carotid disease, as it is likely secondary to fibromuscular dysplasia. Fibromuscular dysplasia may present as renal artery stenosis, which is treated by stent placement. Recurrent disease may be due to myointimal hyperplasia. The presence of stroke following a CEA requires re-exploration; stroke hours after a CEA may be due to microembolisms and requires a CT of the head for diagnosis and staging. The most commonly injured nerve following a CEA is the vagus, and leads to hoarseness. Dissection of the carotid artery is treated with anticoagulation.

What is the most common acute complication of popliteal aneurysms?

A. Development of thromboembolisms distally
B. Formation of an arteriovenous fistula
C. Ischemic compression of adjacent tissue
D. Rupture of the aneurysm
E. Thrombosis of the aneurysm

The best answer is <u>Development of thromboembolisms distally</u>. The most common peripheral aneurysm is a popliteal aneurysm, and occurs in some 70% of all cases. Femoral aneurysms are next in incidence. Popliteal aneurysms tend to be bilateral in half of all patients, and occur with an abdominal aortic aneurysm in 1/3 of patients. The most common acute complication is thromboembolism leading to a distal occlusion, and tends to occur in 40% of all cases. Rupture of the aneurysm is rare.

A 62 year old male with longstanding vascular disease presents with claudication of his calf muscles. The patient presents with warm feet but significant erythema. Femoral pulses are 2+, but the dorsalis pedis and posterior tibial arteries are only dopplerable as biphasic signals. What is the next best step in treating this patient?

A. Aggressive ambulation therapy
B. Anticoagulation
C. Below knee amputation
D. Femoral arteriography
E. Femoral-popliteal bypass graft

The best answer is <u>Aggressive ambulation therapy</u>. This is a patient who likely has progressive vascular disease leading to femoral-popliteal occlusive disease. This is the most common lower extremity arterial occlusive disease, and occurs in up to 50% of all cases of vascular disease. The major indications for surgery include significant lifestyle limitation in the setting of endangered limb. This patient does not meet these criteria, as the presence of dopplerable pulses indicates that the limb is still being perfused. An aggressive walking regimen and amelioration of other risk factors is the recommended therapy. In the setting of continued compromise, arteriography is a veritable course of action.

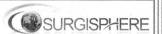

GASTROINTESTINAL SURGERY

CHAPTER CONTENTS

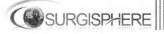

GENERAL CONCEPTS

ANATOMY

STOMACH

The stomach is composed of three smooth muscle layers. The outer longitudinal muscle, the middle circular muscle, and inner oblique muscle layers work in tandem to assist with digestion. The longitudinal layers are found predominantly along the lesser and greater curvatures. The circular muscle is found throughout the stomach, but is especially found at the pylorus. Like the remainder of the gastrointestinal tract, stimulation is primarily by the parasympathetic fibers. At the stomach, these fibers emanate from the vagus nerve. These fibers initiate normal stomach contractions via a pacemaker located in the greater curvature at the body. The phases of contraction are similar to that of the MMC, discussed below. Relaxation of the stomach occurs with CCK, distention of the duodenum, and the presence of glucose in the duodenum. Atonic gastritis and abnormal distention and failure to empty can occur in the postoperative patient due to electrolyte disturbances, hyperglycemia, and uremia.

SMALL INTESTINE

The layers of the small intestine are similar to that of the rest of the gastrointestinal tract. They include the innermost mucosa, submucosa, muscularis propria, and the serosa. The nerve plexuses throughout the GI tract include the subserosal Auerbach plexus and the submucosal Meissner plexus. Peyer's patches, located within the small intestine, are the local source of IgA production. They are an important part of maintaining immunity and are a reason that many surgeons will begin to feed patients. Some studies have shown that this helps to promote an overall immune system response and may play a role in promoting resistance to overall infection.

INTESTINAL FLORA

The most common bacterium within the colon is *B. fragilis*. *E. coli* and *Enterococcus spp.* are the next most common.

HEPATODUODENAL LIGAMENT

The hepatoduodenal ligament contains the porta hepatis: portal vein, hepatic artery, and common bile duct. The Pringle maneuver is used to clamp this ligament shut in the event of injury to the right hepatic artery during a cholecystectomy. The common bile duct is approximately 8cm long within this ligament and is located to the right of the hepatic artery and anterior to the portal vein.

Hepatoduodenal ligament: portal vein, hepatic artery, CBD.

VASCULAR

The blood supply to the gastric pouch following esophagogastrectomy is carried by the right gastroepiploic artery. The SMA crosses at the junction of D3 and D4. The branches of the gastroduodenal artery (GDA) are the superior pancreaticoduodenal artery (which separates into an anterior and posterior branch), the supraduodenal artery, the right gastroepiploic artery, and retroduodenal artery. The right gastric artery arises from the hepatic artery, but is sometimes a branch of the GDA. The most common anomalous artery related to the liver is the common hepatic artery, which may arise from the SMA. The right hepatic artery also sometimes arises from the SMA. The left hepatic artery may arise from the left gastric artery. The blood supply to the duodenum consists of the superior and inferior pancreaticoduodenal arteries (from GDA and SMA, respectively), and part of the gastroduodenal artery and its branches. The right gastroepiploic and right gastric artery also send collaterals to the duodenum.

PHYSIOLOGY

SALIVA

Saliva, gastric acid, and small intestine fluid have very high levels of potassium. Overall, **saliva** has the **highest amount** of **potassium** at 1170mg, followed by gastric acid at 1120mg.

MUCUS

Epithelial cells located in the gastric mucosa secrete mucus. This secretion, along with the secretion of bicarbonate, are inhibited by aspirin. Therefore, the mechanism by which aspirin could potentially contribute to damage to the gastric lining is through inhibition of production of protective factors.

GASTRIN

The release of gastrin is **inhibited by antral and duodenal acidification** as part of a feedback reaction.

SECRETIN

Secretin leads to the release of bicarbonate-rich and chloride-poor fluid from the pancreas. This is due to the exchange of bicarbonate for chloride; the effect is neutralization of the acidic contents entering into the duodenum from the stomach. Secretin also stimulates the release of pepsin and the inhibition of gastrin release, and mediates its effects through the second messenger cAMP. Without stimulation, the normal constituents of pancreatic fluid are sodium and potassium at a concentration iso-osmolar to that found in the serum.

CCK

CCK is a 33 amino acid peptide hormone that stimulates fat and protein digestion. It is produced by the I-cells of the duodenum, and also leads to the secretion of **digestive enzymes** by the **pancreas** and **bile** through **gallbladder contraction**. CCK suppresses hunger, and it has recently been implicated as playing a significant role in drug tolerance to opioids. CCK may be involved in the hypersensitivity to pain experienced during opioid withdrawal. CCK also relaxes the sphincter of Oddi, stimulates secretin release, and stimulates intestinal motility. CCK production is stimulated by long-chain lipids entering the duodenum. Trypsin inactivates CCK.

 Secretin: Bicarbonate-rich pancreatic fluid and enzymes. CCK: GB contraction, pancreatic enzyme secretion.

SUBSTANCE P

Substance P has been implicated in playing a role in **inhibiting small bowel motility**.

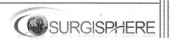

ACID PRODUCTION

Gastric acid is produced by the parietal cells in the stomach. Parietal cells release bicarbonate into the blood stream, known as the alkaline tide, during this process. Carbonate anhydrase plays a role in catalyzing the reaction between CO_2 and H_2O, forming carbonic acid that later dissociates into hydrogen ions and hydrogen carbonate ions. Gastric acid secretion has three phases - the cephalic phase that releases 30% of the total acid in anticipation of eating, the gastric phase that releases 60% of the total acid during digestion, and the intestinal phase that releases 10% of the acid during the secretion of chyme into the small intestine.

INTRINSIC FACTOR

Parietal cells produce intrinsic factor, which plays a role in binding to **vitamin B12** and promoting its absorption in the **ileum**.

IGA PRODUCTION

IgA is an antibody found in **mucous secretions** such as tears, saliva, intestinal juice, vaginal fluid, prostate secretions, and the respiratory epithelium. Secretory IgA is resistant to degradation by enzymes and provides protection against infections that rely on body secretions.

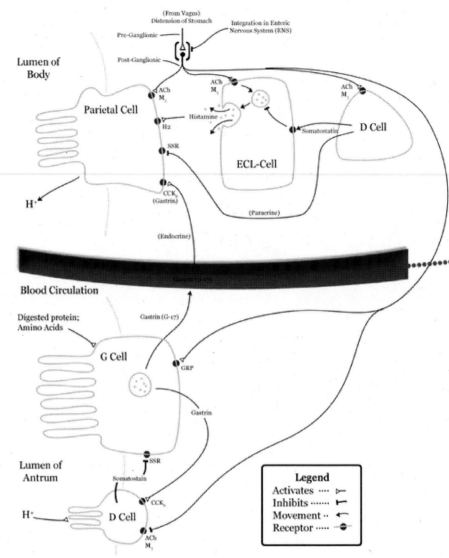

PANCREATIC ENZYMES

Centroacinar cells of the pancreas secrete bicarbonate, and are stimulated by secretin. Basophilic cells of the exocrine pancreas secrete pancreatic amylase, lipase, trypsinogen, chymotrypsinogen, and other digestive enzymes. These cells are stimulated by CCK. Trypsinogen is activated by enterokinase, an enzyme found in the intestinal brush border. Trypsin is the active form of trypsinogen, and activates pancreatic enzymes in the duodenum. High flow pancreatic duct secretions tend to be low in chloride, due primarily to the stimulation by secretin. Amylase and lipase are secreted in active forms by the pancreas. Amylase hydrolyzes carbohydrates in the jejunum. It is cleared rapidly by the kidneys when found in the serum.

MIGRATING MOTOR COMPLEX

The MMC is composed of cyclic waves of activity that regularly sweep through the intestines during a fasting state. The MMC triggers peristaltic waves, starting in the stomach once every 90 minutes between meals. The MMC is partially regulated by **motilin**, starting in the stomach as a response to vagal stimulation. The MMC is independent of other extrinsic nerve activity. The MMC has four phases: Phase I has little electrical activity; phase II has intermittent activity; phase III has maximum activity leading to a regular contraction; phase IV has a brief transitional activity. The MMC starts in the distal esophagus and goes through the entire small intestine. Intermittent contractile activity occurs with eating.

MOTILIN

Motilin is a polypeptide hormone secreted by M cells in the small intestine. Motilin increases the **migrating myoelectric complex** through stimulation of erythromycin receptors, therefore stimulating gastrointestinal motility. Motilin also stimulates the production of pepsin. Alkaline pH in the duodenum appears to stimulate its release. At low pH, motilin inhibits gastric motor activity; while at high pH motilin stimulates gastric motor activity.

NUTRIENT ABSORPTION

Fat, water, sodium, folic acid, proteins, and calcium are absorbed by the jejunum. Nutrients and fluid are absorbed by the ascending colon. Colonic cells receive their energy from short change free fatty acids, typically butyrate acids. Lipids are not directly converted to carbohydrates as acetyl CoA cannot be reversed to create pyruvate. Steatorrhea following ileal resection is typically due to the loss of bile salts from chronic loss. Bile salts are absorbed in the ileum. Micelles are composed of lecithin and cholesterol. Long chain fatty acids are absorbed as chylomicrons by central lacteals. Medium chain fatty acids are absorbed via portal venous blood. The ascending colon reabsorbs most of the water.

Protein absorption is an active process that uses sodium cotransporters. Proteins are absorbed throughout the duodenum and jejunum. The ileum plays only a small role in protein absorption.

PHARMACOLOGY

ANTIHISTAMINES – H1

Table 178 Antihistamines – H1

DRUG	INDICATIONS	MECHANISM OF ACTION	COMPLICATIONS	CONTRAINDICATIONS	NOTES
Diphenhydramine	Sedative Allergic reactions	H1 receptor blocker; reduces smooth muscle contraction	Anticholinergic effects	Severe muscarinic acetylcholine antagonism that may lead to MI in overdose	
Promethazine	Antiemetic Sedative	H1 receptor blocker	Sedation and confusion with anticholinergic effects Fatal respiratory depression in infants	Closed angle glaucoma Alcohol, Hypotension Coma, Hepatic disease BPH	Given with codeine to suppress cough reflex

ANTIHISTAMINES – H2

Table 179 Antihistamines – H2

DRUG	INDICATIONS	MECHANISM OF ACTION	CONTRAINDICATIONS
Ranitidine	GERD, PUD	H2 receptor antagonist to prevent stomach acid production	Hepatic disease

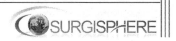

PROTON PUMP INHIBITORS

Table 180 Proton Pump Inhibitors

DRUG	INDICATIONS	MECHANISM OF ACTION	COMPLICATIONS	CONTRAINDICATIONS	NOTES
Omeprazole	PUD GERD ZE syndrome *H. pylori* infection	Proton pump inhibitor that prevents hydrochloric acid secretion from parietal cells	Xerostomia, insomnia	Do not give with antacids due to decreased absorption Prevent antifungal absorption	**Given with clarithromycin, amoxicillin (or metronidazole) and bismuth for *H. pylori* treatment**

MOTILITY AGENTS

Table 181 Motility Agents

DRUG	INDICATIONS	MECHANISM OF ACTION	COMPLICATIONS	CONTRAINDICATIONS	NOTES
Metoclopramide	Gastroparesis N/V	Antidopaminergic effect increases GI motility Prokinetic agent to empty stomach	Sedation, diarrhea, EPS including PD and TD, dystonia	GI obstruction, seizure, pheochromocytoma	Used in anesthesia to tighten LES and avoid aspiration Renal clearance

OSMOTIC AGENTS

Table 182 Osmotic Agents

DRUG	INDICATIONS	MECHANISM OF ACTION	COMPLICATIONS	CONTRAINDICATIONS
Mannitol	Reduce ICP Oliguric renal failure Sweetener for diabetes	Hypertonic solution to increase water and salt excretion in distal tubule Opens BBB through shrinking the endothelial cells	Rare	Few
Lactulose	Constipation Hepatic encephalopathy	Produces ammonia by bacterial flora to reduce body ammonia levels Osmotic reaction draws fluids into the lumen and leads to bowel movements	Diarrhea → dehydration Hypernatremia	Those requiring low galactose diets

STOMACH / DUODENUM

CONGENITAL AND STRUCTURAL

GASTRIC OUTLET OBSTRUCTION

Gastric outlet obstruction presents with a hypochloremic, hypokalemic metabolic alkalosis leading to dehydration. Due to worsening dehydration, sodium conservation occurs with the kidney, leading to a renal tubular acidosis with subsequent aciduria.

AFFERENT LIMB OBSTRUCTION

Afferent limb obstruction (also known as blind loop syndrome) is a complication associated with a Billroth II procedure in which a distal gastric resection followed by a gastrojejunal anastomosis is formed. Afferent limb obstruction is typically due to ulcer formation or technical error. The location of the obstruction is at the limb associated with the gastric remnant going to the duodenum. It presents as severe epigastric pain following eating and leads to a bilious emesis without food. Definitive treatment involves conversion of the Billroth II to a roux-en-Y gastric bypass. A Bilroth II procedure does not delay emptying, while a Roux-en-Y gastric bypass does.

GASTROPARESIS

PATHOPHYSIOLOGY AND PRESENTATION

Gastroparesis is the delay in the normal emptying rate of the stomach, leading to food and liquids being present in the stomach for prolonged periods of time and diminished gastric digestive function. Gastroparesis presents with early satiety, nausea, and vomiting due to defects in gastric emptying. Gastroparesis is most commonly due to degeneration of the innervation to the stomach, chiefly the vagus nerve. The most likely cause of this degeneration is due to **diabetic neuropathy** in patients with longstanding diabetes. Loss of phase 3 activity is the end result. Delayed gastric emptying can also be the result of a truncal vagotomy; however, a paroxysmal easier emptying of liquids can occur due to loss of receptive relaxation.

DIAGNOSIS AND TREATMENT

Diagnosis of gastroparesis is made through radiolabeled studies that gauge the digestive function of the gastrointestinal tract. Metoclopramide to minimize the symptoms of nausea and vomiting is often the treatment of choice. To avoid the problems associated with a truncal vagotomy, a highly selective vagotomy through transection of the criminal nerve of Grassi can be performed.

Table 183 Gastroparesis

Gastroparesis	
Pathophysiology	Delay in normal emptying rate of stomach due to degeneration of stomach nerves.
Presentation	Early satiety, nausea, vomiting.
Diagnosis	Radiolabeled studies that gauge digestive function of the GI tract.
Treatment	Metoclopramide.

METABOLIC AND DEGENERATIVE

GASTRIC BYPASS SURGERY

DUMPING SYNDROME

PATHOPHYSIOLOGY

Dumping syndrome occurs following gastrointestinal surgeries such as bariatric surgery and PUD repair that destroy the normal digestive function. In dumping syndrome, digested food and liquids accumulate in the small intestine, causing

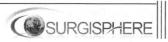

circumferential expansion, additional accumulation of fluids emptying from the stomach into the duodenum, and sudden expulsion of the food through the gastrointestinal system.

PRESENTATION AND DIAGNOSIS

Dumping syndrome presents most commonly after ingesting a fatty or carbohydrate-laden meal. The sudden shift in electrolytes and fluids, and increased sudden blood flow to the small intestine leads to dizziness, lightheadedness, diaphoresis, nausea, and vomiting. Fatty meals tend to present with symptoms within about half-an-hour, while meals rich in carbohydrates present after an hour. Diagnosis is made on clinical presentation.

TREATMENT

Treatment of dumping syndrome requires decreasing fluid intake to small, but frequent amounts that typically should not immediately follow a meal. Fatty foods and simple sugars should be avoided, and meals should be smaller in size. Other complications following bypass is the development of cholecystitis approximately six months following surgery; on the differential is a marginal ulcer. As a result, standard management is to conduct an endoscopy for all patients with clinically significant complaints.

Table 184 Dumping Syndrome

Dumping Syndrome	
Pathophysiology	Occurs after GI surgery & PUD repair.
Presentation	Usually occurs after eating fatty meals. Dizziness, nausea, vomiting, sudden expulsion of food through GI system.
Treatment	Decrease fluid intake to small, frequent amounts. Small meals. Avoid fatty foods, simple sugars.

INFLAMMATORY AND INFECTIOUS

PEPTIC ULCER DISEASE

OVERVIEW

ETIOLOGY AND EPIDEMIOLOGY

PUD is divided into gastric ulcers and duodenal ulcers. Generally, PUD is best thought of as a disruption in the protective barrier of the stomach or duodenum, leading to erosion and subsequent damage to the underlying epithelium. PUD is twice as common in men and has been tied to more stressful personality types ("Type A" personality). The incidence of PUD increases with age, and the largest positive predictors of risk for ulcer development are alcohol use and smoking.

PATHOPHYSIOLOGY

PUD is a consequence of the loss of integrity of the normal mucosal barrier that protects the stomach and duodenum from the hydrochloric acid secreted by parietal cells in the antrum of the stomach. Overall, the most common cause of PUD is *H. pylori*, the same bacterium responsible for type B chronic gastritis.

PRESENTATION

PUD can present as either a gastric ulcer, or a duodenal ulcer. The pathophysiology, presentation, diagnosis, treatment, and complications of each are presented below.

Table 185 Peptic Ulcer Disease

Peptic Ulcer disease (PUD)	
Epidemiology	Twice as common in men and related to Type A personality. PUD increases with age. Predictors-- alcohol use and smoking.
Pathophysiology	Normal mucosal barrier is broken down.

GASTRIC ULCERS

PATHOPHYSIOLOGY

Gastric ulcer formation is most commonly associated with *H. pylori* infection and overuse of NSAIDs or steroidal medications. However, *H. pylori* infection remains a higher predictor of duodenal ulcer formation. Gastric ulcers occur due to a diminished protective barrier against stomach acid, including a thinner mucosal gel and decreased secretion of bicarbonate into the mucosal gel.

PRESENTATION

Gastric ulcers present with a sharp, burning pain in the epigastrium shortly following the consumption of food. The lag time is typically between 10-30 minutes, during this time the stomach increases acid production and additional insult occurs to the protective barrier of the stomach and the underlying epithelium. Gastric ulcers often lead to nausea and vomiting, and the pain may lead to weight loss and anorexia. Due to possible susceptibility from protein similarities, individuals with type A blood are more susceptible to gastric ulcers. Nearly one-quarter of all individuals with gastric ulcers will experience significant hemorrhaging. As a result, gastric ulcers carry a significantly higher risk of complications and death than do duodenal ulcers.

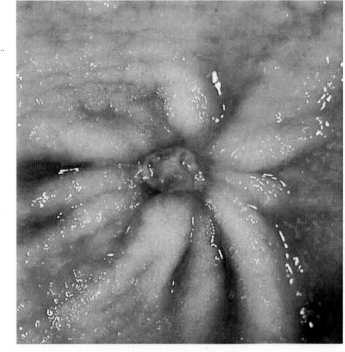

DIAGNOSIS

Diagnosis of gastric ulcer is by **endoscopy** and **biopsy**. Biopsy is mandatory for all endoscopal explorations of gastric ulcer due to the increased association of gastric ulcer with stomach cancer. The presence of *H. pylori* can also be detected using noninvasive tests such as a **urease breath test** and serology, while invasive tests such as a rapid urease test, biopsy, and culture can be utilized as confirmatory tests. Gastric ulcers **most likely to bleed tend to have a visible vessel** (50% of the time). Benign gastric ulcers are usually located along the greater curvature. Gastric ulcer disease due to H. pylori typically is diagnosed by biopsy. These biopsy samples can be taken randomly throughout the corpus and antrum.

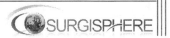

CLASSIFICATION

Type I ulcers occur on the lesser curvature of the stomach and are associated with type A blood. Type II ulcers occur along the lesser curvature and in the duodenum. Type III ulcers are prepyloric. Type IV ulcers are located cranially on the lesser curvature. Type V curvatures are associated with NSAID abuse.

TREATMENT

Treatment options for gastric ulcer primarily involve the eradication of *H. pylori* through a triple therapy, including **bismuth salts, metronidazole, and amoxicillin**. For individuals allergic to penicillins, amoxicillin can be substituted with clarithromycin. These agents are given for a period of several weeks to ensure eradication, and a repeat biopsy afterwards is often

 Treat H. pylori with bismuth salts, metronidazole, and amoxicillin. Eradication is sufficient for MALToma Rx.

done. A proton pump inhibitor such as omeprazole and lanzoprazole is also standard of care, along with antacids and H2 blockers. Examples of antacids include aluminum hydroxide and magnesium hydroxide; examples of H2 blockers include cimetidine, famotidine, nizatidine, and ranitidine. Prostaglandin E in the form of misoprostol is given to buttress the mucosal barrier, and artificial substrates are occasionally given to coat the stomach, such as sucralfate. Symptoms may also be reduced through lifestyle changes such as discontinuing alcohol use and cessation of smoking, and reducing the use of offending medications such as NSAIDs and steroids.

FIRST LINE TREATMENT

The first line treatment for PUD is to eradicate *H. pylori*, followed by the administration of H2 receptor blockers and / or proton pump inhibitors. Prevention is best done by instituting misoprostol therapy for PUD prophylaxis.

COMPLICATIONS

The complications of gastric ulcer disease are numerous, with the most serious including a risk of hemorrhage leading to death. The presence of **H. pylori** has also been tied to the development of lymphoproliferative disease in the form of mucosa-associated lymphoid tissue (**MALT**) lymphoma. Chronic superficial gastritis can also occur, along with chronic atrophic gastritis. The latter condition can lead to the development of gastric adenocarcinoma. Complications may also arise as side effects of treatment. Cimetidine in particular is the only H2 blocker that can cause testicular degeneration and gynecomastia. Cimetidine is not recommended for use in patients on warfarin, phenytoin, or theophylline due to its inhibition of liver enzymes such as cytochrome P450. **Eradication of H. pylori is acceptable management of a MALToma.**

Table 186 Gastric Ulcer Disease

Gastric Peptic Ulcer	
Pathophysiology	*H. pylori* , overuse of NSAIDs and steroids.
Presentation	Sharp, burning pain in epigastrium shortly after eating. Nausea, vomiting, anorexia.
Diagnosis	Endoscopy and biopsy, presence of *H. pylori*.
Treatment	Triple therapy. Proton pump inhibitors, antacids, H2 blockers.

DUODENAL ULCERS

PATHOPHYSIOLOGY

Duodenal ulcers are distinct from gastric ulcers in that they are commonly due to increased gastric acid production. Combined with the insult to the protective mucosal barrier from *H. pylori* infection found in nearly all cases of duodenal ulcers, the two factors combine to cause epithelium destruction and subsequent ulcer formation. *H. pylori* is able to exert its negative effects on the protective lining by degrading the mucous barrier through the production of urease. Other complicating factors include degradation of the mucosal lining through overuse of NSAIDs and steroids, and elevated gastric acid production through high levels of gastrin found in Zollinger-Ellison (ZE) syndrome. ZE syndrome is discussed in the section below. 20% of patients with *H. pylori* develop symptomatic PUD, and 90% of patients with ZE syndrome develop PUD.

PRESENTATION

Duodenal ulcers typically become symptomatic several hours after ingesting a meal. Late dinners often lead to symptoms around midnight, forcing the patient to wake up with severe epigastric pain with a strong burning sensation. Duodenal ulcers are relieved by ingesting additional food, which commonly causes the acidic stomach contents to be retained within the stomach and thereby give the bicarbonate secretion within the proximal duodenum a chance to neutralize the high level of acid. Duodenal ulcers are more common in patients with type O blood.

DIAGNOSIS

Diagnosis of duodenal ulcer is made through endoscopy. Due to the significantly diminished risk of malignancy, biopsy is usually not performed, and the entire diagnosis may even be made following history and physical exam. *H. pylori* infection in duodenal ulcers is diagnosed in the same manner as for gastric ulcer, including through serology, a urease breath test that detects carbon isotopes after ingesting radiolabeled urea.

TREATMENT

Duodenal ulcers require treatment with the triple therapy, including bismuth salts, metronidazole, and amoxicillin, with clarithromycin substituted for amoxicillin in patients with allergies to penicillins. The treatment is otherwise similar to that for gastric ulcers, including cessation of smoking and alcohol, avoiding NSAIDs and steroid medications, using antacids, H2 blockers, proton pump inhibitors, enhancers of the mucosal protective barrier such as prostaglandin E and sucralfate, and surgery when indicated. Surgery becomes the best option for the treatment of duodenal ulcers when the ulcer is refractory to medical management after three months, or there is increasing hemorrhage, obstruction, or even perforation. Perforation of a duodenal ulcer requires prompt surgical attention. The presence of duodenal ulcers does not imply the same risk of a concomitant cancer as it does for gastric ulcers.

Table 187 Duodenal Ulcer

Duodenal Ulcer Disease	
Pathophysiology	Due to increased acid production & *H. pylori*
Presentation	Severe epigastric pain several hours after eating.
Diagnosis	Endoscopy, history, physical exam. Test for *H .pylori*
Treatment	Triple therapy, stop smoking & alcohol consumption, no NSAIDs or steroids, surgery.

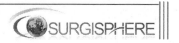

CURLING AND CUSHING ULCERS

Table 188 Curling and Cushing Ulcers

Curling and Cushing Ulcers	
Curling Ulcers	Peptic ulcers formed after sever burn injury.
Cushing Ulcers	Peptic ulcers formed after severe brain damage.

CANCER

VIPOMA

EPIDEMIOLOGY AND ETIOLOGY

Vasoactive intestinal peptide (VIP) is a 28 amino acid peptide that leads to vasodilation, inhibition of gastric acid secretion, and stimulation of pancreatic secretion. VIPomas are a rare (one in ten million persons per year) endocrine tumor that typically originate from the pancreas (the source of vasoactive intestinal peptide). It is caused by non-beta islet-cell tumors and is sometimes associated with MEN.

PATHOPHYSIOLOGY AND PRESENTATION

The high excretion of VIP can lead to significant chronic watery diarrhea, leading to dehydration, hypokalemia, and achlorhydria (WHDA: watery diarrhea, hypokalemia, dehydration, and achlorhydria, also known as Verner-Morrison syndrome). Acidosis, vasodilation with concomitant flushing and hypotension, hypercalcemia, and hyperglycemia are other presenting symptoms. Diarrhea can lead to over 5L of fluid output leading to a non-anion gap acidosis.

DIAGNOSIS AND TREATMENT

Serial levels need to be drawn in order to make an appropriate diagnosis, as VIP production tends to be episodic. Staging of tumor burden is done with a contrasted CT scan; both thoracic and abdominal scans may be necessary. An octreotide scan is also appropriate diagnostic therapy to detect intrapancreatic tumors. VIPoma can be treated with somatostatin (octreotide) or lantreotide. Surgical excision is necessary as the majority of VIPoma are malignant. The most common location they are found is the distal pancreas; hence, a distal pancreatectomy is the definitive procedure. Metastasis to the liver, retroperitoneum, and adrenal glands are the most common sites. Chemotherapy using streptozocin also has some positive effect. Other tumors that secrete VIP include small cell lung cancer, pheochromocytoma, carcinoid, mastocytoma, and ganglioneuroblastoma.

SEROTONINOMA

A serotoninoma is a small bowel tumor that can cause flushing. It is a rare presentation of carcinoid.

ZOLLINGER-ELLISON SYNDROME

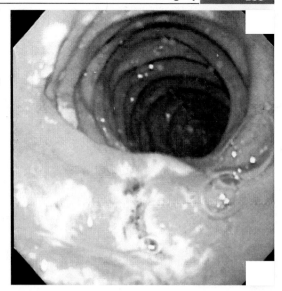

PATHOPHYSIOLOGY

Zollinger-Ellison (ZE) syndrome is due to the uncontrolled production of gastrin, leading to excessive production of hydrochloric acid by the parietal cells of the stomach antrum and thereby exacerbating PUD. Gastrinomas are typically found in the head of the pancreas, but may be located almost anywhere in the gastrointestinal (GI) tract, including the stomach, duodenum, and even spleen. The gastrinoma triangle is where 90% of all tumors are found; the bounds are the junction of the cystic and common bile duct, the confluence of the second and third segments of the duodenum, and the junction of the body and neck of the pancreas.

PRESENTATION

Gastrinoma often presents with PUD, diarrhea with steatorrhea, and other symptoms of mild malabsorption. The PUD is often refractory to medical and surgical interventions as the continuing elevations in hydrochloric acid from the gastrin secretion lead to repeated ulcer formation. Gastrinomas are one of the tumors that sometimes appear in the multiple endocrine neoplasia (MEN) type I disorder, which includes pancreatic tumors (the gastrinoma), pituitary tumors, and parathyroid tumors; approximately one-quarter of all affected individuals will have the full-fledged MEN type I disorder. In those individuals with MEN type I, hypercalcemia may also be part of the presentation. The majority of gastrinomas are malignant tumors.

 Gastrinoma: Positive secretin stimulation test. Presents with multiple ulcers. Resect if not part of MEN I (i.e. sporadic). Else PTHectomy and monitor.

DIAGNOSIS

Diagnosis of ZE syndrome is made through blood tests that find fasting elevations of gastrin of nearly 1 mg/L. The diagnosis is confirmed through the secretin stimulation test. In this test, secretin, the natural inhibitor to gastrin, is administered IV to determine the change in gastrin levels. There is a paradoxical rise in gastrin levels to very high levels following the administration of secretin due to the presence of secretin receptors on the surface of gastrinoma cells. Patients with MEN I typically present with multiple gastrinomas, often located in the duodenum. Intraoperative ultrasound is an invaluable diagnostic tool, given the small size of some of the tumors. The octreotide uptake scan (also known as the somatostatin receptor scintigraphy analysis) is the diagnostic test of choice.

TREATMENT

Treatment of ZE syndrome is best made through surgical resection of the affected region. Medical management is then typically used to control the symptoms, such as the use of proton pump inhibitors.

Table 189 Zollinger-Ellison Syndrome

Zollinger-Ellison Syndrome	
Pathophysiology	Uncontrolled production of gastrin. Gastrinomas often found in head of pancreas.
Presentation	Gastrinomas often with PUD, diarrhea, steatorrhea, malabsorption symptoms.
Diagnosis	Fasting blood tests revealing elevated gastrin titers, secretin stimulation test.
Treatment	Surgical resection of affected area. Proton pump inhibitors.

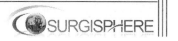

GASTRIC LYMPHOMA

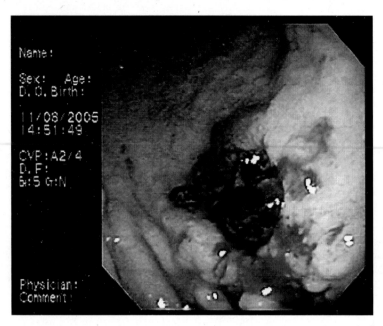

Primary gastric lymphoma accounts for less than 15% of gastric malignancies and about 2% of all lymphomas. The stomach, however, is a common extranodal site for lymphomas. Primary gastric lymphoma usually affects the elderly. It typically presents with epigastric pain, early satiety, weight loss, and malaise.

MALT lymphoma is a form of non-Hodgkin lymphoma (NHL) that involves the mucosa-associated lymphoid tissue (MALT), typically of the stomach. MALTomas are cancers originating from B cells in the marginal zone of the MALT. Gastric MALT lymphoma is frequently associated (72-98%) with chronic inflammation due to H. pylori infection. Patients with a MALToma should be treated for H. pylori presumptively. Chemotherapy is equivalent to surgery for the treatment of gastric lymphoma. Surgery is reserved for cases that have significant comorbidities, such as gastric outlet obstruction.

GASTRIC ADENOCARCINOMA

Gastric adenocarcinoma spreads intramurally and at least 6cm margins should be available with resection. Risk factors include the presence of an adenoma larger than 2cm, type A blood, and the presence of pernicious anemia leading to atrophic gastritis. H. pylori has been attributed as a cause of adenocarcinoma of the stomach.

SMALL BOWEL

CONGENITAL AND STRUCTURAL

SMALL BOWEL OBSTRUCTION

A small bowel obstruction (SBO) is attributed to a mechanical obstruction preventing forward flow of gastrointestinal contents. A partial obstruction permits some flow forward but still leads to distention, nausea, and vomiting. A complete obstruction is a surgical problem that requires intervention and monitoring. The most common cause of an SBO is prior abdominal surgery, due to the presence of adhesions and inflammation. Treatment of a partial obstruction is with nasogastric tube decompression, bowel rest, and if necessary, TPN. Over 2/3s of cases will resolve with this conservative management. Only 1/5 cases of complete obstruction will resolve. The remainder requires operative management with a lysis of adhesions and possible small bowel resection. Extreme care must be taken to avoid making the situation worse with enterotomies leading to enterocutaneous fistulae, or resecting too much bowel and causing short bowel syndrome. The old adage "never let the sun rise or set on a small bowel obstruction" is no longer common practice – it is perfectly reasonable to observe and conservatively treat a complete bowel obstruction so long as the surgeon is ready to take the patient to the operating room at the first sign of distress. Those indicators include a rise in white count, fever, worsening abdominal exam, evidence of clinical deterioration, or evidence of perforation. Most practitioners will take a patient to the OR if their symptoms have not resolved in about 48 hours – others may wait up to one week.

ENTEROCUTANEOUS FISTULA

An enterocutaneous fistula (ECF) is the result of an enterotomy leading to leakage of toxic gastrointestinal contents into the abdomen. Through containment of the abscess, the body naturally shunts this content to the outside by the development of a fistula between the small intestine and skin. Treatment is to remove all foreign bodies, minimize the effects of inflammatory bowel surgery (i.e. infliximab therapy), resolve any distal obstructions, stabilize the patient, and start TPN. Octreotide may also have some benefit.

INTESTINAL PERFORATION

The treatment of a duodenal perforation without prior symptoms or complications can be treated primarily by a Graham patch repair and proton pump inhibitors.

SMALL BOWEL RESECTION

A small bowel resection as a response to a local adenocarcinoma (the most likely site being the duodenum) or a small bowel obstruction leads to a significant morbidity depending on the area and length that is resected. Resection of the terminal ileum leads to a decrease in conjugated bile salt absorption (unconjugated bile salts are absorbed in the jejunum), leading to a decrease in water absorption by the colon and subsequent diarrhea. As intrinsic factor, released by parietal cells in the stomach, binds to vitamin B12 and is absorbed by the terminal ileum, megaloblastic anemia can develop. Decreased binding of oxalate also leads to an increase in oxalate absorption in the colon with subsequent development of oxalate stones in the kidney and gallbladder. Oxalate normally binds to calcium in the bowel to form calcium oxalate, which is excreted with feces. However, the precipitation of fatty acids with calcium in the colon following resection of the terminal ileum prevents this binding, with subsequent absorption of oxalate. Resection of the small intestine to such an extent that less than 100cm remain can lead to the development of short bowel syndrome.

SHORT BOWEL SYNDROME

Short bowel syndrome occurs with resection of the small intestine so less than 100-150cm remains. Severe malabsorption can occur with resection of the terminal ileum or with greater than 50% of the intestine removed. Unless congenital in origin, most cases are acquired due to abdominal surgery leading to complications. Although physiologic changes occur in the small intestine, including expansion of villi, an increase in bowel diameter, and a decrease in the rate of peristalsis, extensive resection leads to lifelong dependence on TPN due to the inability to absorb sufficient nutrients enterally. Patients who are on lifelong TPN have a significant complication rate, with one study estimating that only70% continue to do well after just 2 years. Due to the increased morbidity and mortality, selected patients may be eligible for an intestinal transplant – a procedure that itself carries enormous morbidity and mortality (4 year survival of 60%). Step procedures exist at specialized institutions where duplication of the small intestine can be attempted – the overall success is controversial.

OGILVIE SYNDROME

ASSESSMENT

Ogilvie syndrome is a **distention of the bowel leading to obstruction**. It tends to occur following non-abdominal procedures, especially following cardiac surgery. It is thought to be due to neurologic dysfunction, abnormalities in electrolytes, and related to age.

 Ogilvie Rx = neostigmine. Have atropine for bradycardia. Tends to perforate at cecum.

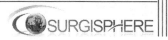

MANAGEMENT

Ogilvie syndrome is treated with nasogastric tube decompression and intravenous **neostigmine** to stimulate the parasympathetic system. **Atropine** should be on hand in the event of significant bradycardia. Decompression with **colonoscopy** has a 90% success rate but a 40% recurrence rate. In the worst circumstance, an **exploratory laparotomy** with bowel resection or cecostomy is required. The **cecum** is at the greatest risk of perforation.

METABOLIC AND DEGENERATIVE

MALABSORPTION SYNDROMES

ETIOLOGY

Malabsorption syndromes are defined as the alterations in intestinal absorption of vital fluids, vitamins, and nutrients. The small bowel is the site of many of these malabsorption problems, which may include selective deficiencies in monosaccharides, lipids, lipid-soluble vitamins, amino acids, nucleic acids, fluids, water-soluble vitamins, bile salts, and electrolytes. Malabsorption syndromes commonly occur due to defects in digestion, poor distribution of emulsifying bile acids, changes to the anatomy of the bowel, obstruction to the lymphatic drainage of the bowel, decreased function or surface area available for absorption, alterations in hormones, and infection.

PATHOPHYSIOLOGY – MONOSACCHARIDE

Defects in absorption related to **monosaccharides** involve the **entire small bowel**. In this scenario, only monosaccharides are absorbed due to defects in the degradation of complex carbohydrates, poor transport with the sodium cotransporter due to low amounts of sodium in meals, or excess fructose in the diet that overwhelms the fructose transporters and causes an osmotic diarrhea.

PATHOPHYSIOLOGY – LACTOSE INTOLERANCE

Lactose is a major sugar digested by many people who consume dairy products, but some patients have an inherent deficiency in lactase that usually worsens with age. It is especially common in adult patients from Africa, Asians, and a minority of Caucasians. This congenital defect in lactase leads to symptoms including abdominal cramps, flatus, and diarrhea.

> **Duodenum**: Water-soluble vitamins except B12. Chloride, iron, calcium.
> **Jejunum**: Amino acids.
> **Ileum**: B12, bile salts, lipids
> **Ascending colon**: Water

PATHOPHYSIOLOGY – LIPIDS

The absorption of lipids and **lipid-soluble vitamins** such as vitamins D, E, K, and A typically affects the **ileum** more often than in the other parts of the small intestine. For proper absorption to occur, pancreatic lipase must be present in appropriate amounts to hydrolyze triglycerides, bile salts must be present to emulsify fats and form micelles, and digestive products must be reabsorbed in the ileum and not sooner. In addition, sufficient micelles must be present to permit proper absorption of the fat-soluble vitamins.

PATHOPHYSIOLOGY – AMINO ACIDS AND NUCLEIC ACIDS

The absorption of **amino acids** occurs more often in the **jejunum** than in other parts of the small intestine. Protein digestion starts in the stomach and must continue without problems in the duodenum, with the proper functioning of pancreatic enzymes such as trypsin, chymotrypsin, and elastase. **Cotransport of most amino acids requires sodium**, but there are also various sodium-independent transporters available for certain amino acids. **Nucleic acid transport** involves the **entire small intestine** and requires pancreatic nucleases to cleave nucleic acids into **pentoses** for **passive transport** through diffusion.

PATHOPHYSIOLOGY – FLUIDS

Fluids are absorbed mostly in the jejunum, followed by the ileum and then colon. The small intestine secretes an additional 7 L to the 2 L ingested daily, with only 200 mL remaining for defecation after absorption by the intestines. Water moves parallel to the osmotic gradients, and thus any defect in fluid absorption requires a search for shifts in these gradients.

PATHOPHYSIOLOGY – VITAMINS AND BILE SALTS

The transport of **water-soluble vitamins** primarily occurs in the **duodenum** through passive diffusion. **Vitamin B12** is an exception to this rule because it requires intrinsic factor to be produced by the parietal cells in the stomach for absorption in the **terminal ileum**. Bile salts are reabsorbed through an active transport process in the ileum for recycling.

PATHOPHYSIOLOGY – ELECTROLYTES

Sodium, potassium, chloride, calcium, and iron ions are absorbed and secreted throughout much of the small intestine. The majority of **chloride, calcium, and iron transport occur in the duodenum**. Sodium ions are absorbed through an active and a passive mechanism, while secretion of sodium ions into the intestinal lumen occurs through the Na+-K+-ATPase transport system. Potassium ions are absorbed in the small intestine, and secreted in the colon. Chloride ions are secreted in small amounts, but overall, they are absorbed, especially in the duodenum. Calcium ions are actively transported with the assistance of 1,2,5-dihydroxycholecalciferol and further assisted by protein absorption. A diet high in phosphates or oxalates inhibits calcium ion transport. Finally, iron ion transport is generally poor and is best done when iron is in the Fe2+ form, as this ferrous form freely diffuses through the mucosa and binds to the iron storage molecule, apoferritin. The iron then moves from apoferritin to the transport protein known as transferrin. Proper iron ion absorption thereby requires the reduction of the dietary form of iron (Fe3+, or ferric iron) to ferrous iron (Fe2+) by stomach acid, binding to adequate amounts of apoferritin, and subsequent binding to proper amounts of transferrin.

PRESENTATION

The signs and symptoms of malabsorption syndromes are numerous and depend on the particular etiology of the disorder. Generally, malabsorption syndromes present with steatorrhea (which is in especially large amounts with pancreatic defects), deficiencies in one or more vitamins and/or minerals, weight loss, bloating and abdominal pain, osteoporosis with poor calcium absorption, diarrhea, flatus, amenorrhea, anemia and platelet defects leading to easy bruising, and neuropathy.

DIAGNOSIS AND TREATMENT

Diagnosis of malabsorption syndromes is made using a Sudan stain to confirm the presence of steatorrhea, confirming the nature of the malabsorption through a challenge test, and finally doing a biopsy of the small bowel to determine the presence of certain malabsorptive diseases. Treatment for malabsorptive disorders is accomplished by treating diseases that are causing the defect or correcting for deficits in the body through replacement of particular nutrients or replacing pancreatic enzymes that are not functioning properly. All malabsorptive syndromes require vitamin replacement due to normal losses experienced with the diarrhea. Lactose intolerance is treated by avoiding dairy products and administering lactase supplements.

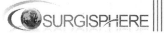

Table 190 Malabsorption Syndromes

Malabsorption Syndromes	
Etiology	Alteration in intestinal absorption of vital fluids, vitamins, and nutrients.
Monosaccharides	Involve entire SI. Defect in degradation of complex carbohydrates, excess fructose.
Lactose intolerance	Inherited deficiency in lactase.
Lipids & Vitamins A, D, E, K	Occurs more often in the duodenum. May be lipase, or bile salt deficient.
Amino & nucleic acids	Occurs more often in jejunum. May be deficient in trypsin, chymotrypsin, and elastase.
Water soluble vitamins & bile salts	Vitamin transport occurs in the duodenum. Bile salts are reabsorbed in the ileum.
Electrolytes	Na, K, Ca, and Fe ions are absorbed and secreted through much of the SI.
Presentation	Generally present with steatorrhea, deficiencies in one or more vitamins/minerals, weight loss, bloating, abdominal pain, neuropathy, easy bruising.
Diagnosis & treatment	Sudan stain, malabsorption challenge tests, biopsy. Replace nutrients & vitamins.

INFLAMMATORY AND INFECTIOUS

APPENDICITIS

ETIOLOGY

Appendicitis is attributed to the formation of an **appendicolith** in **adults**, leading to bacterial overgrowth with subsequent development of pain, fever, chills, and overlying abdominal tenderness in the right lower quadrant. In **children**, the most common cause of appendicitis is **lymphoid hyperplasia**. Tumors such as **carcinoid** and adenocarcinoma can also lead to appendicitis.

PATHOPHYSIOLOGY

The most common mechanisms are fecalith for adults and lymphoid hyperplasia for children. Carcinoid is the most common tumor causing appendicitis (90%), followed by adenocarcinoma.

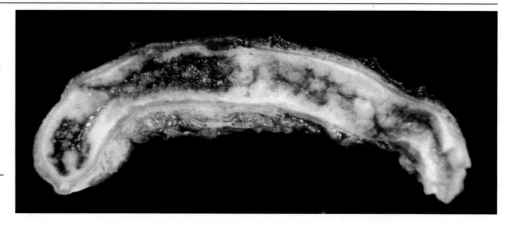

DIAGNOSIS

A clinical diagnosis is sufficient to take a patient to the OR for an appendectomy. However, many times, a CT scan of the abdomen is typically completed. Findings on CT scan include periappendiceal inflammation including stranding, incomplete contrast filling of the appendix, a diameter greater than 6mm, wall thickening, and enhancement with IV contrast.

TREATMENT

Treatment of appendicitis is by appendectomy. The presence of perforation and a walled-off **abscess** can be treated with **interval drainage** of the abscess followed by scheduled appendectomy. **Carcinoid** less than 2cm in size at the tip of the appendix can be treated by appendectomy alone. A carcinoid that is larger than 2cm or at the base of the appendix must be treated by a right hemicolectomy. The presence of an ovarian cyst that is likely leading to the

Carcinoid < 2cm at tip of appendix = appendectomy. Carcinoid > 2cm or at base of appendix = right hemicolectomy.

signs and symptoms of what was originally thought to be appendicitis should be treated by removing the appendix and pursuing treatment for the cyst afterwards. The presence of terminal ileitis but a normal cecum and appendix should also prompt the surgeon to remove the appendix. The presence of a cystic mass at the base of the appendix is likely a cystadenocarcinoma and must be treated by a right hemicolectomy. Due diligence is required to avoid spilling the contents as seeding of the tumor will occur. The presence of a walled-off abscess can be treated with a CT-guided drain placement followed by interval appendectomy.

TRAUMA

DUODENAL HEMATOMA

A duodenal hematoma is the result of blunt abdominal trauma leading to nausea, vomiting, and a right upper quadrant mass. It is diagnosed by an upper GI study that indicates filling of the duodenal lumen with a coiled spring in the second and third portions due to compression from the hematoma. Amylase tends to be elevated. Treatment is to make the patient NPO, insert an NG tube, and start TPN. Drainage of the hematoma can be successfully done after seven days if the patient does not improve clinically.

COLON AND RECTUM

CONGENITAL AND STRUCTURAL

PROCIDENTIA

A diagnostic sign of procidentia is the presence of concentric folds. It is more common in **women** who have given birth. Symptoms include constipation, incontinence, and the presence of a prolapse. Treatment is **tacking** the rectum to the presacral fascia; barring this treatment, **resecting** redundant rectosigmoid intestine is required.

VOLVULUS

SIGMOID VOLVULUS

Sigmoid volvulus is an acquired disorder due to redundant sigmoid colon. It tends to occur in the **elderly** and is the most common type of colonic volvulus. A KUB is diagnostic, and a barium enema shows a **bird's beak narrowing**. Distention with obstipation are the presenting signs, followed by fever and peritoneal signs. Treatment is **sigmoidoscopy** for decompression followed by resection.

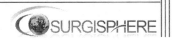

CECAL VOLVULUS

This is the next most common type of volvulus, making up 10% of all colonic volvulus. Diagnosis is made by KUB and shows a dilated loop of colon with a point. While a sigmoid volvulus typically points to the RUQ, a cecal volvulus points to the LUQ. Treatment is by **resection of the right colon**.

INTUSSUSCEPTION

Intussusception in adults is likely due to the presence of cancer. A partial or complete SBO typically ensues, along with cramping abdominal pain and, occasionally, bloody diarrhea.

HEMORRHOID

There are two types of hemorrhoids: internal hemorrhoids tend to lead to prolapse and painless rectal bleeding. External hemorrhoids tend to present with pain, burning, and itching. Treatment is with Sitz baths, stool softeners, and hemorrhoidectomy.

ANAL FISSURE

Anal fissures are linear tears in the anal mucosa. They tend to occur in the posterior midline; the presence of additional fissures should raise the suspicion for inflammatory bowel disease or HIV. It presents with pain and bleeding. Treatment is with Sitz baths, stool softeners, and **lateral internal sphincterotomy** if refractory to maximum medical management after three weeks.

FISTULA-IN-ANO

A fistula-in-ano tends to be present in about half of all cases with a perianal abscess. **Anterior fistulas** tend to connect with the rectum **linearly**. **Posterior fistulas** tend to **curve** into an **internal opening** within the rectum. Treatment is with **fistulotomy** or Seton placement.

CONSTIPATION

PRESENTATION AND DIAGNOSIS

Constipation is defined as the passage of stools less than 3 times every 7 days unless this is a normal bowel habit. Constipation is often secondary to a diet low in fiber with poor oral fluid intake. Constipation may also occur due to complications associated with diabetes, secondary to medications, obstruction, pregnancy, Hirschsprung disease, Chagas disease, or hypothyroidism. Medications such as narcotics, anticholinergics, iron, and calcium-channel blockers can also cause constipation.

TREATMENT

Treatment of constipation is by increasing fluid intake, either orally or intravenously. A diet high in fiber, up to 30 grams per day, often ameliorates most cases of constipation. Laxatives that lead to increased bulk and emollient laxatives may be prescribed as needed.

Table 191 Constipation

Constipation	
Causes	Low fiber and fluid diets. Complications of diabetes, medications (iron, narcotics, anticholinergics, calcium channel-blockers) hypothyroidism, pregnancy.
Treatment	High fiber and liquid diets, laxatives (emollients and/or bulk increasers).

INFLAMMATORY AND INFECTIOUS

DIARRHEA

OVERVIEW

ETIOLOGY

Diarrhea may be due to a number of disparate causes, including infectious, medication-induced, inflammatory, osmotic, secretory, and altered intestinal motility etiologies. The most common causes of infectious diarrhea include *E. coli* (ETEC), *Vibrio cholerae*, *E. coli* (O157:H7), *Giardia lamblia*, rotavirus, Norwalk agent, *Salmonella*, and *Clostridium difficile*. The most common causes of bloody diarrhea include *Campylobacter*, *E. coli* (EHEC), *E. histolytica*, *Salmonella*, and *Shigella*. Inflammatory diarrhea is commonly secondary to inflammatory bowel disease and infections from AIDS. Osmotic diarrhea is most commonly due to lactase deficiency and celiac sprue disease. Secretory diarrhea may occur from carcinoid syndrome and gastrinoma due to ZE syndrome. Altered intestinal motility leading to diarrhea may be secondary to irritable bowel syndrome.

PATHOPHYSIOLOGY

Diarrhea is defined as increase in stool weight over 200 grams per day or abnormally frequent passage of stools. Eight of the 9 liters of fluids that enter the gastrointestinal tract are absorbed in the small intestine, and only about 1 liter passes into the large intestine. Of that liter, about 4/5's of it are reabsorbed and the remainder goes towards the formation of stool. Any alteration in that absorption either through poor absorption, increased secretion, or increased production may lead to diarrhea. Most cases of diarrhea lasting less than two weeks are infectious in etiology, while chronic diarrhea lasting more than a few weeks is typically due to lactase deficiency.

Table 192 Diarrhea

Diarrhea	
Epidemiology	Medication induced, pathogens, inflammatory, osmotic and secretory causes. Chronic diarrhea lasts more than a few weeks, infectious diarrhea less than two weeks.
Pathophysiology	Stool weight over 200g/day or abnormally frequent defecation.
Diagnosis	Fecal analysis for ova and parasites.
Treatment	When infectious agents ascertained, Bactrim. Hydration therapy.

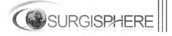

INFECTIOUS DIARRHEA

Infectious diarrhea from *E. coli* may be enterotoxigenic (ETEC) such as traveler's diarrhea, or enteroinvasive (EIEC) or enterohemorrhagic (EHEC) that presents with fever and bloody diarrhea. The most common bacterial diarrhea in North America is *Campylobacter*, which may also lead to a seronegative arthropathy known as reactive arthritis. Diarrhea in day care centers that is commonly transmitted through impure food or water is commonly due to *Shigella*. *Salmonella* is a cause of diarrhea in patients who consumed improperly prepared poultry or dairy products. Diarrhea that presents similar to appendicitis but with joint pain and a skin rash should lead to a clinical suspicion for *Yersinea*. Poorly cooked beef and unpasteurized dairy products may lead to poisoning with *E. coli* O157:H7 and concomitant thrombotic thrombocytopenic purpura (TTP) or hemolytic uremic syndrome (HUS). Diarrhea from viral agents are very common, especially Norwalk agent on cruise ships and rotavirus through oral-fecal infection. *Shigella* infection leads to diarrhea after several hours or days. *Staphylococcus aureus* infection leads to rapid diarrhea within a few hours. Most infectious diarrhea occurs within one day. Common microorganisms found in diarrhea in immunocompromised individuals include *Mycobacterium avium*, *Cryptosporidium*, and *Isosporium*.

Table 193 Infectious Diarrhea

Infectious Diarrhea	
Types	ETEC, EIEC, EHEC (presents with fever and bloody diarrhea).
Causes	*Campylobacter*, *Shigella* (in impure water or food), *Salmonella* (improperly prepared poultry or dairy products), *E. coli* (improperly prepared beef and dairy products). Viral agents (Norwalk, Rota virus, etc.).

IATROGENIC DIARRHEA

Diarrhea may be induced through the consumption of a number of medications. These include laxatives, antibiotics such as penicillins, cephalosporins, clindamycin, and tetracycline, antacids that contain magnesium, colchicine, beta blockers such as propranolol, quinidine, theophylline, diuretics such as furosemide or thiazide diuretics, angiotensin-converting enzyme (ACE) inhibitors, and antidepressants such as fluoxetine and sertraline. Diarrhea following digoxin and lithium is typically an early sign of toxicity, and diarrhea following consumption of medications is typically a sign that the offending drug should be stopped.

Table 194 Medication-Induced Diarrhea

Medication-Induced Diarrhea	
Causes	Laxatives, antibiotics, antacids with magnesium, beta blockers, diuretics.
Treatment	Cease offending medication(s).

INFLAMMATORY DIARRHEA

Inflammatory diarrhea is associated with intestinal changes in inflammatory bowel disease such as Crohn disease and ulcerative colitis, and in infections associated with AIDS. Ulcerative colitis tends to present with a bloody diarrhea, while Crohn disease tends to present with a diarrhea that contains more mucus and pus, and smaller amounts of blood.

Table 195 Inflammatory Diarrhea

Inflammatory Diarrhea	
Causes and presentations	Crohn disease (mucus and pus filled diarrhea), ulcerative colitis (bloody diarrhea), infections associated with AIDS.
Pathophysiology	Intestinal changes in inflammatory bowel disease.
Treatment	Treat underlying cause.

OSMOTIC DIARRHEA

Table 196 Osmotic Diarrhea

Osmotic Diarrhea	
Cause	Indigestible solutes and high carbohydrate content (mannitol, sorbitol, fructose).
Presentation	Watery diarrhea which abates after expulsion of offending solute.
Treatment	Eliminate offending nutrient(s).

SECRETORY DIARRHEA

Secretory diarrhea is often a result of gastrinoma, as in ZE syndrome and in carcinoid syndrome. High levels of vasoactive intestinal peptide (VIP) from pancreatic adenomas and irritation from certain laxatives (such as phenolphthalein) may also result in secretory diarrhea. Secretory diarrhea tends to be very high in volume, and resolves with treatment of the underlying disorder or cessation of the offending medication. Secretory diarrhea is the diagnosis if the stool osmotic gap is negative. A positive osmotic gap indicates malabsorptive diarrhea.

$$Stool\ Osmotic\ Gap = 2Na^+ + K^+ - Osmolality$$

PSEUDOMEMBRANOUS COLITIS

ETIOLOGY AND PATHOPHYSIOLOGY

Pseudomembranous colitis is diarrhea caused by *Clostridium difficile* that overgrows within the colon and disrupts the normal bacterial flora, leading to impaired absorption. *C. difficile* releases a toxin that may lead to damage to the mucosa and further contributes to the diarrhea. Pseudomembranous colitis commonly occurs **between a week and a month** after stopping antibiotics, and the most commonly implicated antibiotics are **clindamycin**, vancomycin, and cephalosporins.

PRESENTATION AND DIAGNOSIS

Pseudomembranous colitis presents with watery diarrhea that contains scant, if any blood, abdominal cramping, fever, and leukocytosis. Diagnosis is made by searching for the *C. difficile* toxin in stool samples. The majority of patients with actual *C. difficile* infection will have a positive test after testing three separate stool samples. Sigmoidoscopy or colonoscopy clinches the diagnosis with the visualization of **yellow membranous plaques** on the mucosa, but this test is rarely used.

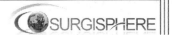

TREATMENT

Treatment of *C. difficile* requires cessation of the antibiotics leading to the demise of the bowel flora, and the use of **metronidazole or vancomycin** to treat the *C. difficile*. **Oral** metronidazole is preferred unless the strain is resistant, then oral vancomycin becomes the preferred regimen. Toxin can be bound with cholestyramine. Inhibitors of motility such as loperamide should be avoided. Treatment for up to two weeks is necessary. If treatment is not started in a timely manner, severe inflammation and infection can occur throughout all layers of the colonic epithelium, leading to severe diarrhea, sepsis, and toxic megacolon. Plain films of the abdomen demonstrate long loops of colon with signs of edema in the bowel wall (known as a positive "thumb printing" sign). The standard of care, if these complications arise, is colectomy.

Table 197 Pseudomembranous Colitis

Pseudomembranous Colitis	
Etiology	*Clostridium difficile*. May occur a week to a month after stopping antibiotics.
Presentation	Watery diarrhea that contains little or no blood, abdominal cramps, fever.
Diagnosis	Positive *C. difficile* test, sigmoidoscopy or colonoscopy showing yellow plaques.
Treatment	Metronidazole or vancomycin; if severe, colectomy.

IRRITABLE BOWEL SYNDROME

ETIOLOGY AND EPIDEMIOLOGY

Irritable bowel syndrome is the most common outpatient complaint with regard to the gastrointestinal system. Irritable bowel syndrome is defined as a change in bowel habits due to a change in intestinal motility, which itself may be secondary to a number of causes. Irritable bowel syndrome is most common in young adults up to the age of 40, and affects females twice as much as males.

PRESENTATION AND DIAGNOSIS

Irritable bowel syndrome presents as continuous transitions between diarrhea and constipation with frequent abdominal pain and a sense of bloating and distention relieved by defecation. Diagnosis is made by clinical history, and requires the presence of intermittent symptoms for more than three months with no night time symptoms. The lack of systemic symptoms and the presence of stress typically clinch the diagnosis. The symptoms must include two elements from the Rome criteria, which are altered passage of stool, abnormal frequency, change in consistency, mucus in stool, and abdominal distention. The differential diagnosis of irritable bowel syndrome includes *Giardia* infection, inflammatory bowel disease, lactase deficiency, hypothyroidism, and colon cancer. Irritable bowel syndrome is associated with fibromyalgia, interstitial cystitis, fatigue, and depression.

TREATMENT

Irritable bowel syndrome is treated with a **high-fiber, low-fat diet** to promote proper passage of intestinal contents. All gas-forming foods should be eliminated. One of the following medications may also be used in severe cases: psyllium, antispasmodics, anticholinergics, antidiarrheals, tricyclic antidepressants, anxiolytics, or osmotic laxatives.

Table 198 Irritable Bowel Syndrome

Irritable Bowel syndrome	
Presentation	Fluctuation between diarrhea and constipation, frequent abdominal pain for at least 3 months.
Diagnosis	Two elements of Rome criteria. Differential diagnosis--Eliminate Giardia, inflammatory bowel disease, lactase deficiency, hypothyroidism, colon cancer.
Treatment	High fiber, low fat diet. Eliminate gas-forming foods. Psyllium, antispasmodics, anticholinergics, antidiarrheals, osmotic laxatives, anxiolytics.

INFLAMMATORY BOWEL SYNDROME

CROHN DISEASE

ETIOLOGY AND EPIDEMIOLOGY

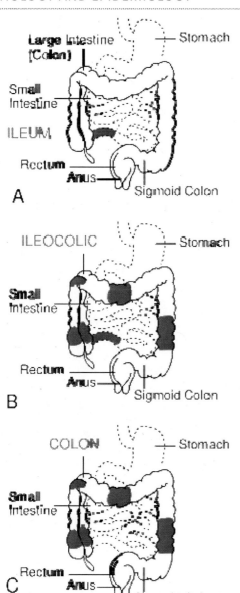

A

B

C

Crohn disease is one of two major inflammatory bowel diseases. Inflammatory bowel disease is significantly more common in the Ashkenazi Jewish and Caucasian populations, and tends to affect young adults up to the age of 35 but may also affect individuals over 60 years of age. There is a strong pattern of family inheritance. Crohn disease has an incidence of approximately 5 in 100,000 individuals, and is more common in men. Crohn disease is three times more likely to cause colon cancer, with the risk increasing over time. Although the precise cause remains unknown, some researchers have implicated the presence of antibodies to alpha-*Saccharyomyces cerevesiae* as prognostic.

Crohn disease: Transmural, fistula, spares rectum but any location within GI tract, aphthous ulcers, cobblestoning, skip lesions, targets terminal ileum, nonbloody diarrhea, calcium oxalate stones.
Rx: remicade, gastrojejunostomy

PATHOPHYSIOLOGY

Crohn disease occurs from an unknown source and leads to inflammation of the intestines. It **affects all of the layers** of the bowel, leading to the formation of **fistulas** and **abscesses**. Crohn disease **spares the rectum** in about half of all patients, but may be found in any location of the gastrointestinal tract. Discontinuous, **skipping lesions** are present with normal bowel located between stretches of diseased bowel. **Thickening** of the submucosal layer in the diseased region also leads to a **cobblestone** appearance that alternates with regions of **ulceration** of the submucosal layer. The most commonly affected regions of the gastrointestinal tract are the **terminal ileum** (1/3 of all cases), the **colon** (1/3 of all cases), or both regions (1/3 of all cases).

PRESENTATION

Crohn disease presents with **nonbloody diarrhea**, unless there is

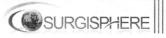

significantly involvement of the rectum. Crampy abdominal pain, weight loss, fever, malaise, and a tender right lower quadrant are typically the signs and symptoms. Crohn disease, like all inflammatory bowel diseases, may also have a number of extraintestinal manifestations such as arthritis, uveitis, iritis, **erythema nodosum**, and **pyoderma gangrenosum**. Nearly 1 in 5 patients may be afflicted with such extraintestinal complications. Occasionally, **calcium oxalate stones** may be present in the kidney. These extraintestinal complications are discussed in their own sections below.

DIAGNOSIS

Crohn disease is diagnosed through colonoscopy (skip lesions, cobblestoning, abscess formation, and fistulas may be pathognomonic). Histology often demonstrates **granulomas**. Laboratory tests that may raise the suspicion of Crohn disease include **iron-deficiency anemia**, **vitamin B12 deficiency**, and high erythrocyte sedimentation rate (ESR).

TREATMENT

The cornerstone of treatment is to reduce inflammation, which is achieved with **sulfasalazine** and **corticosteroids**. Sulfasalazine is a combination of sulfapyridine and 5-aminosalicylic acid (5-ASA). Immunosuppressive therapy is occasionally used, typically in lieu of corticosteroids, and may include the use of 6-mercaptopurine, infliximab, methotrexate, and azathioprine. If Crohn disease primarily affects the small intestine, sulfasalazine is replaced with 5-ASA. Should fistulas complicate the presentation of Crohn disease, administration of metronidazole and ciprofloxacin for three weeks for bowel flora control is the standard of care. Experimental therapies with antibodies or cytokines against tumor necrosis factor (TNF) have also shown some success (**remicade, or infliximab**). **The last bastion of treatment for duodenal Crohn disease is a gastrojejunostomy and vagotomy.**

Table 199 Crohn Disease

Crohn Disease	
Pathophysiology	Affects all layers of bowel leading to fistulas and abscesses. Discontinuous lesions.
Presentation	Nonbloody diarrhea, crampy abdominal pain, fever, malaise, tender RLQ.
Diagnosis	Colonoscopy (skip lesions, cobblestoning, abscesses, fistula). Histology (granulomas), high ESR.
Treatment	Sulfasalazine, corticosteroids, metronidazole for bowel flora control, antidiarrheals.

SUPPORTIVE THERAPY

Supportive therapy for Crohn disease includes the use of antidiarrheals such as loperamide or diphenoxylate for those with diarrhea due to fatty acids, or cholestyramine for those with other causes of diarrhea. Antidiarrheals are absolutely contraindicated in individuals with toxic megacolon or those with severe colitis that may lead to toxic megacolon. Anticholinergics are used to reduce the symptoms of inflammatory bowel disease, including abdominal cramping and urgency. **Diarrhea** following ileocecectomy for Crohn disease is due to a paucity of bile salts. It can be alleviated by the administration of **exogenous bile salts**. The most effective acute treatment for a perirectal fistula secondary to Crohn disease is infliximab. A stricturoplasty is the typical treatment of choice in young patients with multiple, short Crohn's related strictures.

ULCERATIVE COLITIS

ETIOLOGY AND EPIDEMIOLOGY

Ulcerative colitis is the second major inflammatory bowel disease, and is approximately equal to Crohn disease in incidence. Ulcerative colitis affects the same populations and age groups, but is more common in women. In addition, the risk of colon cancer with ulcerative colitis is significantly greater than with Crohn disease: there is a 30 fold increase in risk with ulcerative colitis. In 1 out of 10 persons, ulcerative colitis spontaneously remits. In ¾, symptoms are intermittent. In 1/10, the symptoms are continuous, and in 1/20, death results due to complications. A positive ANCA is associated with ulcerative colitis.

PATHOPHYSIOLOGY

Ulcerative colitis tends to have **continuous lesions** that are **restricted to the mucosa**. This tends to lead to a **rectal discharge** of mostly mucus, blood, and pus. Ulcerative colitis begins with **rectal involvement**, and lesions in the majority of patients extend from the rectum into adjacent gastrointestinal structures.

PRESENTATION AND DIAGNOSIS

Signs and symptoms of ulcerative colitis include **bloody diarrhea** and **rectal pain**. Ulcerative colitis is otherwise similar in presentation to Crohn disease. Diagnosis of ulcerative colitis is made through a **colonoscopy** that demonstrates continuous lesions emanating from the rectum, and a **lead pipe colon** that is secondary to chronic damage leading to scarring. Granulomas are not present. Extraintestinal complications of inflammatory bowel disease are discussed below.

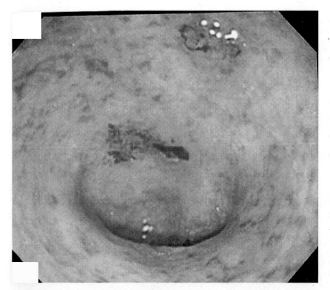

TREATMENT

Treatment of ulcerative colitis is similar to that of Crohn disease, including the use of sulfasalazine, azathioprine, 6-mercaptopurine, and corticosteroids for management of the inflammation. Colectomy is mandatory after 15 years of symptoms to minimize the risk of colon cancer; this is typically curative. The presence of toxic megacolon with ulcerative colitis is treated with fluid resuscitation, high dose steroids, electrolytes, and **total proctocolectomy with ileal pouch-anal anastomosis**. Other surgical interventions include TPC with continent ileostomy, and TPC with end ileostomy. Other indications for surgery include hemorrhage, obstruction, perforation, worsening clinical course, and prophylaxis.

Table 200 Ulcerative Colitis

Ulcerative Colitis	
Pathophysiology	Continuous lesions restricted to the mucosa. Begins in rectum.
Presentation	Bloody diarrhea and rectal pain.
Diagnosis	Colonoscopy shows continuous lesions starting at rectum. No granulomas.
Treatment	Similar to Crohn disease. Colectomy after 15 years of symptoms.

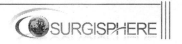

INTESTINAL COMPLICATIONS

Complications of ulcerative colitis include perforation, stricture formation, and toxic megacolon. Hemorrhage can also occur if there is significant damage to blood vessels. Toxic megacolon is especially likely to occur in the face of severe inflammation that leads to dilation of the bowel. Hypotension and septic changes may also occur in long-standing ulcerative colitis.

EXTRAINTESTINAL COMPLICATIONS

Both Crohn disease and ulcerative colitis may be complicated with a number of extraintestinal symptoms. Those that affect the eye include episcleritis and uveitis. Uveitis is more common in Crohn disease. Episcleritis typically presents with the conglomeration of uveitis, erythema nodosum, and colitic arthritis. Dermatologic symptoms include erythema nodosum (especially in Crohn disease), pyoderma gangrenosum (ulcerative colitis), and aphthous ulcers (Crohn disease). Colitis arthritis is more common in Crohn disease, and ankylosing spondylitis is often a progressive feature of ulcerative colitis. Primary sclerosing cholangitis is more common in ulcerative colitis, and renal failure due to amyloidosis is more common in Crohn disease. All forms of inflammatory bowel disease may be complicated with anemia, thromboembolic disorders, steatohepatitis, and cholelithiasis.

Table 201 Complications of Inflammatory Bowel Disease

Complications of Inflammatory Bowel Disease	
Ulcerative colitis	Perforation, stricture formation, and toxic megacolon. Hemorrhage, if there is significant damage to blood vessels. Toxic megacolon is likely to occur, if severe inflammation leads to dilation of the bowel. Hypotension and septic changes may also occur in long-standing ulcerative colitis.
Extraintestinal (Ulcerative colitis & Crohn)	Episcleritis, uveitis, erythema nodosum, colic arthritis, pyoderma gangrenosum, aphthous ulcers, ankylosing spondylitis, primary sclerosing cholangitis, colitis, and renal failure, due to amyloidosis. Note: All forms of inflammatory bowel disease may be complicated with anemia, thromboembolic disorders, steatohepatitis, and cholelithiasis.

DIVERTICULOSIS

ETIOLOGY

Diverticulosis is the development of a saclike outpouching of the colon that herniates in between the teniae coli. Diverticulosis is the most common cause of significant bleeding from the lower gastrointestinal tract in elderly patients. The outpouchings of diverticulosis generally occur in the sigmoid colon, likely due to the higher pressures experienced in this section of the gastrointestinal tract. Diverticulosis is more common in patients who have a diet poor in fiber, and generally affects a majority of the elderly population. The majority tend to occur after the age of 85. 20% of patients will develop diverticulitis. Complications occur in 1/5 of patients.

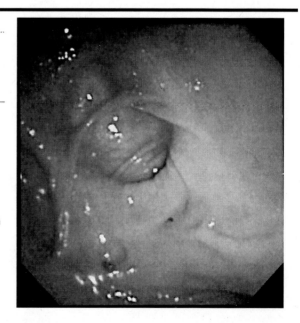

PATHOPHYSIOLOGY AND PRESENTATION

Diverticulosis can lead to a lower gastrointestinal bleed due to inflammation of the mucosa that eventually affects an intestinal artery. Profuse bleeding can occur with this erosion, leading to painless hemorrhage and bright red blood per rectum (BRBPR). The majority of bleeds occur with **right-sided diverticula**, and tend to resolve spontaneously. Most cases of diverticulosis tend to be painless, but abdominal pain relieved by defecation can occur.

DIAGNOSIS

Diagnosis of diverticulosis is made through colonoscopy that detects the outpouching. A more sensitive test is **barium enema**, which is also a safer test as the colonoscopy can lead to perforation of the sac. **Tagged red blood cells** (RBCs) or **angiography** can be used to assess the cause of the lower gastrointestinal bleed and potentially correct it.

TREATMENT

Treatment of diverticulosis is to correct the cause of the lower gastrointestinal bleeding, as discussed in the section on gastrointestinal bleeds. A high fiber diet is recommended in all patients with existing diverticulosis (and generally, in all patients). A complication of diverticulosis is the inflammation of the outpouching, leading to diverticulitis.

Table 202 Diverticulosis

Diverticulosis	
Etiology	Sac-like outpouching of the colon that herniates between the teniae coli.
Presentation	Lower GI bleeding (BRBPR), most cases painless.
Diagnosis	Colonoscopy, (shows outpouching), barium enema, tagged RBCs, angiography.
Treatment	Correct GI bleeding, high fiber diet.

DIVERTICULITIS

PATHOPHYSIOLOGY AND PRESENTATION

Diverticulitis is the inflammation of the outpouching of the colon due to the formation of a fecalith and subsequent proliferation of bacteria within the diverticulum. Diverticulitis presents with lower abdominal pain, typically in the lower left quadrant (the site of most diverticulitis; a **right-sided diverticulitis is typically due to Meckel diverticulitis**). There is generally constipation and increased flatus. Irritation from the diverticulum and the inflammatory process can lead to urinary urgency. Further, as this is an infectious process, there is typically fever and peritonitis can occur with perforation of the diverticulum. A sigmoid mass may be present upon physical examination.

DIAGNOSIS

The presence of pneumaturia and left lower quadrant pain should begin a search for diverticulitis. Diagnosis of diverticulitis requires blood cultures positive for infection, leukocytosis indicating an inflammatory and infectious process underway, and a computed tomographic (CT) scan can be done to confirm the presence of a diverticulum. In diverticulitis, **invasive tests such as barium enema and colonoscopy are contraindicated** due to the increased risk of perforation and subsequent peritonitis and sepsis, especially in the acute phase of diverticulitis.

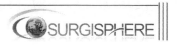

TREATMENT

Treatment of diverticulitis is to prescribe nothing per oral (NPO), hydration to assist in the propulsion of intestinal contents, antibiotics to cover bowel flora, and to control pain symptoms. **Sigmoid resection** should be considered to minimize the ¼ chance of recurrence, especially in older adults. Finally, testing to rule out colon cancer should be undertaken once the acute phase has resolved. A localized abscess is treated with CT-guided drain placement and antibiotics. Perforation requires a Hartmann's procedure.

Table 203 Diverticulitis

Diverticulitis	
Presentation	Inflammation of outpouching of colon due to fecalith and bacterial proliferation. Lower abdominal pain (typically left quadrant), constipation, fever.
Diagnosis	Blood cultures positive for infection, leukocytosis, CT scan (confirm diverticulum).
Treatment	NPO, hydration, antibiotics, sigmoid resection, testing to rule out colon cancer.

RECTUM / ANUS

PROCTITIS AND ANUSITIS

ASSESSMENT

Inflammation of the rectum and anus is commonly secondary to various inflammatory bowel diseases, infection by *Clostridium difficile, Salmonella, or Shigella,* and due to radiation therapy. Inflammation of the epithelial lining leads to rectal bleeding, change in bowel habits, tenesmus, fecal urgency, constipation, and abdominal cramping. Stool cultures, anorectal swabs, and other studies are done for diagnosis.

MANAGEMENT

Proctitis due to IBD is treated with sulfasalazine, 5-ASA, steroids, immunosuppressants, and antibiotics. *Salmonella, Shigella, Yersinia,* and *Campylobacter* infections are self-limited. *E. histolytica* is treated with metronidazole and iodoquinol. *C. difficile* is treated with vancomycin or metronidazole. Pain control, steroids, and 6-mercaptopurine or azathioprine are used for radiation-induced proctitis.

Table 204 Proctitis and Anusitis

Proctitis and Anusitis	
Etiology	Commonly secondary to various inflammatory bowel diseases, infection by *Clostridium difficile, Salmonella, or Shigella,* and due to radiation therapy.
Presentation	Rectal bleeding, change in bowel habits, tenesmus, fecal urgency, constipation, and abdominal cramping.
Diagnosis	Stool cultures, anorectal swabs, and other studies.
Treatment	Proctitis due to IBD is treated with sulfasalazine, 5-ASA, steroids, immunosuppressants, and antibiotics. *Salmonella, Shigella, Yersinia,* and *Campylobacter* infections are self-limited. *E. histolytica* is treated with metronidazole and iodoquinol. *C. difficile* is treated with vancomycin or metronidazole. Pain control, steroids, and 6-mercaptopurine or azathioprine are used for radiation-induced proctitis.

CANCER

CARCINOID

ETIOLOGY AND EPIDEMIOLOGY

Carcinoid syndrome is the result of a neuroendocrine tumor that secretes hormones or neurotransmitters that have an effect on the gastrointestinal system. These active compounds can include **serotonin** (5-HT), adrenocorticotrophic hormone (ACTH), histamine, dopamine, tryptophan, substance P, and bradykinin. Carcinoid is an idiopathic disorder that has no known familial inheritance pattern. It is part of the **MEN type I** disorder, and the incidence of carcinoid syndrome is greater in patients who have Gardner syndrome or Crohn disease.

PATHOPHYSIOLOGY

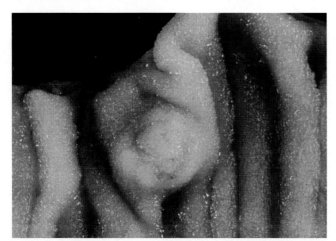

The majority of carcinoids are in the appendix, but the endocrine cells in this location tend not to have any effect. The majority of carcinoids in the ileum are secreting, as are those found in the lung. Carcinoid typically causes most of its effects through the **conversion of tryptophan to serotonin**, and the unchecked production of serotonin may lead to symptoms of niacin deficiency and subsequent pellagra.

PRESENTATION

Many carcinoids are asymptomatic and discovered only incidentally. Those located in the appendix may create symptoms of appendicitis, and any carcinoid in the small intestine may lead to a small bowel obstruction or diarrhea. Carcinoid, like any tumor, may lead to weight loss. The **classic triad of carcinoid** rarely presents with the tripartite symptoms, but it includes **flushing** due to excessive bradykinin production, **diarrhea** from excessive serotonergic effects, and **valvular heart disease** that primarily affects the mitral valve from excess serotonin. Other classic symptoms include hypotension, tachycardia, and alcohol intolerance. Carcinoid may metastasize to the liver, leading to right upper quadrant (RUQ) pain and elevated liver function tests (LFTs) and the lung, leading to wheezing, obstructed bronchus, and pneumonia.

DIAGNOSIS

Diagnosis of carcinoid syndrome is made with a 24 hour 5-hydroxyindolacetic acid (5-HIAA) collection, with elevated titers 100% specific for carcinoid. Point collections through serum or urine samples may also be done. 5-HIAA is the metabolite of serotonin when it is broken down by monoamine oxidase (MAO) and then by aldehyde dehydrogenase. CT of the lung and abdomen are compulsory to detect metastasis. The most common location for carcinoid is in the appendix (50%), followed by the ileum (25%) and rectum (20%). Ileal carcinoid has the highest potential for metastasis; appendiceal carcinoid has the lowest potential for metastasis.

TREATMENT

Carcinoid syndrome is best treated with surgical resection and radiation therapy. With metastasis to the liver, embolization and alpha interferon therapy are often used, in addition to surgical resection. Symptomatic

 Appendiceal Carcinoid: <2cm at distal appendix = appendectomy >2cm or at base = right hemicolectomy

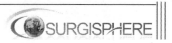

control of carcinoid can sometimes be achieved with the somatostatin analog octreotide. Survival after a diagnosis of active carcinoid syndrome is typically 3 years. Carcinoid primarily located in the appendix carries a very good prognosis, while primary carcinoid outside of the appendix has a 50% 5 year survival. **Appendiceal carcinoids less than 2 centimeters at the distal end can be treated by appendectomy. Carcinoids over 2 centimeters or those at the base require a right hemicolectomy.** A rectal carcinoid less than 1cm can be treated by endoscopic excision; carcinoid between 1-2 cm requires transanal excision; carcinoid over 2cm requires an LAR. Invasive carcinoid requires an LAR or APR. Most rectal carcinoids over 2cm have metastasis to the liver on presentation, and the vast majority has metastasized to local lymph nodes. The presence of a gastric carcinoid receives local excision if less than 1cm; subtotal gastrectomy with omentectomy may be required for carcinoid larger than 1cm.

Table 205 Carcinoid Syndrome

Ulcerative Colitis	
Etiology	Idiopathic.
Pathophysiology	Majority in appendix, those in ileum are secreting, niacin deficiency.
Presentation	Most asymptomatic, possible symptoms of appendicitis, SI blockage, diarrhea.
Diagnosis	24 hour 5-HIAA collection (elevated titers specific for carcinoid) CT lung & abdomen.
Treatment	Surgical resection and radiation therapy.

COLORECTAL CANCER

EPIDEMIOLOGY AND ETIOLOGY

The second most common cause of death due to cancer is from colon cancer, affecting both males and females equally. The most common underlying etiology is the presence of sessile, villous, adenomatous polyps greater than 2 cm in size. Risk factors for colon cancer include a positive family history, the presence of APC gene or p53 gene defects, ulcerative colitis (more than Crohn disease), and smoking. Longstanding infection with *Streptococcus bovis* can also predispose individuals to colon cancer, while chronic aspirin use over a long period of time somewhat reduces the risk of colon cancer. **p53 is a tumor suppressor gene** that regulates cell cycle progression. **APC is a tumor suppressor gene mutated in FAP**. It is one of the first mutations that occur. **DCC is deleted in about 70% of colorectal cancers**. Inflammatory polyps may develop with IBD. They

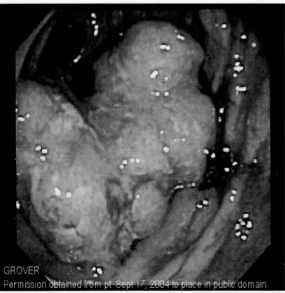

do not have a significant potential for malignancy. Oncogenes function during G1 of the cell cycle. Recall that G1 is followed by S (DNA synthesis), then G2, then M phase (mitosis). The cell has the option of going into a rest phase at G1 (G0).

PATHOPHYSIOLOGY

The polyps present preceding the development of colorectal cancer may be one of three types. A pure villous adenoma occurs about 10% of the time. Tubulovillous adenomas are present about 20% of the time, while an adenomatous polyp is present about 70% of the time. Villous adenomas have the highest risk of becoming cancerous (about 40%). Larger polyps have a greater potential for malignancy. Every attempt should be made to completely remove a polyp via colonoscopy; failure to do so requires an operative intervention for a colectomy. Villous adenomas larger than 4cm with induration have an over 90% risk of being cancerous; transanal excision is recommended in this case with satisfactory margins. Very large adenomas may require a coloanal anastomosis or a total protectomy. Sphincter-saving surgery is not possible with the latter option. Villous adenomas of the small bowel are more rare, but can become quite large with a malignant potential of about 50% at 5cm. Whipple procedure is necessary under these circumstances. Villous adenomas may present with watery diarrhea. A villous adenoma may present with a decrease in bicarbonate, a drop in urine pH.

CLASSIFICATION

Following the diagnosis of colon cancer, classification into one of four Duke's stages is done to determine the prognosis. In stage A disease, the cancer is limited to the mucosa and submucosa, and carries a greater than 90% 5 year survival. In stage B disease, the cancer has invaded the muscularis propria, with a 70% 5 year survival. Stage C disease has invasion into local lymph nodes, with a 30% 5 year survival. Stage D disease has distant metastases with limited survival after a few years.

Table 206 TNM Staging of Colorectal Cancer

TNM Staging of Colorectal Cancer			
T0	In-situ cancer	N0	No nodes affected
T1	Invasion of the **submucosa**	N1	1-3 regional nodes positive
T2	Invasion of the **muscularis propria**	N2	4+ regional nodes positive
T3	Invasion into the **serosa**	M0	No metastasis
T4	Invasion to adjacent structures	M1	Metastasis present

Table 207 Staging of Colon Cancer—Duke's Stages

Staging of Colon Cancer—Duke's Stages	
Stage A	Cancer limited to mucosa and submucosa. 90% 5 year survival.
Stage B	Cancer invades the muscularis propria. 70% 5 year survival.
Stage C	Invasion of local lymph nodes. 30% 5 year survival rate.
Stage D	Distant metastases. Limited survival.

TREATMENT

Colon cancer that falls into Duke's stage A or B is highly amenable to surgery, and wide resection of the colon is typically done along with sampling of nearby lymph nodes to rule out higher stages of disease. Stage C disease is often treated with a combination of surgery and chemotherapy, including agents such as 5-fluorouracil (5-FU) and leucovorin. Stage D disease is treated only with palliation. Radiation therapy is often used for stage B and C disease, and chemotherapy is sometimes employed in stage B disease. 3cm margins are required for resection along with the vascular supply and lymphatic drainage to the entire segment. **Tumors located 5-10cm from the anal verge can be treated with LAR. Tumors less than 5cm from the anal verge require an APR.** Recurrent cancer at the site of an LAR requires an APR. Failure to treat will lead to chemoradiation and likely palliative therapy. Cancer involving the dome of the bladder requires a partial bladder resection, reconstruction, and use of a foley for several weeks. Squamous cell cancer of the anus is typically

Stage A: Resection
Stage B: Resected
Stage C: Chemoradiation, resection
Stage D: Palliation

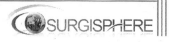

treated with chemoradiation. A sessile villous adenoma with negative margins requires no further therapy. However, masses over 4 cm cannot be treated endoscopically; they require surgical intervention and resection.

COMPLICATIONS

Mild **anastomotic leaks** leading to low grade fever and some discomfort can be treated with antibiotics (i.e. ciprofloxacin and metronidazole). The presence of an abscess larger than 5cm can be drained by a CT-guided procedure. The presence of a multiloculated abscess or clinical deterioration requires a Hartmann's procedure. Radiation proctitis is a side effect and tends to occur 8-12 months after radiotherapy. Formalin is a therapy for radiation proctitis.

Table 208 Treatment of Colon Cancer

Treatment of Colon Cancer	
Stage A & B	Surgery and wide resection of colon, sampling of lymph nodes (radiation and chemo are sometimes used in B).
Stage C	Surgery and chemotherapy (5-FU, leucovorin), radiation may also be utilized.
Stage D	Palliation.

Table 209 Metastatic Colon Cancer

Metastatic Colon Cancer	
Hepatic metastasis	25% 5-year survival once resected; up to 3mm metastases can be detected by intraoperative ultrasound
Pulmonary metastasis	20% 5-year survival once resected
Common sites of metastasis	Prostate, breast, lung, kidney, thyroid, and bone (least likely)

SCREENING

Colon cancer screening guidelines are proposed by the American Cancer Society, and recommends annual digital rectal exam in all individuals age 40 and over. Occult blood tests with the stool (FOBT) are recommended in individuals over the age of 50. In asymptomatic individuals with no risk factors for colon cancer, flexible sigmoidoscopy is done every 5 years starting at the age of 50. Finally, colonoscopy is recommended in any individual with positive stool guaiac (positive FOBT), those with a high risk assessment following sigmoidoscopy, and for those with inflammatory bowel disease and hereditary risk factors. Many practitioners now recommend the use of colonoscopy in lieu of sigmoidoscopy due to the increased sensitivity and specificity, the reach of colonoscopy to the ascending and transverse colon (where half of all colon cancers may lie), and the ability to biopsy polyps with the colonoscope. Digital rectal exam may find up to half of all colon cancers, and many practitioners urge that a digital rectal exam be performed with any abdominal exam.

Table 210 Screening of Colon Cancer

Screening of Colon Cancer
Annual digital rectal exam in all over 40.
FOBT in all over 50.
Flexible sigmoidoscopy every 5 years over 50.
Colonoscopy for those with risk factors.

TUMORS OF THE ANAL CANAL

The presence of squamous cell cancer above the dentate line has its prognosis determined by size. Risk factors include STDs. Treatment is with chemoradiation and cisplatin. An APR is required thereafter. **Melanoma** is treated with a wide local excision but has an overall survival of less than 20%. **WLE has the same survival as an APR**.

Table 211 Tumors of the Anal Margin

Tumors of the Anal Margin		
Bowen disease	Squamous cell carcinoma	Wide local excision
Paget disease	Intraepithelial adenocarcinoma	Non-invasive: wide local excision Invasive to sphincter: APR
Basal cell	Basal cell epithelial cancer	Wide local excision
Squamous cell carcinoma	Squamous cell carcinoma	Wide local excision
Verrucous carcinoma		Wide local excision
Kaposi sarcoma	Secondary to HIV	Wide local excision with chemoradiation

INHERITED NEOPLASIAS

FAMILIAL ADENOMATOUS POLYPOSIS

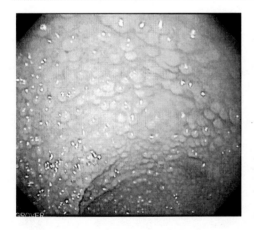

Colon cancer develops over approximately a decade of having large villous or tubulovillous adenomatous polyps. The presence of familial adenomatous polyposis (FAP) syndromes, due to an autosomal dominant gene, is a certain predictor of malignancy. FAP is due to a deletion on chromosome **5q**, and it requires **total colectomy** to avoid colon cancer from the numerous polyps that inevitably form by the age of 25. Without treatment, colon cancer is likely to have occurred in nearly all individuals by the age of 40. FAP is due to loss of the **APC tumor suppressor gene**. It tends to lead to left-sided tumors and is virtually guaranteed to lead to cancer by the mid-30s. Celebrex can be used to decrease the growth of polyps but a **total proctocolectomy with end ileostomy** (or ileal pouch-anal anastomosis with J-pouch) is required.

HEREDITARY NONPOLYPOSIS COLON CANCER

ASSESSMENT

Hereditary nonpolyposis colon cancer (HNPCC) is transmitted via an **autosomal dominant** mechanism and is due to a genetic defect in a **DNA mismatch repair gene**. A strong family inheritance is also relevant. In most cases, early colon cancer develops in several relatives of the patient, and there is a strong risk of the development of other cancers within the family. HNPCC is a strong predictor of future colon cancer development in the patient. In this disorder, also known as Lynch syndrome, the cancer arises spontaneously from the mucosa, and it is a strong predictor of future ovarian or endometrial cancer. **Lynch I tends to lead to right sided colon cancer** that develops in the early 40s. **Lynch II** leads to colon cancer and concomitant cancer of the **ovary, bladder, small intestine, and stomach**. Endometrial cancers are associated with HNPCC. The presence of **microsatellite instability** is likely to be later stage with a worse prognosis.

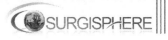

MANAGEMENT

Colonoscopy should be conducted starting at age 20 due to the development of adenomas. A **subtotal colectomy** is required for Lynch I. **Prophylactic TAHBSO** may be required for Lynch II. **CA-125** levels should be tracked for individuals with Lynch II.

>
>
> **HNPCC**: Lynch I – right side CRC in 40s; Lynch II – CRC in 20s, ovary, bladder, SI, and gastric CA; both assoc w/ endometrial CA
> **Gardner**: CRC w/ skull osteomas and extra teeth
> **Turcot**: CRC w/ CNS tumors
> **Peutz-Jeghers**: Hamartomas w/ skin hyperpigmentation
> **JVP**: Benign polyps

GARDNER SYNDROME

Gardner syndrome is the development of **numerous polyps** due to an autosomal dominant disorder. Gardner's syndrome is further complicated by the presence of **fibrous dysplasia** of the skull, osteomas, and extra teeth. Gardner syndrome typically evolves into colon cancer. **Desmoid tumors** also tend to occur.

TURCOT SYNDROME

Turcot syndrome is the development of **polyps** and **tumors within the central nervous system** (CNS). It presents a significant risk for colon cancer.

PEUTZ-JEGHER SYNDROME

Peutz-Jeghers syndrome presents a relatively low risk of developing colon cancer. Many polyps develop within the small and large intestine, but they are typically hamartomas and therefore benign. Peutz-Jeghers syndrome typically leads to **pigmentation** of the cutaneous and mucosa, especially with the development of macules within the oral mucosa. While the risk of colon cancer is low, Peutz-Jeghers should raise the suspicion of cancers that occur in women. These **hamartomas** may bleed. Other associated hamartomatous diseases include Cowden disease (polyps with facial epithelial lesions and breast cancer) and Cronkite-Canada syndrome (polyps with diarrhea, alopecia, and hyperpigmentation).

JUVENILE POLYPOSIS SYNDROME

Juvenile polyposis syndrome is an insignificant cause of colon cancer, with polyps often occurring as a result of benign hamartomas within the intestines. Peutz-Jeghers and juvenile polyposis syndrome are worth keeping on the differential diagnosis of any polyposis syndrome as rapid diagnosis of these two varieties may avoid costly and invasive tests and obviate the need for prophylactic colon resection.

Table 212 Other Colonic Syndromes

Other Colonic Syndromes	
Gardner syndrome	Numerous polyps due to autosomal dominant disorder. Evolves into colon cancer.
Turcot syndrome	Polyps and tumors in CNS. High risk for colon cancer.
Peutz-Jeghers synd.	Many polyps in SI and LI , low cancer risk.
Juvenile Polyposis	Benign hamartomas in intestines.

HERNIAS

FEMORAL HERNIA

The femoral canal is located below the inguinal ligament on the lateral aspect of the pubic tubercle. Inguinal hernias are above and medial to the pubic tubercle, while femoral hernias are inferior and lateral to the pubic tubercle. The femoral canal is bounded by the inguinal ligament anteriorly, the pectineal ligament posteriorly, the lacunar ligament medially, and the femoral vein laterally. The canal typically consists of empty space or rare lymphatics. A node is occasionally located within the femoral canal, known as Cloquet's node. Femoral hernias occur when abdominal contents pass through the femoral canal. **Femoral hernias are located medial to the femoral vein.**

INGUINAL HERNIA

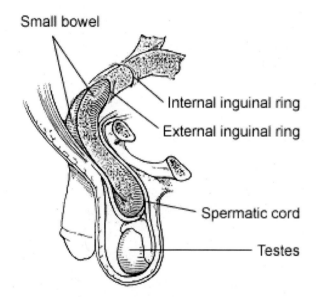

Inguinal Hernia

Small bowel

Internal inguinal ring

External inguinal ring

Spermatic cord

Testes

An indirect inguinal hernia protrudes through the inguinal ring and is typically congenital in nature due to failure to close the internal inguinal ring after the testicle passes through it during development. Indirect inguinal hernias are lateral to the inferior epigastric vessels and are covered by the internal spermatic fascia. Direct inguinal hernias enter through a weakness in the abdominal floor and are acquired. They are located medial to the inferior epigastric vessels and are not covered by the internal spermatic fascia. A reduced incarcerated hernia that presents with a small bowel obstruction requires surgical exploration.

MDs (direct hernia, medial to inferior epigastric vessels) don't Lie (indirect hernia, lateral to vessels). Also, <u>I</u>ndirect = <u>I</u>nfantile.

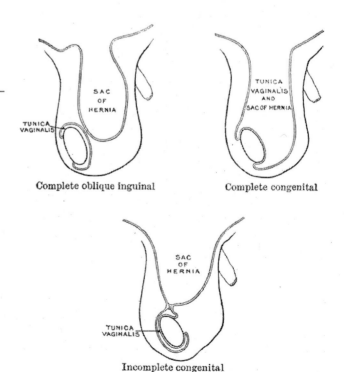

Complete oblique inguinal

Complete congenital

Incomplete congenital

COMPLICATIONS OF HERNIA REPAIR

The presence of oliguria following laparoscopic hernia repair may be due to ureteral injury. The most common nerve injured in the TAPP (transabdominal preperitoneal) approach to hernia repair is the genitofemoral nerve (2%) of the time. This is closely followed by the ilioinguinal nerve (1.1%) and lateral cutaneous nerve of the thigh (1.1%). The ilioinguinal, iliohypogastric, and genitofemoral nerves also go through the region and are often transected intentionally or accidentally. Damage to the genital branch of the genitofemoral nerve leads to loss of the cremaster reflex and loss of sensation to the penis and scrotum. The femoral branch of the genitofemoral nerve provides sensation to the proximal medial thigh. The ilioinguinal provides redundant sensation to this region.

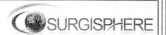

Another complication includes hemorrhage from the obturator artery, deep circumflex iliac artery, external iliac artery, cremaster artery, or inferior epigastric vessels. Constriction of the femoral vein is possible in certain repairs, leading to DVT and possible PE postoperatively. Intentional or accidental transection of the spermatic cord leads to swelling in the testis followed by atrophy in about 1/3 of patients. Orchiectomy is not required following transection of the spermatic cord. Damage to the vas deferens should be repaired primarily.

Damage to the intestines is also possible during a high ligation of the hernia sac, and care must be taken to open the hernia sac and deliberately reduce the contents of the sac prior to ligation. This is more likely to occur with an indirect hernia. Damage to the bladder wall can occasionally occur with a direct hernia, and closure in two layers is required along with foley catheter drainage. Recurrence following indirect or direct inguinal hernia repair is about 5% per year.

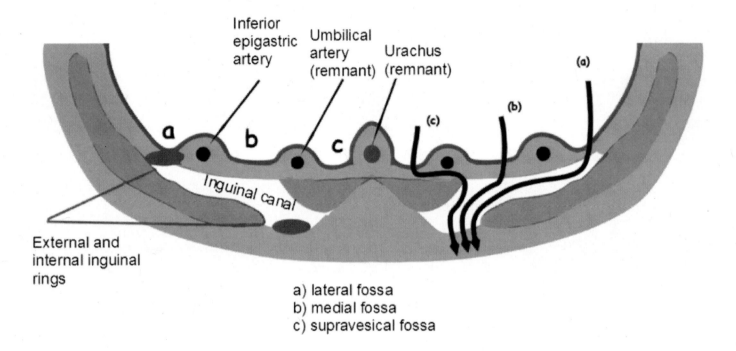

PARASTOMAL HERNIA

Parastomal hernias can be observed until symptoms develop.

SPIGELIAN HERNIA

Spigelian hernias are located at the semilunar line.

PRACTICE QUESTIONS

 What is the source of the gastroduodenal artery?

A. Celiac artery
B. Common hepatic artery
C. Left gastric artery
D. Proper hepatic artery
E. Superior mesenteric artery

The best answer is <u>Common hepatic artery</u>. The gastroduodenal artery is a direct branch of the common hepatic artery before it becomes the proper hepatic artery. Damage to the common hepatic artery typically does not compromise the gastroduodenal artery due to its anastomosis with the superior mesenteric artery via the pancreaticoduodenal branches, and liver function is typically preserved. However, damage to the proper hepatic arteries often leads to liver ischemia.

 A 36 year old female presents to the surgery clinic with a right lower quadrant bulge that is difficult to reduce. She has signs and symptoms of a bowel obstruction and is taken to the OR for reduction and repair. She is diagnosed with a Spigelian hernia. Which of the following best describes the particular anatomy of this hernia?

A. Hernia is anterior to the external oblique and travels between the internal oblique and transversus abdominus
B. Hernia is anterior to the external oblique and travels medial to the internal oblique and transversus abdominus
C. Hernia is posterior to the external oblique and travels between the internal oblique and transversus abdominus
D. Hernia is posterior to the external oblique and travels lateral to the internal oblique and transversus abdominus
E. Hernia is posterior to the external oblique and travels medial to the internal oblique and transversus abdominus

The best answer is <u>Hernia is posterior to the external oblique and travels between the internal oblique and transversus abdominus</u>. A Spigelian hernia commonly leads to an incarcerated hernia that usually requires urgent surgical management for signs and symptoms of bowel obstruction. It travels between the attachment of the internal oblique and transversus abdominus to the rectus sheath and lies posterior to the external oblique muscle.

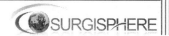

Which of the following is a non-mechanical cause leading to bowel obstruction? It is receptive to therapy with neostigmine.

A.   Colorectal cancer

B.   Crohn disease

C.   Diverticulitis

D.   Ogilvie syndrome

E.   Ulcerative colitis

The best answer is Ogilvie syndrome. Ogilvie syndrome is the acute pseudoobstruction and dilation of the colon in the absence of any mechanical obstruction in severely ill patients. Colonic pseudo-obstruction is characterized by massive dilatation of the cecum (diameter > 10 cm) and right colon on abdominal X-ray. Recent surgery (most common following coronary artery bypass surgery),neurologic disorders, serious infections, cardiorespiratory insufficiency, metabolic disturbances, and drugs that disturb colonic motility (e.g. anticholinergics or narcotics) contribute to the development of this condition. The exact mechanism behind the acute colonic pseudo-obstruction is not fully elucidated. The probable explanation is imbalance in the regulation of colonic motor activity by the autonomic nervous system. It usually resolves with conservative therapy stopping oral ingestions, i.e. nil per os and a nasogastric tube, but may require colonoscopic decompression which is successful in 70% of the cases. A study published in the New England Journal of Medicine showed that neostigmine is a potent pharmacological way of decompressing the colon. According to the American Society for Gastrointestinal Endoscopy (ASGE), it should be considered prior to colonoscopic decompression. The use of neostigmine is not without risk since it can induce bradyarrhythmia and bronchospasms. Therefore atropine should be within immediate reach when this therapy is used. Mortality can be as high as 30% in Ogilvie syndrome.

Which of the following organs utilizes glutamine as its primary nutritional resource?

A.   Esophagus

B.   Large intestine

C.   Rectum

D.   Small intestine

E.   Stomach

The best answer Is Small intestine. The primary source of energy for the small intestine is glutamine. Neoplastic cells also utilize this resource. The large intestine uses butyrate and other small chain fatty acids.

A 28 year old female has a significant family history of colorectal cancer, with numerous first-degree and second-degree relatives diagnosed and treated early for cancer. Which of the following would you consider for this patient?

A.   Colonoscopy to search for proximal tumors in FAP
B.   Genetic testing to determine whether she has autosomal recessive HNPCC
C.   Prophylactic chemotherapy
D.   Prophylactic subtotal colectomy with mucous fistula for Peutz-Jegher syndrome
E.   Prophylactic total abdominal hysterectomy with bilateral salpingo-oopherectomy if she has HNPCC type 2.

The best answer is **Prophylactic total abdominal hysterectomy with bilateral salpingo-oopherectomy if she has HNPCC type 2**. Hereditary nonpolyposis colon cancer (HNPCC) is an autosomal dominant disorder with a strong family inheritance. In most cases, early colon cancer develops in several relatives of the patient, and there is a strong risk of the development of other cancers within the family. HNPCC is a strong predictor of future colon cancer development in the patient. In this disorder, also known as Lynch syndrome, the cancer arises spontaneously from the mucosa, and it is a strong predictor of future ovarian or endometrial cancer. Lynch II syndromes include right sided colon cancer due to mismatch repair. It is typically autosomal dominant. Colon cancer develops over approximately a decade of having large villous or tubulovillous adenomatous polyps. The presence of familial adenomatous polyposis (FAP) syndromes, due to an autosomal dominant gene, is a certain predictor of malignancy. Prophylactic chemotherapy has no role in therapy.

A 62 year old male undergoes a low anterior resection for colorectal cancer. The specimen is sent to pathology, which indicates invasion of the muscularis propria but 0 out of 17 lymph nodes come back as positive. What is the correct staging, therapy, and expected survival?

A.   T1N0M0, no chemotherapy, 5 year survival over 50%
B.   T1N0M0, no chemotherapy, 5 year survival over 90%
C.   T1N1M0, no chemotherapy, 5 year survival over 70%
D.   T2N0M0, chemotherapy, 5 year survival over 70%
E.   T3N0M0, chemotherapy, 5 year survival over 50%

The best answer is **T1N0M0, no chemotherapy, 5 year survival over 90%**. This patient has a T1N0M0 tumor, and therefore does not require chemotherapy. Such tumors have an expected 90% five year survival. In stage A disease, the cancer is limited to the mucosa and submucosa, and carries a greater than 90% 5 year survival. In stage B disease, the cancer has invaded the muscularis propria, with a 70% 5 year survival. Stage C disease has invasion into local lymph nodes, with a 30% 5 year survival. Stage D disease has distant metastases with limited survival after a few years. Colon cancer that falls into Duke's stage A or B is highly amenable to surgery, and wide resection of the colon is typically done along with sampling of nearby lymph nodes to rule out higher stages of disease. Stage C disease is often treated with a combination of surgery and chemotherapy, including agents such as 5-fluorouracil (5-FU) and leucovorin. Stage D disease is treated only with palliation.

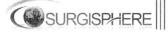

A diagnosis of carcinoid is made after a one centimeter mass is discovered at the distal end of the appendix following an appendectomy. What is the next best step?

A.   Cecectomy with primary anastomosis
B.   No further surgical procedure
C.   Right hemicolectomy with ileostomy
D.   Right hemicolectomy with primary reanastomosis

 The best answer is <u>No further surgical procedure</u>. Carcinoid less than 2cm in size at the tip of the appendix can be treated by appendectomy alone. A carcinoid that is larger than 2cm or at the base of the appendix must be treated by a right hemicolectomy. Metastasis is rare, and nearly ¾ of tumors are located at the distal extent.

 Infliximab (remicade) is used as a therapy for Crohn disease. Which of the following best characterizes the nature of infliximab?

A.   Chimeric anti-TGF antibody
B.   Monoclonal antibody
C.   Protein C inhibitor
D.   Recombinant DNAase
E.   Tumor marker

 The best answer is <u>Monoclonal antibody</u>. Infliximab (brand name Remicade) is a drug used to treat autoimmune disorders. Infliximab is a chimeric monoclonal antibody. The drug blocks the action of TNFα (tumor necrosis factor alpha) by binding to it and preventing it from signaling the receptors for TNFα on the surface of cells. TNFα is one of the key cytokines that triggers and sustains the inflammation response.

 Which of the following organisms is tied to the development of a lymphoma?

A.   Difficile
B.   E. coli
C.   fragilis
D.   H. pylori
E.   S. bovis

 The best answer is <u>H. pylori</u>. The presence of *H. pylori* has also been tied to the development of lymphoproliferative disease in the form of mucosa-associated lymphoid tissue (MALT) lymphoma. Most lymphomas of the stomach tend to be of the non-Hodgkin lymphoma variant. Chronic superficial gastritis can also occur, along with chronic atrophic gastritis. The latter condition can lead to the development of gastric adenocarcinoma. C. difficile leads to colitis. S. bovis has been tied to colorectal cancer.

Which of the following tumor suppressor genes is the first to be mutated in the pathway leading to colorectal cancer?

A. APC
B. DCC
C. hMSH2
D. K-ras
E. p53

The best answer is <u>APC</u>. APC is the earliest change that occurs in the pathway to colorectal cancer. A further dysplastic change occurs in the oncogene K-ras. Later changes leading to carcinoma occur in p53 and DCC.

 Which of the following patients requires a mandatory Hartmann's procedure?

A. 23 year old female with gunshot wound to rectum, 3 hours old
B. 37 year old female with stab wound to left colon, 2 hours old
C. 44 year old male with gunshot wound to transverse colon, 1 hour old
D. 53 year old male with gunshot wound to right colon, 4 hours old
E. 71 year old female with stab wound to transverse colon, 4 hours old

The best answer is <u>23 year old female with gunshot wound to rectum, 3 hours old</u>. Low velocity or stab wounds to the colon less than 4-6 hours old may be primarily repaired after sufficient washout. The patient must be stable and minimal soilage must be the case. However, all extraperitoneal rectal wounds require washout and a diverting colostomy.

 A 64 year old male is diagnosed with a 2cm squamous cell carcinoma of the anus. The tumor is located just 4cm from the anal verge and can be palpated with a finger. The patient presents with itching and bleeding. What is the first step in management?

A. APR
B. APR followed by chemoradiation
C. Chemoradiation
D. Chemoradiation followed by APR
E. LAR

The best answer is <u>Chemoradiation</u>. The initial step in management is chemotherapy with radiation therapy. Chemotherapeutic agents include 5-FU and mitomycin. If this approach fails, the next step is APR.

A 36 year old male presents with an incarcerated inguinal hernia in his left groin. The hernia cannot be reduced, is exquisitely tender, and appears to have overlying skin changes. What is the next best step in management?

A. Inguinal hernia repair
B. Inguinal hernia repair with small bowel resection
C. NPO + NGT and IVF
D. Reduction of hernia in the OR
E. Small bowel resection

The best answer is <u>Inguinal hernia repair</u>. This patient has an incarcerated inguinal hernia with signs of strangulation. This patient requires immediate operative intervention with primary reduction of the hernia and repair of the underlying defect. If ischemic bowel is found, a small bowel resection may also be necessary. Whenever possible, elective repair is preferred due to less morbidity and mortality. Recurrence of a hernia following mesh repair is most likely due to migration of the mesh. Repair of hernias via laparoscopy may lead to damage of the lateral femoral cutaneous nerve, presenting as numbness in the lateral proximal lower extremity. Related to this discussion, a Spigelian hernia is due to a defect in the linea semilunaris between the rectus and transversalis muscles. Repair is required. In the event of infection following hernia repair, the most common offending organism is group A Staphylococcus. Obturator hernias require immediate repair (positive Howship-Romberg test), as do Grynfelt hernia's through the L12 vertebral column. The lateral border of a femoral hernia is the femoral vein; medially is the lacunar ligament; posteriorly the pectineal ligament; anteriorly the inguinal ligament.

A 46 year old alcoholic presents with worsening ascites and a new umbilical hernia. There is evidence of some skin breakdown around the umbilicus. Which of the following is the next best step in management?

A. Antibiotics and observation
B. Liver transplantation
C. Peritovenous shunt with umbilical hernia repair
D. Spironolactone, lasix, and salt restriction
E. Umbilical hernia repair

The best answer is <u>Peritovenous shunt with umbilical hernia repair</u>. This patient has an umbilical hernia due to worsening ascites with new evidence of superficial skin breakdown. This requires an immediate surgical intervention due to the elevated risk of bacterial peritonitis with seeding through the broken skin. Repair of the umbilical hernia alone is insufficient; this patient also requires diversion of his ascites, which is accomplished via a peritovenous shunt. If the patient did not have skin breakdown, treatment with spironolactone, lasix, and salt restriction would be sufficient. The cause of the patient's worsening ascites is likely retention of fluid secondary to elevated aldosterone.

Following an emergent thoracotomy for several stab wounds sustained to the abdomen, an 18 year old teenager has a drop off in urine output and sudden difficulty with ventilation. What is the next best step in management?

A. Cisatracuronium
B. Exploratory laparotomy
C. Increase ventilation settings
D. Succinylcholine
E. Thoracotomy

The best answer is <u>Exploratory laparotomy</u>. This patient has abdominal compartment syndrome until proven otherwise. Signs include the decrease in urine output due to compression of the renal vessels and ureter, and difficulty with ventilation due to the high abdominal pressures precluding ventilation of the lungs. Management includes going to the OR for exploratory laparotomy and decompression. On a related note, a positive DPL includes the presence of over 100,000 RBCs per mm3, over 500 WBCs per mm3, amylase over 175, bile, or urine. These are all indications for an exploratory laparotomy.

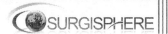

HEPATOPANCREATOBILIARY SURGERY

CHAPTER CONTENTS

GENERAL CONCEPTS

EPIDEMIOLOGY

It is estimated that over 25,000 patients die yearly from liver disease and cirrhosis. This makes liver disease the eighth leading cause of death in the United States, and nearly ¾ of the cases of cirrhosis can be prevented by better treatment of alcohol

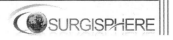

abuse. Hepatitis C contributes to nearly half of all liver disease deaths, and infects nearly 3 million people in the US. Hepatitis B contributes nearly one quarter to all liver disease deaths, with close to 100,000 new cases diagnosed yearly.

ANATOMY

LIVER

LOBES AND DIVISIONS

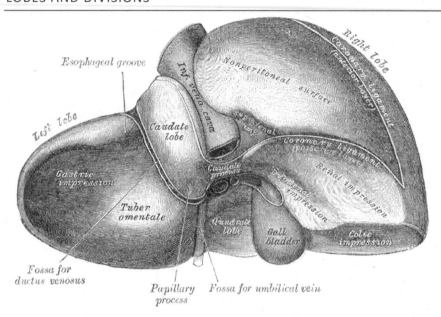

The liver is a three pound, cone-shaped organ that lies in the RUQ. It is divided into two main lobes, each composed of thousands of lobules. The ducts within each of the lobules coalesce to eventually form the hepatic duct, which transports bile produced by the liver to the gallbladder, and then to the duodenum. The liver is supplied by the hepatic artery, which provides oxygenated blood. The hepatic portal vein supplies minerals and nutrients from digestion to the liver. At any particular time, the liver contains over 10% of the body's total blood volume. Nearly ¾ of the liver can be destroyed before it is unable to carry out its functions. The liver is divided into right and left lobes using an artificial demarcation between the inferior vena cava and the gallbladder fossa. As indicated in the above diagram, the liver segment lateral to the gallbladder fossa is segment 5. The common bile duct is located parallel, anterior, and lateral to the hepatic artery (i.e. to the right of the hepatic artery). The portal vein is located posteriorly.

HISTOLOGY

The liver is composed of hepatocytes (50% by number, 80% by volume), Kupffer cells (macrophages), and endothelium. Hepatocytes are divided into three zones. Zone I cells are nearest the periportal blood supply and process incoming nutrients. These cells primarily produce protein. Zone III cells are far from arterial blood and take part in glycogenolysis and Lipogenesis. Formation of urea occurs in zones II and III. Gluconeogenesis predominantly occurs in zone I.

VASCULAR SUPPLY

The central area where the common bile duct, hepatic portal vein, and hepatic artery enter the liver is known as the hilum or porta hepatis. The duct, vein, and artery divide into left and right branches, and the portions of the liver supplied by these branches constitute the functional left and right lobes. The functional lobes are separated by an artificial plane joining the gallbladder fossa to the inferior vena cava. This separates the liver into the true right and left lobes. The middle hepatic vein also demarcates the true right and left lobes. The right lobe is further divided into an anterior and posterior segment by the right hepatic vein. The left lobe is divided into the medial and lateral segments by the left hepatic vein. The fissure for the ligamentum teres or falciform ligament also separates the medial (quadrate lobe) and lateral segments. The functional lobes are further divided into a total of eight subsegments based on a transverse plane through the bifurcation of the main portal vein. The caudate lobe is a separate structure which receives blood flow from both the right- and left-sided vascular branches. The anatomic separation of the liver is based on an artificial plane between the inferior vena cava and gallbladder fossa.

The inferior mesenteric vein and splenic vein combine together and then join the superior mesenteric vein to form the hepatic portal vein. The portal vein travels posterior to the hepatic artery and common bile duct, then divides into the right and left portal veins to supply their respective liver lobes. There are no valves within the portal vein. Venous outflow from the pancreas, stomach, small intestine, large intestine, and spleen flows to the liver. The hepatic veins drain into the inferior vena cava. The hepatic artery is a branch of the celiac trunk. Approximately 3/4s of the blood to the liver comes from the portal venous system, while 1/4 comes from the hepatic artery. Occasionally, hepatic arteries will emanate from the superior mesenteric artery. This tends to be in the form of a displaced right hepatic artery.

BILIARY TREE

The biliary system is composed of the gallbladder, bile ducts, and related transport systems to deliver bile from the liver to the duodenum. The right and left hepatic ducts collect bile produced by the thousands of lobules of the liver and transport it to the common hepatic duct and then the gallbladder for bile storage. The common hepatic duct joins with the cystic duct from the gallbladder to form the common bile duct, which transports bile to the duodenum for emulsification of fats and release of waste products from the liver.

PANCREAS

The pancreas is the abdominal organ located dorsal to the stomach and extends between the right and left upper quadrants. The widest part of the pancreas is known as the head, and is located within the first section of the intestines – the duodenum. The left side tapers and travels somewhat superiorly and is known as the body of the pancreas. The pancreas terminates as the tail near the spleen. The pancreas is composed of exocrine tissue that secretes digestive enzymes into the small intestine and endocrine tissue that secretes hormones into the bloodstream. The blood supply to the head of the pancreas is from the superior and inferior branches emanating from the gastroduodenal artery and superior mesenteric artery, respectively. In the event of a transection of the pancreatic neck, a distal pancreatectomy should be done. The dorsal pancreatic artery is a branch of the splenic artery, and supplies the body and tail of the pancreas along with a bit of the head. It anastomosis with the posterior arcades and left gastroepiploic artery. The transverse pancreatic artery comes from the left gastroepiploic artery. Venous drainage of the pancreas terminates in the portal vein. As a result, splenic vein occlusion leading to gastric varices is possible with pancreatic cancer. Gastric varices occur due to retrograde venous drainage from flow diversion into the short gastric and left gastroepiploic veins.

PHYSIOLOGY

HORMONAL MEDIATORS

GALLBLADDER REGULATION

The liver serves to regulate the concentration of toxic chemicals and byproducts within the body. It also processes ingested minerals and nutrients and converts most ingested substances into a more easily used form. The liver serves to create proteins necessary for coagulation, breaks down waste products and uses bile to carry them to the intestines, serves as a storage organ for glucose in the form of glycogen, controls the concentration of amino acids, forms urea from toxic ammonia, stores iron for use with hemoglobin, and produces a number of factors present in inflammatory and immune reactions for control of infection. Bile itself is composed of waste products, cholesterol, and bile salts and is responsible for the dark color of feces. Impaired bile secretion leads to clay-colored stools. Bile is released from the gallbladder through stimulation by

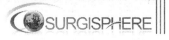

CCK. Emptying of the gallbladder is inhibited by parasympathetic blockade. The gallbladder absorbs a significant amount of water and sodium through sodium diffusion created by a sodium-potassium ATPase. Water absorption is linked to this active sodium transport.

PANCREAS

The exocrine pancreas serves a distinct function from the endocrine pancreas, even though the two tissues are juxtaposed within the same organ. The exocrine pancreas releases a number of enzymes into the pancreatic duct in an inactive form. These digestive enzymes are activated by the acidic environment within the duodenum and break down carbohydrates, proteins, and fats. The exocrine pancreas also secretes bicarbonate to neutralize the hydrochloric acid produced by the parietal cells of the stomach. Nearly 3L of bicarbonate and enzyme-rich fluid are produced every day by the pancreas, and the release of these compounds is facilitated by cholecystokinin (CCK), secretin, and bile salts. The endocrine pancreas secretes insulin and glucagon to regulate the titer of sugar within the bloodstream, and also somatostatin to control the function of the intestines and modulate the concentration of insulin and glucagon. The amount of bicarbonate secretion from the pancreas is inversely related to the amount of chloride secretion.

SERUM-ASCITES ALBUMIN GRADIENT

The SAAG is calculated by comparing the albumin concentration in the serum to that of the ascites fluid. If the difference between the serum and the ascites is greater than 1.1 and portal hypertension is present, it indicates the underlying etiology to likely be due to liver disease such as hepatitis, cirrhosis, liver failure, or HCC; it may alternatively be due to congestion caused by hepatic failure, heart failure, constrictive pericarditis, tricuspid insufficiency, or Budd-Chiari syndrome. A SAAG less than 1.1 with hypoalbuminemia typically indicates that nephrotic syndrome, severe malabsorption with protein loss, or malnutrition with anasarca are the cause. Other conditions that may lead to a SAAG less than 1.1 include ascites of pancreatic, bile, stomach, kidney, bladder, or ovarian origin. A diseased peritoneum can also present with a SAAG less than 1.1 with causes including infection, malignancy, and rarer conditions such as familial Mediterranean fever (FMF), vasculitis, granulomatous peritonitis, and eosinophilic peritonitis.

HEPATIC BIOSYNTHESIS

Proteins created by the liver include albumin, which has a half-life of 3 weeks, prealbumin, which has a half-life of 2 days, and transferrin, which has a half-life of 10 days. Factor VII has the shortest half-life at 5 hours. The cytochrome p450 system in the liver plays a role in toxin metabolism. Phase I reactions lead to oxidation and reduction, while phase II reactions lead to conjugation. Hepatic biotransformation is dependent on the cytochrome P450 system.

BIOCHEMISTRY

BILE SALT METABOLISM

The most important bile acids are cholic acid, deoxycholic acid, and chenodeoxycholic acid. Bile acids are conjugated with either the amino acid glycine or taurine prior to secretion by the liver. Conjugation increases water solubility and thereby

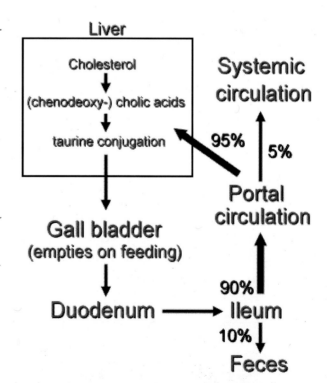

Circulation of Bile Acids

prevents passive reabsorption once secreted into the small intestine. The concentration of bile acids in the small intestine can thereby stay high enough to form micelles and solubilize lipids. Bile acid salts are reabsorbed in the terminal ileum. The primary bile acids are cholic acid and chenodeoxycholic acid. The secondary bile acids are deoxycholic acid and lithocholic acid formed by anaerobic bacteria in the intestine. Biliverdin is the bile pigment formed from the breakdown of hemoglobin. Urobilinogen is produced by bacteria in the intestines. It can be converted to stercobilin, which gives feces their brown color. It may be converted to urobilin, which is absorbed and secreted in urine. Conjugation of bile acids is required for absorption.

The bile salt pool is approximately 2 grams and is recycled half a dozen times a day. Cholesterol synthesis by the liver replenishes this pool. The cholesterol content in bile is entirely derived from that created by the liver. The rate of this production is inhibited by high cholesterol intake. Cholesterol gallstones are the most common type of stone in the gallbladder.

GLUCONEOGENESIS

During an overnight fast, 75gm of liver glycogen is depleted rapidly through glycogenolysis and serum glucose begins to fall. The result is a decrease in insulin and an increase in glucagon, growth hormone, catecholamines, and cortisol. The net effect is stimulation of hepatic gluconeogenesis and glycogenolysis. Gluconeogenesis relies on amino acids as the main carbon source, especially glutamine and alanine. Other sources include lactate, pyruvate, propionate, and glycerol. The primary source of substrate is from proteins, where nearly 75gm of proteins are broken down every day leading to excretion of 10gm of nitrosurea products. This protein breakdown stops about a week after starvation as the body begins to shift to ketoacid use. The fuel source to the body during periods of prolonged starvation (i.e. > 2 weeks) comes from ketone bodies. These ketone bodies are generated by the oxidation of fatty acids. The primary tissues that relay upon glucose are the kidney and liver. The brain, red blood cells, and testes also require glucose.

BILIARY TRACT

CONGENITAL AND STRUCTURAL

CHOLEDOCHOCELE

A choledochocele is treated by resection of the common bile duct followed by a hepaticojejunostomy anastomotic diversion. A choledochal cyst has a risk of cholangiocarcinoma and therefore must be resected. A hepaticojejunostomy is then performed.

CHOLELITHIASIS

PATHOPHYSIOLOGY

Cholelithiasis is the formation of gallstones that may lead to a cessation in bile transport. Cholesterol stones are the most common and are typically located in the gallbladder. Stones in the common bile duct tend to be pigmented stones or calcium bilirubinate stones. Pigmented stones are more common in liver disease, alcohol abuse, and hemolytic anemia. It is several times more common in women, and has a number of risk factors including patients who are in their 40's, fertile, female, overweight, currently fasting, rapid weight loss, Crohn disease, hypertriglyceridemia, a history of cystic fibrosis, a familial tendency, sickle cell disease, diabetes, or use of oral contraceptive drugs (OCDs). These risk factors generally tend to cause an increase in cholesterol content in bile, decreased secretion of bile by the liver, and lead to pooling of cholesterol-laden gallstones within the gallbladder. The sludge that is created has difficulty passing through the ducts and may become lodged within the lumen, leading to obstruction and the signs and symptoms of cholelithiasis.

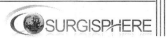

PRESENTATION

Cholelithiasis presents with colicky, RUQ pain that lasts several hours. The pain is severe and worsens with eating. Nausea and vomiting accompany this relentless pain, and there is some tenderness to RUQ palpation but no rebound tenderness.

DIAGNOSIS

Diagnosis of cholelithiasis is made by serum blood tests that demonstrate elevated alkaline phosphatase, direct bilirubin, and signs and symptoms of concomitant hepatitis and pancreatitis. As cholesterol stones tend to be radiolucent and only the minority of stones are radiopaque (pigment stones), ultrasound is the best way to detect gallstones and diagnose cholelithiasis. Stones within the common bile duct are diagnosed and treated with ERCP. Cholesterol stones make up 80% of all gallstones and are composed primarily of cholesterol. Pigment stones are found about 20% of the time and are made of calcium and bilirubin. Risk factors for pigment stones include cirrhosis, biliary tract infections, and red blood cell dyscrasias.

TREATMENT

Treatment of cholelithiasis includes ERCP with sphincterotomy, lithotripsy, and ursodeoxycholic acid (UDCA) and other oral bile acids to dissolve cholesterol stones. A retained stone following a T-tube placement that is not amenable to ERCP should be removed with interventional radiology.

Table 213 Cholelithiasis

Cholelithiasis	
Pathophysiology	Formation of gall stones (cholesterol or calcium bilirubinate) leads to stoppage of bile flow.
Presentation	RUQ pain, pain worse with eating. Nausea/vomiting, tenderness in RUQ.
Diagnosis	Elevated serum alkaline phosphatase, radiolucent cholesterol stones, ERCP.
Treatment	ERCP with sphincterotomy, lithotripsy, UDCA, pain control.

CHOLEDOCHOLITHIASIS

Development or diagnosis of choledocholithiasis following laparoscopic cholecystectomy requires an ERCP to attempt stone removal. The success rate of this procedure is 90% with a 1% mortality. A sphincterotomy is routinely done as part of this procedure. Stones larger than 1.5cm or the presence of multiple stones may require a takeback to the operating room for a choledocholithotomy with choledochoduodenostomy. A contraindication to ERCP is the presence of duodenal diverticula. ESWL is a possible alternative procedure. The development of shock following ERCP may be due to a retroduodenal perforation. A CXR, KUB, and gastrograffin swallow study are mandatory as part of the diagnostic workup.

GALLSTONE ILEUS

In gallstone ileus, the gallbladder can be left behind if significantly inflamed. The presence of small bowel obstruction and pneumobilia typically indicates the onset of gallstone ileus.

CHOLEDUODENAL FISTULA

A cholecystoduodenal fistula typically presents with small bowel obstruction due to gallstone ileus. It tends to occur in the elderly. Treatment is to remove the obstructing stone but to leave the gallbladder and fistula intact to minimize morbidity. The pain response is mediated by thoracic visceral afferent nerves.

METABOLIC AND DEGENERATIVE

JAUNDICE

Jaundice is the deposition of excess bilirubin into the tissues of the body leading to a yellow discoloration of the eyes and skin. Elevated bilirubin also darkens the color of the urine due to high levels of excretion from the kidney. Causes of elevated bilirubin include damage to the liver, inflammation, blockade of bile drainage from the bile ducts, or hemolytic anemia.

INFLAMMATORY AND INFECTIOUS

CHOLECYSTITIS

ETIOLOGY AND PATHOPHYSIOLOGY

Cholecystitis is inflammation and infection that results following cholelithiasis. Nearly ¾ of all presentations of cholecystitis have concurrent infection by enteric bacteria, including *E. coli*, *Klebsiella*, *Enterococcus*, and *Bacteroides* species. Other causes of cholecystitis include abscess and tumors.

PRESENTATION

Charcot's triad is positive in cholecystitis, including fever, jaundice, and RUQ pain. Guarding and rebound tenderness are common, and a positive Murphy's sign is often present (inspiration is suddenly arrested during palpation of the RUQ). Murphy's sign is very sensitive for cholecystitis.

DIAGNOSIS AND TREATMENT

Diagnosis of cholecystitis is best made with a HIDA scan. Elevated PMNs and positive ultrasound findings increase the clinical suspicion of cholecystitis. Cholecystitis is treated with antibiotic administration, pain control with meperidine, and cholecystectomy for refractory cases. Complications of

 Charcot Triad: fever, jaundice, RUQ pain

cholecystitis include the formation of abscesses and fistulas, gallstone ileus, and pancreatitis. One variant of cholecystitis is with acalculus cholecystitis, which occurs in about 10% of all cases. In this situation, there is increased morbidity and mortality. Risk factors for acalculus cholecystitis include increased age, systemic disorders such as diabetes, infections such as HIV, surgery, labor of pregnancy, gallbladder torsion, and vasculitis. Another variant of cholecystitis is emphysematous cholecystitis caused by *Clostridium* infection leading to gangrene and perforation. Immediate antibiotic treatment and surgery is required.

Table 214 Cholecystitis

Cholecystitis	
Pathophysiology	Infection & inflammation after cholelithiasis, infections with enteric bacteria.
Presentation	Charcot's triad, rebound tenderness, Murphy's sign.
Diagnosis	HIDA scan, high PMN, ultrasound findings.
Treatment	Antibiotics, meperidine, cholecystectomy in refractory cases.

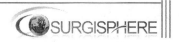

COMPLICATIONS

The morbidity due to a laparoscopic cholecystectomy is about 3%, and the mortality about 1%. Hemorrhage, infection, disability from anesthesia, biliary tree injuries, vascular injury, and organ injury are the most common problems. The use of carbon dioxide insufflation can lead to gas embolism, which may present as a sudden decrease in end tidal CO_2. Treatment is to place the patient in the left lateral decubitus position to facilitate gas bubble absorption by the right atrium. An intraoperative cholangiogram performed following a laparoscopic cholecystectomy with no proximal ducts found should elicit open exploration. If a common bile duct injury occurs during a cholecystectomy, the proper treatment is returning the patient to the operating room and to permit an experienced surgeon perform a hepaticojejunostomy. Indications for converting to an open procedure include poor visualization of the anatomy, bleeding, anomalous anatomy, and the presence of adhesions. The presence of a cystic duct leak can be initially treated with ERCP for stenting. Otherwise, a cystic duct leak with a biloma is treated with a sphincterotomy followed by percutaneous drainage. A patient who undergoes an uncomplicated laparoscopic cholecystectomy but then develops a stricture at the left and right biliary ducts years later has cholangiocarcinoma until otherwise proven.

ASCENDING CHOLANGITIS

ETIOLOGY AND PATHOPHYSIOLOGY

Ascending cholangitis is due to obstruction of the common bile duct leading to obstruction of the biliary tree. This condition is also referred to as choledocholithiasis. Other causes include tumors and strictures that lead to the blockade of the biliary tree.

PRESENTATION

Choledocholithiasis presents with Charcot's triad, including fever, RUQ pain, and jaundice. It is not specific to choledocholithiasis and is present in only some cases. Reynold's pentad may also develop, which includes the tripartite Charcot's triad in addition to altered mental status and shock. Reynold's pentad is an indicator of poor outcome.

DIAGNOSIS AND TREATMENT

Diagnosis of choledocholithiasis is made by ultrasound. It is treated with IV fluids and vasopressors to maintain BP, antibiotics to cover enteric flora to prevent cholecystitis, use of ERCP to remove the biliary tree blockade, and surgery to permit the resumption of bile flow. Ascending cholangitis is an emergency.

Table 215 Ascending Cholangitis

Ascending Cholangitis	
Pathophysiology	Obstruction of common bile duct.
Presentation	Charcot's triad, fever, RUQ pain, jaundice.
Diagnosis	Ultrasound.
Treatment	IVs, vasopressors, antibiotics, ERCP to remove blockage, surgery.

PRIMARY SCLEROSING CHOLANGITIS

PATHOPHYSIOLOGY

PSC is common in patients with ulcerative colitis, and presents as chronic, progressive inflammation and scarring of the bile ducts. It is thought that PSC is due to a hypersensitivity reaction.

DIAGNOSIS AND TREATMENT

Diagnosis of PSC is made by ultrasound (US), ERCP, and PTC. PSC presents with elevated alkaline phosphatase, GGT, bilirubin, and symptoms of cholestasis and liver disease. Treatment is through surgical intervention to decompress the biliary tree.

Table 216 Primary Sclerosing Cholangitis (PSC)

	Primary Sclerosing Cholangitis (PSC)
Pathophysiology	Chronic, progressing, inflammation and scarring of bile ducts.
Presentation	Elevated alkaline phosphatase, GGT, bilirubin.
Diagnosis	US, ERCP, PTC.
Treatment	Surgery.

PRIMARY BILIARY CIRRHOSIS

ETIOLOGY AND EPIDEMIOLOGY

PBC is an autoimmune disorder that causes destruction of the intrahepatic bile ducts. It is more common in women, and is predicted by the presence of AMA and a demonstrable autoimmune response to the epithelium of the biliary tree. PBC leads to the accumulation of waste products commonly dissipated with bile secretion, namely, cholesterol, bile acids, and bilirubin.

PRESENTATION

PBC presents with symptoms similar to other liver diseases, including jaundice, fatigue and weakness and pruritus. In addition, PBC presents with xanthomas from the elevated cholesterol. There is typically an additional autoimmune disorder present with PBC, such as rheumatoid arthritis (RA). Nearly 1/3 of patients are asymptomatic, and the most common initial complaint is fatigue.

DIAGNOSIS AND TREATMENT

Diagnosis of PBC is made by elevated alkaline phosophatase and GGT. AST and ALT are typically normal. There is also a positive AMA. Ultrasound is typically unremarkable. Hyperlipidemia is another feature of PBC. Treatment largely consists of surgical intervention due to the failure of medical management. Liver transplantation is necessary.

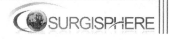

Table 217 Primary Biliary Cirrhosis (PBC)

Primary Biliary Cirrhosis (PBC)	
Epidemiology	Autoimmune disorder which destroy intrahepatic bile ducts. More common in women.
Presentation	Jaundice, fatigue, weakness, pruritus, Xanthomas, RA.
Diagnosis	Elevated alkaline phosphatase and GGT. AST and ALT usually normal. Positive AMA.
Treatment	Surgery, liver transplant.

LIVER

CONGENITAL AND STRUCTURAL

VARICES

Esophageal varices are the result of dilated blood vessels within the distal portion of the esophagus that can become abraded and subsequently hemorrhage. Rupture of varices can lead to significant blood loss, hematemesis, and anemia, and these large bleeds can be fatal in over half of all patients. BP is maintained during acute variceal hemorrhage through normal saline and transfusions, fresh frozen plasma (FFP) to replace clotting factors, vasopressin or somatostatin to decrease mesenteric blood flow, beta blockers to decrease blood flow, sclerotherapy, and band ligation of bleeding vessels.

HEMANGIOMA

An asymptomatic hemangioma can be observed; surgery is not indicated until the development of clinically significant symptoms. These tumors tend to be contrast-enhancing lesions.

METABOLIC AND DEGENERATIVE

HEPATIC ENCEPHALOPATHY

Encephalopathy from liver disease is commonly the result of elevated levels of ammonia leading to central nervous system (CNS) damage. The elevated amino acid content of the blood also leads to an increase in GABA levels and endogenous benzodiazepines. Hepatic encephalopathy is often heralded by signs of impaired consciousness such as drowsiness, confusion, disorientation, or coma, changes in personality, behavior, mood or judgment, changes in speech, asterixis, fetor hepaticus, and cerebral edema. Hepatic encephalopathy is worsened by acute GI bleeds, increased protein intake, and active infection. The differential diagnosis of hepatic encephalopathy includes alcohol intoxication, delirium tremens, dementia, infection, and various systemic disorders.

HEPATIC CIRRHOSIS

ETIOLOGY

Cirrhosis is the development of repeated liver damage leading to cycles of fibrosis, necrosis, regeneration, and eventually, HCC. Causes of cirrhosis include alcohol, viral infection, primary biliary cirrhosis (PBC), Wilson disease, alpha-1-antitrypsin deficiency, and hemochromatosis. The most common cause of cirrhosis in the United States is alcohol abuse leading to fatty liver, and eventually hepatitis and cirrhosis with continued insult.

PRESENTATION

Cirrhosis presents with many of the signs discussed above for liver damage, including jaundice, nausea and vomiting, hepatomegaly, loss of appetite, angiomas, ascites, encephalopathy, palmar erythema, Dupuytren contracture, and portal hypertension. Overall, 15% of alcoholics will develop cirrhosis. There is a 10% mortality from hepatitis, and half of all cases are due to progression to cirrhosis and the other half to fibrosis.

DIAGNOSIS

Diagnosis of cirrhosis is made with abnormal LFTs including an elevated AST to ALT ratio (viral disorders raise the ALT to AST ratio), elevated direct and indirect bilirubin, elevated GGT, prolonged PT, low albumin, and anemia.

TREATMENT

Cirrhosis is treated by avoiding risk factors that can further exacerbate liver injury. Failure to do so, and continued use of alcohol, will likely lead to fulminant hepatic failure or HCC. Unlike some other hepatobiliary conditions, a high protein diet is recommended with vitamin supplements to permit the liver to form the necessary proteins required for normal body function. Medications that can further damage the liver are avoided, including acetaminophen and isoniazid (INH). Inflammatory changes can often be halted with the use of colchicine and glucocorticoids. Other complications of cirrhosis such as ascites should be treated as necessary. Alpha 1-antitrypsin deficiency is a defect in alpha 1-antitrypsin production leading to excess deposition of abnormal A1AT protein in lung and liver. The result is COPD and cirrhosis. Treatment involves a lung and liver transplant, whenever possible.

PROGNOSIS

The prognosis of cirrhosis is made by the Child-Pugh score, which examines the levels of bilirubin, albumin, PT, the presence of hepatic encephalopathy, and the grade of ascites. The score for each category is summed, and a Child class assigned based on the range of the scores. Child class A is a score between 5 and 6, class B with a score between 7 and 9, and class C with a score greater than 9. With serum bilirubin less than 2, a score of 1 is given; bilirubin greater than 3 has a score of 3. Serum albumin more than 3.5 has a score of 1; less than 2.8 has a score of 3. PT of 4 or less is given a score of 1; PT more than 6 has a score of 3. No hepatic encephalopathy has a score of 1, while severe symptoms have a score of 3. No ascites is given a score of 1, while severe ascites has a score of 3. A Child score of A has a 15-20 year survival; Child class C survival has a survival of only a few years.

Table 218 Cirrhosis

Cirrhosis	
Pathophysiology	Repeated liver damage leading to fibrosis, necrosis, regeneration, and HCC.
Cause	Alcohol, viral infection, PBC, Wilson disease, hemochromatosis.
Presentation	Jaundice, nausea/vomiting, hepatomegaly, ascites, encephalopathy, portal hypertension, Dupuytren contracture, palmar erythema.
Diagnosis	Abnormal LFTs, elevated AST to ALT ratio, high bilirubin and GGT, long PT.
Treatment	Avoiding risk factors, high protein diet, vitamins.
Prognosis	Made by Child-Pugh score

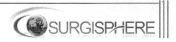

Table 219 Child-Pugh Scoring for Liver Failure

	Child-Pugh Scoring for Liver Failure					
	Bilirubin	Albumin	PT	Ascites	Encephalopathy	Mortality
Child A	< 2	> 3.5	1-3	None	None	7% mortality
Child B	2 – 3	3 – 3.5	4-6	Moderate	Moderate	15% mortality
Child C	> 3	< 3	> 6	Severe	Severe	33% mortality

HEPATORENAL SYNDROME

Hepatorenal syndrome is the development of acute renal failure with worsening oliguria, azotemia, and sodium retention. It is diagnosed by very low urine sodium. It is especially common in later stages of severe hepatic failure. There is no known treatment other than supportive therapy and palliative care. Hepatorenal syndrome is due to the inability to concentrate urine and is associated with portal hypertension. It is attributed to an alteration in blood flow to the splanchnic circulation and kidney. Type I involves a rapid increase in creatinine to over 2.5 mg/dL and a drop in creatinine clearance to less than 20 mL/min. Type II is progressive over a longer period of time and has more gradual worsening of renal function. Type II hepatorenal syndrome is typically due to ascites that is refractory to medical management. Urine sodium is typically less than 10 mEq/dL. IV albumin has been shown to improve outcomes in some studies. Octreotide or midodrine used individually have no beneficial effects.

INFLAMMATORY AND INFECTIOUS

SPONTANEOUS BACTERIAL PERITONITIS

Spontaneous bacterial peritonitis occurs in a subset of patients with longstanding ascites, and is due to infection by enteric gram negative bacteria from the intestinal flora. Spontaneous bacterial peritonitis presents with fever and chills, rebound abdominal tenderness, and sepsis. It is diagnosed with gram stain, culture, and sensitivity following paracentesis of the ascites. The presence of over 250 polymorphonuclear lymphocytes (PMNs) is diagnostic. Spontaneous bacterial peritonitis is treated with cefuroxime to cover the intestinal flora and electrolyte replacement for the ascites.

LIVER ABSCESS

Pyogenic abscesses can be diagnosed by the presence of fever, and a blunting of the costophrenic angle. The presence of a ring-enhancing lesion in the liver with numerous satellite lesions should be treated with abendazole. An amoebic liver abscess is treated with metronidazole. Percutaneous drainage of the abscess can be attempted once therapy is started. Surgical intervention is necessary only if the intestinal phase cannot be adequately controlled. Drainage alone is not likely to be successful.

HEPATITIS

ETIOLOGY

Viral hepatitis is an infectious process due to hepatitis A (HAV), B (HBV), C (HCV), D (HDV), E (HEV), or G (HGV). Longstanding viral hepatitis leads to symptoms of liver damage, including jaundice and dark urine, right upper quadrant (RUQ) pain, weakness and fatigue, anorexia, nausea and vomiting, low-grade fever, and general malaise. Generally, viral hepatitis presents with elevations in ALT. The increases are significant – viral hepatitis is one of three serious causes of transaminases increasing above 1,000; the other two causes are acetaminophen toxicity and septic shock leading to fulminant liver failure. Fulminant liver failure can also occur with infection by any of the hepatitis viruses except HGV. Cirrhosis is most commonly associated with chronic hepatitis, which can occur with HBV and HCV. Finally, all of the causes of viral hepatitis are due to RNA viruses except HBV, which is a DNA virus. The specific hepatitis viruses are discussed below.

Table 220 Viral Hepatitis

Viral Hepatitis	
Cause	HAV, HBV, HCV, HDV, HEV, HGV
Presentation	Jaundice, dark urine, RUQ pain, weakness, fatigue, anorexia, nausea/vomiting, low grade fever, general malaise. Typically has a high ALT

HEPATITIS A VIRUS

PATHOPHYSIOLOGY

HAV is a single-stranded RNA virus in the hepatovirus family. It is predominantly spread by the fecal-oral route and is associated with poor hygiene and contaminated food. Contaminated shellfish in particular have been implicated. HAV is not transmitted vertically from mother to neonate, and there is no chronic carrier state. HAV has a 30 day incubation. A minority of HAV infections lead to fulminant hepatic failure.

DIAGNOSIS

The assessment of HAV infection is made by serology that is positive for IgM antibodies to HAV, which indicates recent exposure, and IgG antibodies to HAV, which indicates exposure in the past and current immunity. In general, the presence of IgM antibodies indicates acute exposure as the immunoglobulin has not yet had a chance to shift to IgG expression.

TREATMENT

Symptomatic management is often the treatment of choice for HAV infection. This is due to HAV often being a self-limited disorder with little chance of progression to a more serious disease. HAV prophylaxis is given to people who are planning to travel to developing nations by way of a vaccine that takes three weeks to take effect. Immunoglobulins against HAV can also be administered in susceptible patients if given within a couple of weeks of exposure. The vaccine and immunoglobulin therapy are typically administered to patients with chronic liver disease to avoid further insult and injury.

Table 221 Hepatitis A (HAV)

Hepatitis A (HAV)	
Pathophysiology	Single-stranded RNA. Spread by fecal-oral route, contaminated food.
Diagnosis	Positive for IgM and IgG to HAV in serum.
Treatment	Symptomatic management. Prophylaxis available.

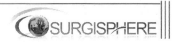

HEPATITIS B VIRUS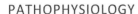

PATHOPHYSIOLOGY

HBV is a DNA virus in the hepadnavirus family. HBV is spread predominantly through sex, blood products, and saliva. It is found in all body fluids. HBV has a 1/10 chance of progressing to chronic hepatitis in adults, and a 90% risk in neonates. Chronic infection significantly increases the risk of hepatocellular carcinoma (HCC) due to repeated cycles of damage and healing. The risk of fulminant liver failure is approximately 1 in 100 patients, and half of all cases of fulminant hepatitis are due to HBV. HBV has a two-six month incubation period.

DIAGNOSIS

A number of markers for HBV infection are used to determine the infectivity and prognosis of the disease. Hepatitis B core antigen (HBcAg) is expressed in infected hepatocytes, but not detectable in the serum. HBcAg is a marker for early infection. IgM antibodies to hepatitis B core (HBcAb IgM) indicates the onset of the window period, and is the time between disappearance of hepatitis B surface antigen (HBsAg) and appearance of antibodies to HBs (HBsAb) in the serum. HBcAb IgM is detectable during the acute phase of infection, which typically occurs 1-6 months after infection. HBsAg is the antigen present on the protein coat of the virus and is a marker of active hepatitis and a carrier state. Ongoing viral replication with a high chance of infectivity is indicated by the hepatitis B "e" antigen. Both HBsAg and HBeAg are expressed between 1-6 months after initial infection. A significantly decreased risk of infection is indicated by the presence of antibodies to HBe (HBeAb), which can take several months to years and are present in the acute phase of resolution. Immunity is signified by antibodies to HBs (HBsAb). Signs of infection in the distant past are indicated by IgG antibodies to HBc (HBcAb IgG), and are detectable for the longest period of time. Essentially, if HBsAg is positive, infection is ongoing. If HBcAb IgM is present, the infection is in the window period. The presence of only HBsAb indicates immunity via vaccination.

TREATMENT

Treatment of HBV is instituted with immunoglobulins to HBV (HBIG), use of alpha-interferon or lamivudine for chronic infections, and liver transplantation in the case of fulminant hepatic failure. Prophylaxis to HBV is the best way to avoid infection, and it is done with a series of three HBV IgG injections and standard precautions to body fluids should be taken. Only the hepatitis B surface antibody is present following vaccination in a hepatitis-naïve person.

HAV: fecal-oral
HBV: body fluids; → HCC
HCV: body fluids; → HCC

Table 222 Hepatitis B (HBV)

Hepatitis B (HBV)	
Pathophysiology	DNA virus spread through sex, blood, saliva.
Diagnosis	HbcAG in hepatocytes but not in serum IgM to HBV. Also HBsAg, HBcAb, HBeAg, HBeAb, HBsAb at various stages (see text).
Treatment	Immunoglobulins to HBV, lamivudine, alpha-interferon, transplant.

HEPATITIS C VIRUS

PATHOPHYSIOLOGY

HCV is a single-stranded RNA virus in the flavivirus family, and is spread in a manner similar to HBV. HCV is now the most common cause of viral hepatitis in the United States due to precautions against blood-borne transmission of HBV instituted earlier than HCV precautions. HCV transmission is especially common in IV drug users and in prisons. Vertical transmission is possible but minimal (5%), as is sexual transmission (5%) and via needles (5%). Like HBV, the incubation period is typically on the order of 1-6 months. About ¾ of HCV infections become chronic and there is up to a 5% risk of HCC. HCV infection can present with symptoms of hepatitis and also polyarteritis nodosa (PAN) and cryoglobulinemias. Only ¼ of patients are symptomatic.

DIAGNOSIS

Diagnosis is made by positive serum titers for antibodies to HCV (HCVAb). HCVAb indicates chronic infection. Repeated infections over time are possible due to poor antibody development.

TREATMENT

HCV is treated with alpha-interferon and ribavirin with a 50% chance of remission. Patients who do not respond to this therapy can be given a course of amantadine or rimantadine. As with HBV, the best treatment is prevention.

Table 223 Hepatitis C Virus (HCV)

Hepatitis C Virus (HCV)	
Pathophysiology	Single-stranded RNA. Spread through sex, saliva, blood.
Presentation	Symptoms of hepatitis, PAN and cryoglobulinemias.
Diagnosis	Positive serum levels of HCVAb.
Treatment	Alpha-interferon and ribavirin, amantidine, rimantadine.

HEPATITIS D VIRUS

PATHOPHYSIOLOGY AND DIAGNOSIS

HDV is the delta agent, and requires the presence of HBV in order to be infective. Elements from HBV are required in order for HDV to propagate and retain its infectivity. In patients with pre-existing HBV, a super-infection may occur with HDV; both HBV and HDV can be simultaneously transmitted to cause a co-infection. HDV infection dramatically increases the risk of liver damage and cirrhosis. HDV is an RNA virus. Superinfection carries the greatest risk of fulminant liver failure. Treatment is to eradicate the HBV infection; the presence of HBsAb indicates immunity to HBV and HDV.

Table 224 Hepatitis D Virus (HDV)

Hepatitis D Virus (HDV)	
Pathophysiology	RNA virus. Requires HBV to be infective.
Treatment	Treat the concurrent HBV infection.

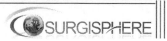

HEPATITIS E VIRUS

PATHOPHYSIOLOGY AND DIAGNOSIS

HEV is a RNA virus with a 1-2 month incubation period. Like HAV, it is transmitted through the fecal-oral route. It is most common in Asia and Africa, and carries a relatively high rate of fulminant liver failure. Pregnant patients are especially susceptible for unknown reasons, and the risk of fulminant liver failure and death is especially worrisome in this population. There is no carrier state with HEV, and no marker for diagnosis.

TREATMENT

Treatment of HEV is primarily supportive therapy and avoidance with good hygienic practices.

Table 225 Hepatitis E Virus (HEV)

Hepatitis E Virus (HEV)	
Pathophysiology	RNA virus. Transmitted by fecal-oral route. Most common in Asia and Africa.
Diagnosis	No marker for diagnosis.
Treatment	Supportive therapy.

VASCULAR

PORTAL HYPERTENSION

Portal hypertension is the elevation of blood pressure (BP) within the portal vein due to elevated back pressure from the flow of blood through the liver. Portal hypertension may present with splenomegaly, hemorrhoids, ascites, esophageal varices, and caput medusa. Collateral vessel development can occur as a measure to alleviate this elevated BP, and this can lead to the development of ascites and varices. The formation of ascites can lead to the build-up of fluid within the abdominal cavity due to fluid leaks. Ascites can present with a significantly distended abdomen and SOB. Portal hypertension is treated with the surgical formation of a transjugular intrahepatic portacaval shunt (TIPS) to bypass the liver, and also via portasystemic shunts. Decreased portal pressure can also be done with beta-blockade. The most common cause of portal hypertension is schistosomiasis infection.

 The presence of a left-sided portal hypertension requires a splenectomy to avoid splenic vein thrombosis.

CANCER

HEPATIC ADENOMA

An adenoma of the liver is most likely to present with shock due to the high risk of bleeding, especially in pregnancy. About 33% are likely to hemorrhage. Treatment is to stop all oral contraceptives; if the adenoma does not improve, resection is necessary.

HEPATIC HEMANGIOMA

No intervention is necessary unless the hemangioma is growing in size and becomes symptomatic. Hemangiomas are not likely to spontaneously rupture.

HEPATIC ANGIOSARCOMA

Angiosarcoma of the liver may develop following exposure to vinyl chloride. This carcinogen also leads to cancer in the brain and lung. Vinyl chloride is used in the manufacture of plastics.

HEPATOCELLULAR CARCINOMA

ETIOLOGY AND PATHOPHYSIOLOGY

Primary hepatocellular carcinoma is a highly morbid and lethal cancer that commonly occurs following chronic liver injury such as cirrhosis. However, up to one quarter of all patients may develop HCC spontaneously. Metastasis from the liver to the bones, brain, and lungs is common in late stage HCC. HCC composes 2% of all cancers and affects some 10,000 new persons annually. Males are more affected than females. The most common causes include chronic alcoholism, HBV, HCV, hemochromatosis, and aflatoxin poisoning.

PRESENTATION AND DIAGNOSIS

HCC presents with signs and symptoms of liver failure, including jaundice, pruritus, hepatosplenomegaly (often with hepatic nodules as in cirrhosis), bleeding diatheses, cachexia, encephalopathy, asterixis, ascites, and varices. LFTs are elevated along with AFP. Biopsy confirms the diagnosis, while imaging studies are used to determine the extent of disease and whether a surgical approach could be beneficial. The presence of a liver mass in a patient with a history of cirrhosis is hepatocellular carcinoma unless otherwise proven. Over 90% of patients will have an elevation in alpha-fetoprotein. All liver metastases must have an arterial supply and so are susceptible to chemoembolization. A liver tumor with a central, stellate scar is focal nodular hyperplasia.

TREATMENT

Vaccination for HBV and HCV is protective, and avoiding alcohol is important. Complications of hepatic failure are treated to minimize patient discomfort. Paracentesis and diuretics are often used to treat ascites. Lactulose is used to reduce the symptoms of hepatic encephalopathy. Ursodiol is used for the treatment of significant pruritus. Band ligation is used to cease variceal hemorrhage. Prophylactic antibiotics to avoid SBP may also be used. Chemotherapy is used but has poor response. Use of chemoembolization techniques to provide targeted tumor therapy is beneficial in some patients. Surgical resection with clear margins is the definitive care, but this approach can only be done in only a small percentage of patients; due to missed metastases, there is a high relapse rate even with this aggressive procedure. Transplantation is also an option for localized disease. The most common site of metastasis is the lung. Long term survival from a single colorectal liver metastasis has a 25-50% 5 year survival.

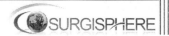

Table 226 Hepatocellular Carcinoma

Hepatocellular Carcinoma	
Etiology	Chronic alcoholism, HBV, HCV, hemochromatosis, and aflatoxin poisoning.
Presentation	Jaundice, pruritus, hepatosplenomegaly (often with hepatic nodules as in cirrhosis), bleeding diatheses, cachexia, encephalopathy, asterixis, ascites, and varices.
Diagnosis	Biopsy confirms the diagnosis. LFTs are elevated along with AFP.
Treatment	Avoiding alcohol, vaccination is important. Complications are treated to minimize patient discomfort. Paracentesis and diuretics, lactulose, ursodiol, band ligation, and, prophylactic antibiotics. Surgical resection with clear margins is the definitive care. Transplantation is also an option for localized disease.

PANCREAS

STRUCTURAL AND CONGENITAL

PANCREATIC DIVISUM

Pancreatic divisum is the failure of the minor pancreatic duct to become confluent with the major duct. The result is pancreatitis with failure of ERCP. Failure of these two ducts to fuse is treated by stenting the minor papilla.

ANNULAR PANCREAS

An annular pancreas wraps around the entire duodenum and is due to failure of normal clockwise rotation of the ventral pancreas during ontogeny. The eventual presentation is a partial small bowel obstruction, developing of peptic ulcer disease, and chronic pancreatitis. Treatment involves a duodenojejunostomy; resection of the pancreas is not indicated.

PANCREATIC FISTULA

The formation of a pancreatic fistula typically results between the pancreas and transverse colon. Greater than 200 ml / day output is classified as a high output fistula. Treatment involves conversion to TPN, use of somatostatin, and time to permit spontaneous closure. Failure of a high output fistula to close requires a roux-en-Y diversion to the fistula. A distal pancreatectomy can also be performed if the fistula is located in the body or tail.

PANCREATIC PSEUDOCYST

A pseudocyst is typically the result of either pancreatitis or trauma. It is known as a pseudocyst as there is no true capsule surrounding the fluid collection. Treatment is external drainage in the case of infection. Internal drainage can be completed for large cysts. Most simple cysts can be observed with CT scan.

INFLAMMATORY AND INFECTIOUS

GALLSTONE PANCREATITIS

ASSESSMENT

Gallstone pancreatitis is the development of pancreatitis due to an obstructing gallstone. This gallstone is typically located in the distal common bile duct, which shares its passageway with the main pancreatic duct. About 5% of patients with cholelithiasis present with gallstone pancreatitis. An intraoperative cholangiogram that indicates no emptying into the duodenum when performed for gallstone pancreatitis can be checked by giving glucagon to the patient.

MANAGEMENT

Therapy involves supportive care until amylase and lipase return to normal. An ERCP with sphincterotomy and stone retrieval is typically indicated in patients who do not spontaneously pass the stone and return to their baseline quickly. The presence of choledocholithiasis on gallbladder ultrasound necessitates an ERCP prior to operative intervention. A patient who has had resolution of gallstone pancreatitis should be treated with a laparoscopic cholecystectomy with a cholangiogram within the same hospitalization. The risk of recurrent disease is as high as 50% within a month without cholecystectomy.

ACUTE PANCREATITIS

ETIOLOGY AND PATHOPHYSIOLOGY

Acute pancreatitis is the result of direct damage from prematurely activated pancreatic enzymes digesting the parenchyma of the organ. Severe disease can lead to systemic inflammatory response syndrome (SIRS) and subsequently progress to severe septic shock, multi-organ system failure, and adult respiratory distress syndrome (ARDS). Causes of acute pancreatitis include perforation of a alcoholism, peptic ulcer, neoplastic disorders, cholelithiasis, end stage renal disease (ESRD), endoscopic retrograde cholangiopancreatography (ERCP), malnutrition leading to anorexia, direct trauma to the pancreas, certain infections, use of drugs that lead to toxic byproducts, burn injuries, surgery, and scorpion bites. The most common causes are alcohol abuse and gallstones. Metabolic conditions that predispose to pancreatitis include very high hypertriglyceridemia, and hypercalcemia. Medications that can lead to pancreatitis include oral hypoglycemic agents, thiazide diuretics, furosemide, pentamidine, TMP-SMX, and DDI.

PRESENTATION

Acute pancreatitis presents as severe epigastric pain that radiates to the back. The pain worsens after consumption of food and may improve if the patient leans forward. Nausea and vomiting are common, as is fever, tachypnea (to avoid deep breaths that may lead to further irritation of the already inflamed pancreas), a positive Cullen sign, and a positive Turner sign. Cullen sign is the presence of a bluish hue to the umbilicus due to hemorrhaging within the peritoneum – it is most commonly found in necrotizing pancreatitis. Turner sign is a bluish discoloration in the flanks due to hemoglobin deposition and decomposition in the soft tissue. Abdominal exam typically reveals tenderness and involuntary guarding, but no rebound tenderness. Metabolic derangements in pancreatitis include a decrease in calcium, magnesium, and hematocrit. An increase in WBC, BUN/Cr, bilirubin, LFTs, and glucose can occur.

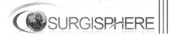

DIAGNOSIS

Acute pancreatitis is diagnosed primarily by blood tests that indicate elevations in amylase and lipase. Neither of these two enzymes are 100% specific to the pancreas, and they may be elevated in a number of other conditions. Perforation of the gastrointestinal system may lead to elevations in amylase; this enzyme is also found in the salivary glands, small intestine, reproductive organs such as the testes and ovaries, and in striated muscle. Renal disease and hypertriglyceridemia also lead to elevations in amylase. Lipase is found throughout the gastrointestinal system and the liver. Notwithstanding, very high elevations in both amylase and lipase are often pathognomonic for acute pancreatitis. Overall, the most specific test for pancreatitis is lipase levels, while the most sensitive test is amylase titers. The presence of acute pancreatitis with hyponatremia may be due to significant hypertriglyceridemia.

DIAGNOSTIC IMAGING TESTS

The diagnosis of acute pancreatitis can be confirmed through various imaging tests. As acute pancreatitis progresses, various anatomical changes can occur including the development of a pseudocyst, abscess, phlegmon, splenic vein thrombosis, and clear evidence of pancreatic necrosis. These changes are detectable on a CT scan. The earliest changes that can be detected are the development of a phlegmon, which is typically obvious within a couple of days. Pancreatic necrosis and pseudocyst formation are typically apparent within a couple of weeks. Abscess formation is clear within a month or two. Plain films are also of some value in diagnosis. Chest X-rays (CXR) are taken to determine pancreatitis-induced pleural effusions or elevations in part of the diaphragm. Abdominal X-rays (AXR) are taken to detect calcification within the pancreas, which is actually a better predictor of chronic pancreatitis instead of acute pancreatitis. Ultrasound is used to identify gallstones as the causative agent of pancreatitis, and once identified; they may be removed with ERCP. Amylase has a sensitivity of 90%.

TREATMENT

Treatment of acute pancreatitis is to cease the progression of reversible causes such as alcoholism and gallstones (treat with ERCP). Complications of acute pancreatitis such as pseudocyst or abscess formation may be drained with CT-guided aspiration. Most cases are self-limited, and so the standard of care is to provide supportive therapy, IV fluids, pain control with meperidine, nothing by mouth (NPO), and bowel rest. A nasogastric tube is used to decompress the GI system. Morphine is not used with pancreatitis due to the risk of sphincter of Oddi spasms and needless worsening of the pain. Surgical debridement is used in cases refractory to standard management. Gastric varices following acute pancreatitis require splenectomy to avoid splenic vein thrombosis.

Table 227 Acute Pancreatitis

Acute Pancreatitis	
Epidemiology	Direct damage from prematurely activated pancreatic enzymes.
Etiology	Perforation form PUD, alcoholism, cancer, cholelithiasis, ESRD, ERCP, direct trauma, infections, toxic drugs, burn injuries, surgery.
Presentation	Severe epigastric pain radiating to back. Pain is worse after eating. Nausea/vomiting, fever, tachypnea, Cullen and Turner signs, tender abdomen.
Diagnosis	Blood tests (elevated amylase & lipase), CT scan, CXR, AXR, ultrasound.
Treatment	Treatment for alcoholism, ERCP, surgical debridement.
Prognosis	Ranson criteria scores: Mortality low if under 3 factors; 1/6, 3-4 risk factors; 2/5, 5-6 factors, more than 6, 100%.

PROGNOSIS

The prognosis of acute pancreatitis is gauged by Ranson criteria. Mortality depends on the number of risk factors present. The risk factors are divided into those present on admission and those that develop after two days. Risk factors that increase the risk of mortality and may present on admission include age over 55, elevations in blood sugar over 200, elevated white blood cell (WBC) counts over 16,000, elevated aspartate transaminase (AST) over 250, and elevated lactate dehydrogenase (LDH) over 350. Risk factors present after two days include a decrease of more than 10% in the hematocrit (HCT), increase in BUN over 5, calcium less than 8, PO2 less than 60 mmHg, a base deficit greater than 4, and a fluid deficit of more than 6 L. The risk of mortality is low if less than two risk factors are present. Two through four risk factors carries a 1/6 risk of death. Five or 6 risk factors increase the mortality to 2/5, and more than 6 risk factors have a mortality that approaches 100%.

Table 228 Ranson Criteria for Pancreatitis

Ranson Criteria for Pancreatitis		
Criteria on Admission	**Criteria Within 48 Hours**	**Mortality Estimate**
Age over 55	Hct decrease over 10%	Less than 2 criteria: 1% mortality
WBC over 16,000	BUN increase over 5	2-4 criteria: 16% mortality
Blood glucose over 200	Serum calcium less than 8	5-6 criteria: 40% mortality
AST over 250	PO2 less than 60mmHg	More than 6 criteria: Nearly 100%
LDH over 350	Base deficit greater than 4	
	Fluid deficit more than 6L	

CHRONIC PANCREATITIS

ETIOLOGY AND PATHOPHYSIOLOGY

Repeated episodes of acute pancreatitis can lead to chronic injury and scarring to the pancreas, thereby inducing the development of chronic pancreatitis. The most common cause of chronic pancreatitis is continued abuse of alcohol. Approximately ¾ of patients with chronic pancreatitis have their disease from alcohol abuse, the remainder tend to be generally idiopathic in nature. Presentation of chronic pancreatitis in younger patients may be a result of cystic fibrosis.

PRESENTATION

Chronic pancreatitis presents with signs and symptoms similar to acute pancreatitis, including epigastric pain that radiates to the back, diarrhea with steatorrhea, signs and symptoms of malabsorption including vitamin deficiencies, elevated blood sugars and polyuria due to damage to the endocrine pancreas and subsequent diabetes, and chronic liver disease.

DIAGNOSIS

Diagnosis of chronic pancreatitis is made by history and blood tests that indicate normal amylase and lipase levels but decreased pancreatic enzyme levels such as trypsin deficiencies. Calcifications are seen on abdominal plain films, which strongly raise the clinical suspicion for this disorder. Finally, the secretin stimulation test is used to stimulate bicarbonate production by the pancreas. The pancreatic duct is typically dilated, and calcification with atrophy of the pancreas is a common finding in late disease.

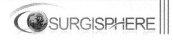

TREATMENT

Treatment for chronic pancreatitis is primarily supportive with modification of risk factors and avoidance of exacerbating activities. Replacement of pancreatic enzymes is often required in addition to dietary changes such as decreased fat intake, vitamin supplements, and use of spontaneously absorbed medium-chain fatty acids. Again, use meperidine instead of morphine for pain control. Diabetes induced by chronic pancreatitis should be controlled carefully due to the decrease in both insulin and glucagon. A dilated, tortuous pancreatic duct in the setting of chronic pancreatitis should be treated with the Peustow procedure.

Table 229 Chronic Pancreatitis

Chronic Pancreatitis	
Cause	Alcohol abuse (3/4), idiopathic (1/4), cystic fibrosis.
Presentation	Similar to acute pancreatitis.
Diagnosis	History, blood tests (amylase, lipase levels), calcification on plain films, secretin stimulation test.
Treatment	Primarily supportive, modification of risk factors, replacement of enzymes.

PANCREATIC NECROSIS

The development of pancreatic necrosis may occur following the onset of acute pancreatitis, sustained chronic pancreatitis, infection, or trauma. Early signs on imaging tests may include gas within the pancreas on CT scan, sometimes referred to as a "soap bubble" sign. CT scan is the gold standard for imaging. Failure to diagnose and treat early may lead to sepsis and ARDS with abdominal findings on physical exam. Amylase tends to be elevated in the early stage of disease, along with an elevation in WBC. Treatment typically involves surgical debridement (necrosectomy) and is done for symptomatic patients with clinical findings. Patients that are not stable for an operation can be treated with a CT-guided drain placement with broad spectrum antibiotics such as imipenem. Alternatives for necrosectomy include laparotomy with wide drainage and laparotomy with open packing. Pancreatectomy is not typically indicated.

CANCER

PANCREATIC LYMPHOMA

Primary lymphoma of the pancreas, such as from NHL, is rare. When present, a CT-guided biopsy is typically used for diagnosis. Staging with bone marrow biopsy and pan-CT scan is necessary. Patients with clinical symptoms, including anorexia, jaundice, and abdominal pain, may need biliary decompression via percutaneous transhepatic catheterization. Localized disease can be successfully treated with local resection. Chemotherapy with doxorubicin has been shown to be successful for more advanced disease.

PANCREATIC ADENOCARCINOMA

ETIOLOGY AND PATHOPHYSIOLOGY

Pancreatic cancer has a dismal prognosis, with over 90% of the patients dead within 1 year. The majority of adenocarcinomas are located at the head of the pancreas, with a concomitant rise in CA 19-9 and CA-50 levels. More advanced disease metastasizes to the liver. A point mutation in K-ras is attributed as the underlying cause for most pancreatic adenocarcinomas.

TREATMENT OF RESECTABLE CANCER

For cancer located in the head of the pancreas without extensive metastasis, a Whipple procedure is the surgery of choice. A Whipple procedure consists of an antrectomy, cholecystectomy, choledochectomy, pancreaticoduodenectomy, proximal jejunectomy, excision of all regional lymph nodes, followed by reconstruction by a gastrojejunostomy, pancreaticojejunostomy, and choledochojejunostomy. Mortality following a Whipple surgery is about 5-10%. A fully resected tumor still requires 5-FU and radiation.

TREATMENT OF UNRESECTABLE CANCER

The criteria for unresectable pancreatic cancer include the presence of distal metastasis (i.e. liver, pelvis, ligament of Treitz), regional metastasis to celiac nodes or lymph nodes posterior to the common bile duct, and locally invasive tumor into the portal vein or superior mesenteric vein. The presence of unresectable pancreatic cancer in the setting of worsening pain may be treated with a double pancreatic bypass and injection of the splanchnic bed. Chemoradiation with 5-FU is typically used as a palliative measure. Treatment is centered on reducing the clinically-significant symptoms, including jaundice, gastric obstruction, and pain. A cholecystojejunostomy or choledochojejunostomy can both be done for palliation. Gastrojejunostomy can be done for bowel obstruction. Pain can be treated through destruction of the celiac plexus with ethanol.

OPERATIVE MANEUVERS

The operation begins with an examination of all structures to ensure that the cancer is resectable. The Kocher maneuver is performed to evaluate the retropancreatic space and to ensure that the pancreas can be separated from the underlying portal vein, SMV, IVC, and aorta. The uncinate process is examined in relation to the SMA. The distal stomach and pylorus are mobilized and the anchoring ligaments (hepatogastric and hepatoduodenal) examined, along with the portal triad. The base of the transverse mesocolon is examined to ensure that the root of the mesentery is intact without deformities, and that the blood supply is intact without evidence of invasive cancer. The lesser sac is explored to examine the anterior pancreas. Resection proceeds with transection of the common hepatic duct and clearing of the local nodes along the celiac axis. The stomach is then transected at the body and antrum and a truncal vagotomy performed. The neck of the pancreas is then transected just left of the portal vein. Reconstruction then occurs by way of gastrojejunostomy, pancreaticojejunostomy, and choledochojejunostomy.

SPLEEN

CONGENITAL AND STRUCTURAL

SPLENECTOMY

Splenectomy can lead to overwhelming sepsis (OPSI) especially with encapsulated organisms due to inability to opsonize organisms and permit complement-mediated destruction. Splenectomy in patients with ITP is advisable as a means to reduce the destruction of platelets due to the presence of antibodies against platelets and their subsequent destruction by macrophages in the spleen.

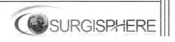

TRAUMA

SPLENIC INJURY

Children with splenic injuries require surgical exploration if significant blood products are required for resuscitation. They may be observed if hemodynamically stable.

PRACTICE QUESTIONS

 What is the source of the superior anterior pancreaticoduodenal artery?

A. Celiac artery
B. Common hepatic artery
C. Gastroduodenal artery
D. Proper hepatic artery
E. Superior mesenteric artery

 The best answer is <u>Gastroduodenal artery</u>. The superior anterior and posterior pancreaticoduodenal arteries are a branch of the gastroduodenal artery. The inferior anterior and posterior pancreaticoduodenal arteries are a branch of the superior mesenteric artery. As the gastroduodenal artery is also removed during a Whipple procedure, the duodenum is also removed due to the loss of its blood supply.

 What is the source of the gastroduodenal artery?

A. Celiac artery
B. Common hepatic artery
C. Left gastric artery
D. Proper hepatic artery
E. Superior mesenteric artery

 The best answer is <u>Common hepatic artery</u>. The gastroduodenal artery is a direct branch of the common hepatic artery before it becomes the proper hepatic artery. Damage to the common hepatic artery typically does not compromise the gastroduodenal artery due to its anastomosis with the superior mesenteric artery via the pancreaticoduodenal branches, and liver function is typically preserved. However, damage to the proper hepatic arteries often leads to liver ischemia.

Which of the following best describes the anatomy of the common bile duct?

A. The CBD is formed by the cystic duct and hepatic duct in the gastroduodenal ligament, and lies posterior to the portal vein

B. The CBD is formed by the cystic duct and hepatic duct in the hepatoduodenal ligament, and lies anterior to the portal vein

C. The CBD is formed by the cystic duct and hepatic duct in the hepatoduodenal ligament, and lies posterior to the portal vein

D. The CBD is formed by the cystic duct and hepatic duct in the hepatoduodenal ligament, and lies lateral to the portal vein

E. The CBD is formed by the cystic duct and hepatic duct, and is supplied by the cystic artery

 The best answer is <u>The CBD is formed by the cystic duct and hepatic duct in the hepatoduodenal ligament, and lies anterior to the portal vein</u>. The common bile duct is formed by the cystic duct and hepatic duct, lies within the hepatoduodenal ligament, lies anterior to the portal vein, and is supplied by the right hepatic artery. Damage to this structure, along with the right hepatic artery, is an unfortunate complication during a laparoscopic cholecystectomy and necessitates a hepaticojejunostomy as the drainage procedure for bile from the liver.

 The right hepatic artery is a branch of which of the following?

A. Celiac trunk
B. Common hepatic artery
C. Gastroduodenal artery
D. Proper hepatic artery
E. Superior mesenteric artery

 The best answer is <u>Proper hepatic artery</u>. The right hepatic artery is a branch of the proper hepatic artery, which itself comes off the common hepatic artery after it gives rise to the cystic artery and gastroduodenal artery. The common hepatic artery is a branch of the celiac artery.

Which of the following is a benign hepatic tumor with significant potential for bleeding and malignancy?

A. Adenoma
B. Cavernous hemangioma
C. Focal nodular hyperplasia
D. Hamartoma
E. Nodular regenerative hyperplasia

 The best answer is <u>Adenoma</u>. Adenomas of the liver have significant potential to transform into a malignant tumor. They also have a significant risk of bleeding, and are the only one of the five listed that may require surgical intervention for resection.

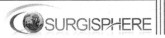

Which of the following laboratory tests is not used as part of Ranson's criteria for predicting mortality in acute pancreatitis?

A. Amylase
B. AST
C. Glucose
D. LDH
E. WBC

 The best answer is <u>Amylase</u>. The prognosis of acute pancreatitis is gauged by Ranson criteria. Mortality depends on the number of risk factors present. The risk factors are divided into those present on admission and those that develop after two days. Risk factors that increase the risk of mortality and may present on admission include age over 55, elevations in blood sugar over 200, elevated white blood cell (WBC) counts over 16,000, elevated aspartate transaminase (AST) over 250, and elevated lactate dehydrogenase (LDH) over 350. Risk factors present after two days include a decrease of more than 10% in the hematocrit (HCT), increase in BUN over 5, calcium less than 8, PO2 less than 60 mmHg, a base deficit greater than 4, and a fluid deficit of more than 6 L.

 A 36 year old male is diagnosed with hepatocellular carcinoma. Which of the following markers should be tested first?

A. AFP
B. CA19-9
C. CEA
D. hCG
E. p53

 The best answer is <u>AFP</u>. Alpha-fetoprotein is associated with 80% of all hepatocellular carcinomas, and should be tested first as a prognostic indicator for disease.

 A 46 year old male comes to you for painless jaundice nearly a decade after having his gallbladder removed laparoscopically. Delta-bilirubin is elevated. You make the diagnosis of cholangiocarcinoma. Which of the following is the next best step?

A. Common bile duct resection with roux-en-y hepaticojejunostomy
B. ERCP
C. Percutaneous transhepatic cholangiography
D. Right hepatic lobectomy
E. Whipple procedure

 The best answer is <u>Whipple procedure</u>. This patient has cholangiocarcinoma, which leads to biliary disease, obstruction, and presentation as painless jaundice. It can happen to people who have had their gallbladders taken out. Diagnosis is made by ERCP and PTC, and definitive treatment is excision via a Whipple procedure.

A 26 year old female presents with significant right upper quadrant pain, fever, chills, nausea, and elevated liver function tests. A diagnosis of acute cholangitis is made. The patient is admitted to a stepdown unit, started on fluids and antibiotics, and has an ERCP the following day after an ultrasound shows an obstructing common duct stone. The ERCP is unsuccessful. What is the next step in management?

A. Common duct exploration in the OR
B. HIDA scan
C. Laparoscopic cholecystectomy
D. Percutaneous cholecystostomy tube
E. Percutaneous transhepatic catheter

 The best answer is <u>Common duct exploration in the OR</u>. This patient has failed an ERCP and will likely not improve on her own at this point. She requires a trip to the operating room for a common duct exploration. It is possible that she may require a hepaticojejunostomy and cholecystectomy. The findings of black stones is due to calcium bilirubinate secondary to Crohn disease, hemolytic disease, or resection of the terminal ileum; brown stones consist of calcium palmitate and are due to bacterial infection; yellow stones are composed primarily of cholesterol.

 A 56 year old woman with acute on chronic cholecystitis goes to the OR for a laparoscopic cholecystectomy. She is found to have frank pus within her gallbladder and goes to the ICU after the case for some intraoperative hypotension. Which of the following is the most appropriate antibiotic regimen?

A. Ampicillin and gentamicin
B. Linezolid
C. Piperacillin / Tazobactam
D. Vancomycin, Piperacillin / Tazobactam
E. Vancomycin, Piperacillin / Tazobactam, Fluconazole

 The best answer is <u>Piperacillin / Tazobactam</u>. This patient likely has a gallbladder infection from one of the PECKS bacteria: Proteus, Enterobacter or E. coli (most common), Clostridium, Klebsiella, or Streptococci. The best antibiotic to begin initial therapy is piperacillin / tazobactam. Additional agents can be added based on culture data and patient status.

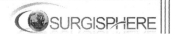

A 32 year old male with signs and symptoms of acute cholecystitis and gallstone pancreatitis undergoes an ERCP. A small stone is removed from the common bile duct, but it is noted that a fusiform cyst exists the duct near the stone. Which of the following is the next best step in management?

A. Cholecystectomy
B. Cholecystectomy with resection and roux-en-y hepaticojejunostomy
C. Cholecystectomy with stent placement in the CBD
D. HIDA
E. Observation

The best answer is <u>Cholecystectomy with resection and roux-en-y hepaticojejunostomy</u>. This patient has a fusiform cyst within the common bile duct. The presence of any type of a cyst is typically an indication for resection. A fusiform cyst is the most common type of cyst found within the CBD, and is treated with complete resection followed by a hepaticojejunostomy. As this patient also has signs and symptoms of gallbladder disease, he also has to undergo a cholecystectomy. If these cysts are located in the liver, a transplant or lobectomy may be required.

A 51 year old female who had a diverting loop ileostomy at a young age after resection of much of her large intestine secondary to Crohn disease is found to have an incidental parastomal hernia during a laparoscopic cholecystectomy. Which of the following is the best step in management?

A. Abort the cholecystectomy and repair the parastomal hernia
B. Abort the entire operation to obtain informed consent
C. Complete the laparoscopic cholecystectomy only
D. Do both the cholecystectomy and parastomal hernia repair
E. Redo the colostomy at another site after the cholecystectomy

The best answer is <u>Complete the laparoscopic cholecystectomy only</u>. This patient has an asymptomatic parastomal hernia. She should have her laparoscopic cholecystectomy at this time and be monitored as an outpatient for signs and symptoms of obstruction related to her parastomal hernia. An immediate repair at this time is not indicated, and there is no reason to abort the cholecystectomy. In the event of symptoms or complications later, redoing the colostomy may be required.

Which of the following is the most common cause of a bacterial liver abscess?

A. Bacteroides
B. E. coli
C. Klebsiella
D. Pseudomonas
E. Streptococcus

The best answer is <u>E. coli</u>. E. coli is the leading cause of bacterial liver abscess formation. Treatment with IV antibiotics and percutaneous drainage is needed.

Which of the following hormones stimulates the flow of bile the most?

A. CCK
B. Gastrin
C. Secretin
D. Somatostatin
E. VIP

 The best answer is <u>Secretin</u>. Secretin leads to the greatest increase in the flow of bile, while CCK predominantly leads to gallbladder contraction.

 A 38 year old longtime alcoholic begins to develop cirrhosis and ascites. Which of the following is the earliest mediator of the ascites?

A. Aldosterone
B. Angiotensin II
C. Nitric oxide
D. Renin
E. Substance P

 The best answer is <u>Nitric oxide</u>. Nitric oxide release from vasodilation leads to the release of renin and activation of the RAA axis. The effect is an increase in aldosterone, leading to salt and fluid retention. A normal portal pressure is between 3-5; when this level rises to over 12, variceal bleeding can ensue. Treatment is with a TIPS procedure, but the common side effect of this procedure is encephalopathy. In the event of failure with a TIPS, a H-type shunt can be completed. The ultimate therapy is liver transplantation. The best measure of synthetic function by the liver is protime. Metastasis of colon cancer to the liver can be diagnosed by an elevated CEA and LDH.

 Which of the following pancreatic enzymes are secreted in their active form?

A. Alpha-reductase
B. Chymotrypsin
C. Enterokinase
D. Lipase
E. Trypsin

 The best answer is <u>Lipase</u>. Lipase and amylase are two pancreatic enzymes secreted in their active forms. All other pancreatic enzymes are secreted in their inactive form until they are activated by enterokinase in the duodenum, trypsin in the duodenum, or the acidic pH of the duodenum. Secretion of pancreatic enzymes is stimulated by CCK and acetylcholine. Secretin leads to stimulation of pancreatic fluid laden with bicarbonate.

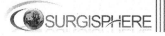

A 38 year old female who has taken birth control pills for many years develops sudden hypotension. She is taken to the ICU, where her hematocrit is 14. After stabilizing her, an exploratory laparoscopy is done, which indicates evidence of bleeding from a rupture located in her liver. What is the underlying etiology?

A. Amebic abscess
B. Focal nodular hyperplasia
C. Hemangioma
D. Hepatic adenoma
E. Hepatocellular carcinoma

The best answer is <u>Hepatic adenoma</u>. This patient has a hepatic adenoma which developed due to long-term birth control medication. The most significant and dangerous risk of hepatic adenoma is rupture leading to bleeding and death. Hepatic adenoma can also lead to carcinogenesis. Once detected, birth control pills should be stopped and the adenoma closely monitored. Failure of the adenoma to regress requires resection. A hemangioma does not require operative intervention due to the low risk of rupture. FNH also does not require operative intervention unless it is changing size; it can be evaluated via a technetium 99 scan. Amebic liver abscesses require metronidazole and percutaneous drainage. Hepatocellular carcinoma can be resected if it is the fibrolamellar type, but typically requires chemoembolization, RFA, and possible liver transplant for definitive cure.

During an intraoperative cholangiogram performed as part of a laparoscopic cholecystectomy, a stricture in the right hepatic duct is noted. Of note, the patient has had multiple bouts of pancreatitis, which is believed to be the underlying cause of this stricture. What is the next best step?

A. ERCP and brush biopsy with metal stent placement
B. Liver transplantation
C. Monitoring with CT scan
D. Percutaneous transhepatic catheter placement
E. Roux-en-y hepaticojejunostomy

The best answer is <u>ERCP and brush biopsy with metal stent placement</u>. While it is likely that this hepatic duct stricture is benign, a definitive diagnosis is required prior to an operative intervention. Therefore, the best step is to complete the cholecystectomy, close the patient, and obtain an ERCP with brush biopsy. A metal stent may be required if the stricture cannot be dilated safely. If the pathology returns as negative, this patient is eligible for a roux-en-y hepaticojejunostomy. A PTC can also be completed, especially if the ERCP is not successful.

A 38 year old male is diagnosed with a pancreatic head cancer and is taken to the OR for resection. He is found to have tumor extension to his SMA and SMV. His expected survival is at least one month. **What is the next step in management?**

A. Abort the operation
B. Duodenal stent placement
C. Gastrojejunostomy and choledochojejunostomy
D. Pancreatic head resection
E. Whipple procedure

The best answer is <u>Gastrojejunostomy and choledochojejunostomy</u>. This patient has unresectable pancreatic cancer with at least two weeks of expected survival. A palliative surgery is necessary, and the best option is to bypass the affected region with a gastrojejunostomy and provide drainage of bile via a choledochojejunostomy. Invasion of a pancreatic mass into the SMA, SMV, or portal vein means a Whipple procedure cannot be completed.

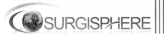

ENDOCRINE SURGERY

CHAPTER CONTENTS

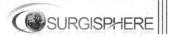

PITUITARY

GENERAL CONCEPTS

ANATOMY

The pituitary is situated below the hypothalamus and is suspended by the hypophyseal stalk. The hypothalamus receives input from the external environment and the internal environment. In addition it receives negative feedback from hormones such as glucocorticoids, estrogen, testosterone, and thyroid hormone. Thus, the hypothalamus integrates sensory and hormonal inputs and provides coordinated responses. These responses include responses to the anterior and posterior pituitary, among many other areas.

The pituitary is divided into two parts, the anterior (adenohypophysis) and posterior (neurohypophysis) sections. The posterior portion is directly innervated from the hypothalamus and releases oxytocin and vasopressin. The anterior portion is controlled by the releasing factors of the hypothalamus. Each anterior pituitary hormone has its own unique hypothalamic releasing factor (hormone). The main releasing hormones are: thyrotropin-releasing hormone, corticotropin-releasing hormone, lutenizing hormone-releasing hormone, growth hormone-releasing hormone, prolactin-releasing peptide, gonadotropin-releasing hormone.

PHYSIOLOGY

Antidiuretic hormone (ADH) is synthesized in the hypothalamus and released by the posterior pituitary as a response to hypotension or increased osmolarity. The response to hypotension is mediated by a decrease in left atrial filling pressure, leading to activation of baroreceptors. ADH increases permeability of the collecting duct, leading to reabsorption of free water and an increase in intravascular volume. However, an increase in osmolality is the more potent stimulus for ADH secretion.

METABOLIC AND DEGENERATIVE

Table 230 Hyperprolactinemia

Hyperprolactinemia	
Etiology	Prolactinomas and dopamine inhibition.
Presentation	Amenorrhea, gynecomastia and galactorrhea, bitemporal hemianopsia.
Diagnosis	Exclusion of other conditions and excluding medication-induced hyperprolactinemia. Prolactin greater than 100 ng / mL.
Treatment	Reversing elevated levels of prolactin. Disease refractory to medical management requires surgical excision or radiation therapy.

HYPOPITUITARISM

Table 231 Hypopituitarism

Hypopituitarism	
Etiology	Lesions may be the result of trauma or damage from tumor overgrowth. Infarction of a pituitary tumor, infection by TB and syphilis, along with sarcoid and various autoimmune disorders.
Presentation	Inability to lactate in pregnant women; amenorrhea, infertility, decreased sexual desire, impotence, loss of sexually-mature hair patterns, insulin-sensitivity, growth failure in children, symptoms of hypothyroidism, symptoms of AI.
Diagnosis	Insulin-challenge test to see if GH increases, measuring the titers of cortisol, LH, FSH, and either estrogen or testosterone, measuring thyroid hormones.
Treatment	Replacement of the lost hormones, especially cortisol. Reversal of any underlying etiology should be undertaken immediately.

DIABETES INSIPIDUS

ETIOLOGY AND PATHOPHYSIOLOGY

Diabetes insipidus (DI) may be due to either decreased production of antidiuretic hormone (ADH) by the posterior pituitary or hypothalamus, or decreased renal response to ADH. Central DI occurs with decreased hormone production and is commonly the result of secondary damage to the endocrine gland, while nephrogenic DI is due to a lack of renal response and may be due to electrolyte imbalances, sickle cell anemia, sarcoid, or various medications (lithium, demeclocycline, colchicine).

PRESENTATION AND DIAGNOSIS

Central DI presents with concomitant loss of anterior pituitary hormones due to tumor infiltration. The result is the inability to concentrate urine and loss of salt excretion, leading to inordinate amounts of dilute urine secretion and increase water intake due to the hypernatremia. Diagnosis of DI is made by comparing urine to plasma osmolarity, but a careful history often yields clues to the correct diagnosis. Nephrogenic DI is the diagnosis if there is no change in osmolarity following administration of ADH.

TREATMENT

Central DI is treated with ADH replacement along with any other missing pituitary hormones. Either vasopressin or desmopressin (DDAVP) may be used as synthetic analogues. Increased ADH secretion can be induced by chlorpropamide, clofibrate, and carbamazepine. Nephrogenic DI is best treated with hydrochlorothiazide (HCTZ), amiloride, or chlorthalidone.

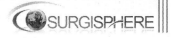

Table 232 Diabetes Insipidus (DI)

Diabetes Insipidus (DI)	
Etiology	Secondary damage to the endocrine gland, while nephrogenic DI is due to a lack of renal response.
Presentation	Concomitant loss of anterior pituitary hormones. The inability to concentrate urine and loss of salt excretion, inordinate amounts of dilute urine secretion and increased water intake.
Diagnosis	Comparing urine to plasma osmolarity.
Treatment	Central DI is treated with ADH replacement along with any other missing pituitary hormones. Increased ADH secretion can be induced by chlorpropamide, clofibrate, and carbamazepine. Nephrogenic DI is best treated with HCTZ, amiloride, or chlorthalidone.

SECRETION OF INAPPROPRIATE ANTIDIURETIC HORMONE

ETIOLOGY AND PATHOPHYSIOLOGY

Secretion of inappropriate antidiuretic hormone (SIADH) may occur with ectopic ADH secretion (the result of endocrine activity by tumors such as oat cell carcinomas of the lung, pancreatic tumors, infections such as TB or pneumonia), CNS trauma, by various medications (chlorpropamide, clofibrate, various chemotherapeutic agents, and carbamazepine) and normally in hypovolemic states leading to hypoperfusion.

PRESENTATION AND DIAGNOSIS

SIADH presents with increase in the ECF and dilutional hyponatremia with hypernatriuria. Edema in the torso is generally not seen; in severe cases, central edema may lead to CNS symptoms. Concentrated urine is formed in SIADH with sodium concentration over 20 mEq / L. The renin-angiotensin system (RAS) is also suppressed. Normal renal, adrenal, and thyroid function is necessary before making this diagnosis.

TREATMENT

SIADH is treated with fluid restriction to minimize the dilutional hyponatremia, the use of demeclocycline to cause a water diuresis, and saline infusion as indicated in when sodium concentration falls below 110 mEq/L (rarely used to avoid CPM). The rate of correction should not exceed 1 mEq / L / hr for the first 24 hours. Cerebropontine myelinolysis can lead to seizure, coma, and death.

Table 233 Secretion of Inappropriate Antidiuretic Hormone (SIADH)

Secretion of Inappropriate Antidiuretic Hormone (SIADH)	
Etiology	Result of endocrine activity by tumors, infections, CNS trauma, by various medications and normally in hypovolemic states leading to hypoperfusion.
Presentation	ECF and dilutional hyponatremia with hypernatriuria. Concentrated urine is formed and the RAS is also suppressed.
Diagnosis	Concentrated urine with sodium concentration over 20 mEq / L. The RAS is also suppressed.
Treatment	Fluid restriction, demeclocycline.

PITUITARY TUMORS

PITUITARY ADENOMA

ASSESSMENT

Tumors of the pituitary comprise some 10% of all intracranial tumors. The majority are benign and slow growing, but over time, may manifest as impingements on the optic nerve (leading to bitemporal hemianopsia) and various endocrinologic effects. The anterior pituitary is the only portion that develops primary tumors, including adenomas and craniopharyngiomas. Craniopharyngiomas develop from the remnants of Rathke's pouch and occur primarily in children; they are typically suprasellar, solid calcified tumors. Adenomas may have abnormal formation of various hormones with expected side effects. Microadenomas are found in a significant number of women, but tend to be asymptomatic. Pituitary tumors present with headache, compression of the optic chiasm, and the endocrinologic effects of the adenoma. Diagnosis is by plain films, CT, and MRI. Hormone studies identify the nature of the endocrinologic excess. The sudden onset of acne, hirsutism, hypertension, amenorrhea, and hypertension may be attributed to a pituitary adenoma.

MANAGEMENT

Pituitary tumors are treated by medical management to decrease hormone production, radiation therapy, or surgical excision.

Table 234 Pituitary Tumors

Pituitary Tumors	
Etiology	Adenomas, craniopharyngiomas,
Presentation	Headache, compression of the optic chiasm, and endocrinologic effects.
Treatment	Decrease hormone production, radiation therapy, or surgical excision.

THYROID

GENERAL CONCEPTS

ANATOMY

 The thyroid gland consists of two lobes connected by a narrow isthmus. It is under the influence to the pituitary TSH (itself under the influence of the hyopothalmic THRH). The thyroid produces thyroxine in two forms (T3 & T4). These iodine based hormones are responsible for controlling the metabolism of the body. The thyroid also produces calcitonin (also secreted by many malignancies) which helps to regulate calcium levels. Calcitonin is antagonistic to PTH. The recurrent laryngeal nerve is located near the inferior thyroid artery and must be preserved during thyroid surgery.

PHYSIOLOGY

Follicular cells of the thyroid are involved in iodine uptake.

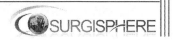

METABOLIC AND DEGENERATIVE

HYPERTHYROIDISM

EPIDEMIOLOGY

Hyperthyroidism most commonly presents in the form of Graves disease, which contributes to nearly 80% of all cases of thyrotoxicosis. About 1 person in 1000 is affected, and the majority of patients are Caucasian young adults. Morbidity and mortality associated with thyrotoxicosis include the development of arrhythmia such as atrial fibrillation (and a subsequent risk of thromboembolism), anorexia, anxiety, heat intolerance, palpitations, osteoporosis, and CHF.

ETIOLOGY

Hyperthyroidism leads to excessive amounts of triiodothyronine (T3) and / or thyroxine (T4) leading to thyrotoxicosis. Common causes include Graves disease, toxic multinodular goiter (also known as Plummer disease), toxic adenomas, and subacute thyroiditis. Less common types of thyrotoxicosis emanate from iodide-induced

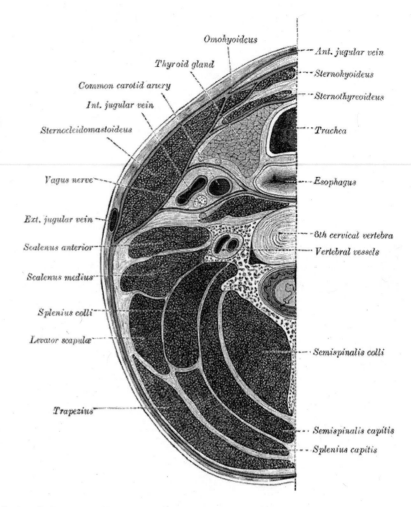

disease, excess beta-human chorionic gonadotropin (B-hCG), factitious disease, pituitary adenomas that produce an excess of thyroid stimulating hormone (TSH), metastatic cancer from the thyroid, and struma ovarii.

PATHOPHYSIOLOGY

Thyrotoxicosis exerts its effects systemically through excess production of T3 and T4. Basal metabolic rate (BMR) increases significantly leading to increased cardiovascular work and heat production. This increase leads to the symptoms of sweating, heat intolerance, and palpitations. Anxiety often occurs as a sympathetic response. Tremor and tachycardia are also common due to activation of the sympathetic nervous system (SNS). Graves' disease is the most common cause, and is the result of an autoimmune complex that produces antibodies against various thyroid proteins, antithyroperoxidase (anti-TPO), and antibodies against TSH. The result of this antibody is thyroid hormone synthesis and thyroid hypertrophy. Subacute thyroiditis, a cause of thyrotoxicosis in about 20% of patients, is discussed separately below. Plummer disease occurs in a subset of patients, and is the development of a toxic multinodular goiter.

PRESENTATION AND DIAGNOSIS

Hyperthyroidism presents with anxiety, anorexia, heat intolerance, diaphoresis, tremor, hyperactivity, palpitations, and oligomenorrhea. HTN may occur. On physical exam, the thyroid may be diffusely enlarged and firm as in Graves disease. Graves' disease itself may present with the triad of proptosis, exophthalmos, and pretibial myxedema. Signs of thyrotoxicosis include tachycardia, atrial fibrillation, HTN, smooth skin, diaphoresis, lid lag, tremor, and hyperkinesis. Diagnosis involves a full thyroid panel, including TSH, T3 (measured by T3 resin uptake) and T4 (measured by the free T4 index), and detecting the presence of any thyroid autoantibodies. Imaging involves the use of a nuclear thyroid scintigraphy with iodine 123 or technetium-99m. Graves' disease will have elevated uptake with those isotopes.

TREATMENT

Hyperthyroidism involves the use of beta-blockers (or calcium-channel blockers in asthmatics) to reduce the activity of the SNS. Oral rehydration may also be necessary. Methimazole and propylthiouracil (PTU) block thyroid hormone synthesis over a period of weeks with remission in some patients over a year. PTU is also useful in preventing the conversion of T4 to the more potent T3. Iodine, in the form of potassium iodide, can be given as a temporary measure to block the release of TH. Radioactive iodide can be administered, and is the most common method of reducing the formation of TH. Over time, hypothyroidism occurs and requires supplemental TH. Finally, surgical options are available in refractory cases, and include surgical excision of part of the thyroid gland with care taken to avoid the parathyroid glands. It is commonly employed in severe cases, pregnancy, and those with serious cardiac manifestations of thyrotoxicosis. Thyroid storm can occur following surgery, and treatment requires propranolol, iodine, steroids, oxygen, and glucose. Thyroid storm presents with tachycardia, hyperthermia, hypertension, followed by systemic decompensation leading to hypotension and death. Hyperthyroidism in pregnancy that is refractory to medical management should be treated with surgery in the 2nd trimester. The most common complication of radioactive iodine ablation of the thyroid is hypothyroidism.

Table 235 Hyperthyroidism

Hyperthyroidism	
Etiology	Graves disease, toxic multinodular goiter, toxic adenomas, and subacute thyroiditis.
Presentation	Anxiety, anorexia, heat intolerance, diaphoresis, tremor, hyperactivity, palpitations, & oligomenorrhea
Diagnosis	Thyroid may be diffusely enlarged and firm. May present with the triad of proptosis, exophthalmos, and pretibial myxedema. Signs of thyrotoxicosis include tachycardia, atrial fibrillation, HTN, smooth skin, diaphoresis, lid lag, tremor, and hyperkinesis. Full thyroid panel and detecting the presence of any thyroid autoantibodies. Imaging involves the use of a nuclear thyroid Scintigraphy.
Treatment	B-blockers, oral rehydration. Methimazole and PTU, iodine, radioactive iodide. Over time, supplemental TH, surgical excision.

THYROTOXICOSIS

ASSESSMENT

Thyroid storm is the sudden release of significant amounts of TH leading to a thyroid crisis, and can occur following surgery on the thyroid for hyperthyroidism. Symptoms include rising fever, elevated anxiety, delirium, tachycardia, restlessness, nausea, vomiting, and diarrhea. Coma can result. Stressors to the body or psyche can result in a thyroid storm.

MANAGEMENT

Treatment of thyroid storm involves supportive treatment, glucose, antithyroid agents, and **beta-blockers**. Dexamethasone is sometimes given to block further release of TH.

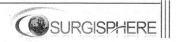

Table 236 Thyroid Storm (Thyrotoxic Crisis)

Thyroid Storm (Thyrotoxic Crisis)	
Etiology	Stressors to the body or psyche.
Presentation	Rising fever, elevated anxiety, delirium, tachycardia, restlessness, nausea, vomiting, and diarrhea. Coma can result.
Diagnosis	Hyperpyrexia out of proportion to other findings, elevated T3, T4, and FT4, suppressed TSH
Treatment	Antithyroid medications, steroids, volume infusions, high-dose steroids

SUBACUTE THYROIDITIS

ASSESSMENT

Inflammation of the thyroid gland can lead to low iodine uptake thyrotoxicosis. Subacute thyroiditis is sometimes referred to as de Quervain thyroiditis. The most common cause is viral injury, but it can also occur in various autoimmune conditions, following release of excessive interferon alpha or beta, cellular injury mediated by amiodarone, in trauma, in a postpartum state, or following radiation therapy. Presentation is similar to that of hyperthyroidism but without the triad of Graves' disease. Diagnosis is made in a similar pathway.

MANAGEMENT

Treatment of subacute thyroiditis involves pain control with **NSAIDs**, corticosteroids to decrease the inflammatory reaction, glucocorticoids to treat the symptoms of thyrotoxicosis, and beta-blockers to manage the SNS activation.

Table 237 Subacute Thyroiditis

Subacute Thyroiditis	
Etiology	Viral injury, various autoimmune conditions, following release of excessive interferon alpha or beta, cellular injury mediated by amiodarone, trauma, postpartum state, or following radiation therapy.
Presentation	Similar to that of hyperthyroidism but without the triad of Graves disease.
Diagnosis	Similar to hyperthyroidism.
Treatment	NSAIDs, corticosteroids, glucocorticoids.

HYPOTHYROIDISM

EPIDEMIOLOGY

Hypothyroidism affects some 20,000 patients, especially from lack of iodide (an international concern). Thyroid disease is up to 8 times more common in women. The incidence increases with age, but there is little mortality attached to this disorder. Hypothyroidism as a congenital condition is known as cretinism.

ETIOLOGY AND PATHOPHYSIOLOGY

Hypothyroidism is commonly due to congenital disease, autoimmune disease, inflammation leading to transient symptoms, medications leading to thyroid toxicity, prior injury from correction of hyperthyroidism, postpartum hypothyroidism, and a variety of central causes leading to decreased hormone production. Low production of TH leads to decreased BMR, myxedematous infiltration of tissue leading to decreased cardiac function, pericardial effusions, decreased CO, decreased GI transit with achlorhydria, delayed puberty, infertility, and worsening of the lipid profile.

PRESENTATION AND DIAGNOSIS

Hypothyroidism presents with asymptomatic goiter (especially in Hashimoto thyroiditis) that may lead to local impingement. Weight gain commonly occurs with concomitant lethargy and decreased energy. Cold intolerance and constipation are commonly present. Dry coarse hair is typically seen along with myxedema. Diagnosis is made by examination and a full thyroid panel to identify deficiencies. TSH is typically elevated but T4 and T3 are decreased.

TREATMENT

Hypothyroidism is treated by supportive therapy and by hormone replacement using levothyroxine. Goiter resection may be necessary.

Table 238 Hypothyroidism

Hypothyroidism	
Etiology	Congenital disease, autoimmune disease, inflammation leading to transient symptoms, medications, prior injury from correction of hyperthyroidism, postpartum hypothyroidism, and a variety of central causes leading to decreased hormone production.
Presentation	Asymptomatic goiter, weight gain with lethargy and decreased energy. Cold intolerance and constipation are commonly present. Dry coarse hair with myxedema.
Diagnosis	Examination and a full thyroid panel to identify deficiencies.
Treatment	Supportive therapy and by hormone replacement. Goiter resection may be necessary.

THYROID TUMORS

PAPILLARY THYROID CANCER

ETIOLOGY AND PATHOPHYSIOLOGY

Papillary carcinoma of the thyroid (PTC) makes up some 70% of all thyroid cancers and presents in the 30s and 40s. Papillary carcinoma is highly amenable to treatment and has a low morbidity and mortality due to its slow growing nature. Caucasian females are more affected than other groups. A dysfunction (possibly hereditary) with the tyrosine kinase receptors has been noted in some patients. Increased risk of papillary thyroid cancer is found in patients exposed to radiation and iodine deficiency. The most common causative factor is with prior radiation exposure to the neck.

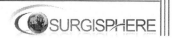

PRESENTATION AND DIAGNOSIS

PTC presents as a subclinical disease, but a mass may be palpable on exam. A painless, hard nodule may be present on exam. Mass effects, such as impingement upon the esophagus or trachea, may occur. Metastasis to the lungs and bones through the lymphatic drainage may occur. Elevated thyroid function tests are found in some patients, but thyroid derangements are not common. Scintigraphy using radioisotopes of iodine are the diagnostic test of choice; CT and MRI are used only to identify distant metastases. Fine needle aspiration biopsy (FNAB) is universally used to identify this type of cancer. Psammoma bodies are present on histologic analysis. The appearance of normal thyroid structure in a cervical lymph node fine needle aspirate heralds a diagnosis of papillary cancer.

TREATMENT

Treatment of PTC involves thyroidectomy, the use of radioactive iodine, and levothyroxine replacement. Radiation is used against metastases; chemotherapy is helpful in only a fraction of patients. Surgical intervention centers around one of two approaches. The first approach is a thyroid lobectomy with isthmectomy to preserve thyroid function. However, I-131 scanning for recurrence or metastasis is not possible following this procedure. The second approach is a total thyroidectomy, which preserves the ability to use I-131 scanning but requires the patient to take thyroid hormone supplements daily. Lymph node dissection is indicated only with invasive tumor, and ipsilateral modified radical neck dissection is required with positive lymph nodes. Cure rate is over 90%. Follow up requires I-131 scanning and monitoring of thyroglobulin levels with CT and MRI as indicated. Locally recurrent tumors can be resected, treated with radiation, or ablated with radioactive I-131. Patients who will receive I-131 scanning are transitioned from T4 to T3 due to its shorter half-life and less inhibition of TSH. A patient with known papillary cancer with metastatic disease requires a total thyroidectomy, nodal dissection, and radioactive iodine therapy. The presence of a hot, hyperactive thyroid nodule may be treated with only medical therapy if the long-term risks of surgery are not indicated, such as in the elderly. Stridor following thyroidectomy requires opening of the wound to protect the airway due to the presumption of a wound hematoma.

Table 239 Indications for Total Thyroidectomy in PTC

Indications for Total Thyroidectomy in PTC
Age > 50 in women or age > 40 in men
Poorly differentiated tumor
Insular, mucoid, or tall cell histology
Invasion into adjacent tissues
Lesion > 4cm

Table 240 Papillary Thyroid Cancer (PTC)

Papillary Thyroid Cancer (PTC)	
Etiology	Radiation, iodine insufficiency, possibly hereditary
Presentation	Subclinical disease, but a mass may be palpable on exam.
Diagnosis	A painless, hard nodule may be present on exam. Elevated thyroid function tests are found in some patients. Scintigraphy is the diagnostic test of choice. FNAB is used to identify this type of cancer.
Treatment	Thyroidectomy, the use of radioactive iodine, and levothyroxine replacement. Radiation is used against metastases.

FOLLICULAR THYROID CANCER

ETIOLOGY AND PATHOPHYSIOLOGY

Follicular thyroid carcinoma (FTC) makes up 15% of all thyroid cancers with a very good morbidity and mortality. Caucasian women are affected more than other groups. FTC is highly differentiated and is similar to the normal thyroid parenchyma; the precise cause is unknown but exposure to radiation is a risk factor. It has also been postulated that a long-standing goiter may predispose certain individuals to developing FTC. Mutations in ras and dysfunction in various cytokines may lead to FTC as well. Spread is hematogenous, with the most common sites being to the bone, lung, and liver.

PRESENTATION AND DIAGNOSIS

FTC tends to be subclinical with only a single hard nodule typically found on exam. Elevations in thyroid function tests may be found. Hormone production by the tumor may be independent of control by TSH; as a result, a TSH suppression test will not change T3 and T4 production by malignant cells. Diagnosis of FTC is made in a method similar to PTC: echography to identify the presence and location of nodules, followed by thyroid scintigraphy, then FNAB. Definitive diagnosis requires a lobectomy. Hurthle cell tumors are a variant but somewhat more aggressive.

TREATMENT

Treatment of FTC includes thyroidectomy with hormone replacement, radiation beam therapy (RT), and occasionally chemotherapy. I-131 ablation is possible with metastatic disease. Total thyroidectomy is the definitive therapy. Suppression of TSH is also beneficial. 10 year survival is 45-90%. Followup is the same as in PTC. Follicular cells on a fine needle aspiration requires a total thyroidectomy. Postoperative radioactive iodine therapy is also indicated. Indeterminate fine needle aspiration results should be repeated; if still no results, then surgery is indicated.

Table 241 Follicular Thyroid Cancer (FTC)

Follicular Thyroid Cancer (FTC)	
Etiology	Unknown but radiation a risk factor.
Presentation	Subclinical with only a mass palpable on physical exam.
Diagnosis	Elevations in thyroid function tests may be found. Made in a method similar to PTC: echography to identify the presence and location of nodules, followed by thyroid scintigraphy, FNAB.
Treatment	Thyroidectomy with hormone replacement, RT, occasionally chemotherapy.

MEDULLARY THYROID CANCER

ETIOLOGY AND PATHOPHYSIOLOGY

Medullary thyroid carcinoma (MTC) arises from derangements in the parafollicular C cells that produce calcitonin. MTC is associated with MEN 2 and MEN 3, but the majority of patients have spontaneous disease. Unilateral disease arises spontaneously, while bilateral disease is more common in those with a familial heritage. Less than 10% of all thyroid carcinomas are MTC, and it is most likely to occur in older adults. The familial form occurs in younger adults. Derangements in ret have been identified in some cases of MTC.

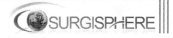

PRESENTATION AND DIAGNOSIS

MTC presents as an asymptomatic thyroid mass that may occasionally present with carcinoid syndrome, diarrhea from elevations in calcitonin, and symptoms from distant metastases. Diagnosis is made by abnormal calcitonin levels, and a pentagastrin-induced increase in calcitonin is diagnostic. Ret oncogene testing is also used. FNAB confirms the diagnosis.

TREATMENT

MTC is treated with thyroidectomy with hormone replacement and treating any secondary disease from MEN 2 or MEN 3. Central lymph node dissection is required, and if positive, lateral neck dissection. Sporadic tumors and those associated with MEN II have a higher survival compared to those from MEN III, with a ten year survival between 30 and 60%. Followup includes monitoring of serum calcitonin, with recurrence managed by resection.

Table 242 Medullary Thyroid Cancer (MTC)

Medullary Thyroid Cancer (MTC)	
Etiology	Unilateral disease arises spontaneously, while bilateral disease is more common in those with a familial heritage.
Presentation	Asymptomatic thyroid mass that may occasionally present with carcinoid syndrome, diarrhea, and symptoms from distant metastases.
Diagnosis	Abnormal calcitonin levels and a pentagastrin-induced increase in calcitonin are diagnostic. Ret oncogene testing is also used. FNAB confirms the diagnosis.
Treatment	Thyroidectomy, hormone replacement and treating any secondary disease from MEN 2 or MEN 3.

ANAPLASTIC THYROID CANCER

ETIOLOGY AND PATHOPHYSIOLOGY

Anaplastic thyroid cancer (ATC) is an aggressive thyroid cancer with a significantly high mortality rate. It comprises only a few percent of thyroid cancer cases. Early spread and rapid progression occurs in ATC leading to a variety of systemic symptoms. It is related to C-myc, H-ras, and other oncogenes, and may be the end result of a longstanding papillary or follicular thyroid cancer.

PRESENTATION AND DIAGNOSIS

ATC presents with a rapidly growing neck mass that impinges upon other structures, and distant metastases that lead to local and systemic effects. FNAB is necessary to definitively diagnose this condition. It typically presents in the 60s.

TREATMENT

By the time ATC is diagnosed, there is little curative potential. Thyroidectomy with chemotherapy and radiotherapy may be attempted in some cases, but the majority of therapy is palliative. Doxorubicin and cisplatin are used as chemotherapeutic agents, but radiotherapy has a higher success rate.

Table 243 Anaplastic Thyroid Cancer (ATC)

Anaplastic Thyroid Cancer (ATC)	
Etiology	Related to oncogenes, and may be the end result of a longstanding papillary or follicular thyroid cancer.
Presentation	Rapidly growing neck mass that impinges upon other structures, and distant metastases that lead to local and systemic effects.
Diagnosis	FNAB
Treatment	Thyroidectomy with chemotherapy and radiotherapy may be attempted in some cases, but the majority of therapy is palliative. Chemotherapeutic agents.

PARATHRYOID

GENERAL CONCEPTS

ANATOMY

The parathyroids are embedded in the thyroid gland and are under the control of the pituitary gland. The parathyroids release PTH which removes calcium from the bones and releases it into the bloodstream to maintain calcium homeostasis. The superior parathyroid glands are located near the recurrent laryngeal nerve and inferior thyroid artery. The inferior parathyroids are derived from the third pouch, along with the thymus. The blood supply to the parathyroid glands emanates from the inferior thyroid artery.

PHYSIOLOGY

PARATHYROID HORMONE

Parathyroid hormone increases the concentration of calcium in the blood by stimulating its release from bones, increasing reabsorption in the distal tubules and thick ascending limb of Henle in the kidney, and increasing the production of vitamin D to promote intestinal absorption. Due to its effect on the kidney, phosphate excretion is stimulated. Paradoxically, osteoblasts are actually stimulated as prolonged osteoblastic stimulation actually stimulates the osteoclasts of the bone to promote calcium release.

CALCITONIN

Calcitonin reduces the concentration of serum calcium by decreasing the absorption of calcium from the intestines, promoting the mineralization of bones by stimulating osteoblasts, and increases its elimination from the body through the kidney. Calcitonin also decreases phosphate reabsorption.

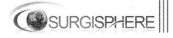

METABOLIC AND DEGENERATIVE

PRIMARY HYPERPARATHYROIDISM

ETIOLOGY AND PATHOPHYSIOLOGY

Primary hyperparathyroidism is the excess production of PTH leading to derangements in calcium homeostasis. Excessive calcium resorption from bone and reabsorption from the kidney lead to hypercalcemia and phosphaturia. Hyperplasia of the parathyroid glands and reset of the normal PTH set point are causes of hyperparathyroidism. Primary hyperparathyroidism may be related to MEN 1 and MEN 2, although the majority of cases are isolated. Multigland disease may occur in 1/10 of all cases.

PRESENTATION AND DIAGNOSIS

Hyperparathyroidism presents with bone pain, nephrolithiasis, metastatic calcification, osteopenia and osteoporosis, fatigue, and other constitutional symptoms. Diagnosis is made by examining total calcium and ionized calcium levels, PTH titers, and a 24 hour urine calcium excretion. The latter test is used to rule out familial hypocalciuric hypercalcemia (FHH). The most common presentation of hyperparathyroidism is asymptomatic hypercalcemia. Diarrhea associated with hyperparathyroidism is likely due to concomitant MEN syndrome leading to a gastrinoma.

TREATMENT

Treatment of primary hyperparathyroidism involves calcium supplements, volume expansion, loop diuretics, and surgical intervention that excises the abnormal tissue. Only glands with an identified adenoma are excised; in the event of four gland disease, a subtotal parathyroidectomy is performed. Resection of ectopic glands may also be necessary. The majority of tumors are cured by excision; if there is incomplete treatment, care must be taken to identify any aberrant glands through ultrasound and sestamibi scans. The most common site of ectopic glands are those higher in the pharynx due to failure to descend (i.e. near the base of the tongue), along the carotid sheath, near the thymus, or elsewhere within the mediastinum. A sternotomy should not be done during initial surgery. Blind thyroid lobectomy is not recommended due to the rare occurrence of intra-thyroid parathyroid glands. Four gland hyperplasia is managed by a total resection followed by reimplantation of a single gland.

Table 244 Primary Hyperparathyroidism

Primary Hyperparathyroidism	
Etiology	Hyperplasia of the parathyroid glands and reset of the normal PTH set point. May be related to MEN 1 and MEN 2, although the majority of cases are isolated.
Presentation	Bone pain, nephrolithiasis, metastatic calcification, osteopenia and osteoporosis, fatigue, and other constitutional symptoms.
Diagnosis	Examining total calcium and ionized calcium levels, PTH titers, and a 24 hour urine calcium excretion. Rule out FHH.
Treatment	Calcium supplements, volume expansion, loop diuretics, and surgical intervention that excises the abnormal tissue.

SECONDARY HYPERPARATHYROIDISM

ASSESSMENT

Secondary hyperparathyroidism is the increased production of PTH due to CRF, vitamin D deficiency, and other secondary causes. It is commonly found in patients receiving dialysis leading to metastatic calcification, osteitis fibrosa cystica, bone erosions (leading to a ground-glass appearance in the skull), hyperphosphatemia, and normal calcium. Bone pain with fractures, peptic ulcer disease, and metastatic calcification are all presenting signs.

MANAGEMENT

Treatment of secondary hyperparathyroidism includes use of calcium supplements, calcitonin, and controlling phosphate levels with phosphate binders and diet. Severe secondary hyperparathyroidism may lead to surgical treatment via total parathyroidectomy with autoimplantation or subtotal parathyroidectomy.

Table 245 Secondary Hyperparathyroidism

Secondary Hyperparathyroidism	
Etiology	Due to CRF, vitamin D deficiency, and other secondary causes. Commonly found in patients receiving dialysis.
Presentation	Metastatic calcification, osteitis fibrosa cystica, bone erosions leading to a ground-glass appearance in the skull, hyperphosphatemia, and normal calcium.
Diagnosis	High CRF and PTH levels
Treatment	Calcium supplements, calcitonin, and controlling phosphate levels with phosphate binders and diet. May lead to surgical treatment.

TERTIARY HYPERPARATHYROIDISM

ASSESSMENT AND MANAGEMENT

Tertiary hyperparathyroidism is the development of ectopic PTH secretion that is especially common following hypertrophy of glands in secondary hyperparathyroidism. Elevations in phosphate occur and diffuse calcinosis occurs. Treatment of tertiary hyperparathyroidism involves parathyroidectomy with hormone supplementation.

Table 246 Tertiary Hyperparathyroidism

Tertiary Hyperparathyroidism	
Etiology	Following hypertrophy of glands in secondary hyperparathyroidism.
Presentation	Elevations in phosphate occur and diffuse calcinosis also occurs.
Treatment	Parathyroidectomy with hormone supplementation.

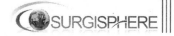

HYPOPARATHYROIDISM

ETIOLOGY AND PATHOPHYSIOLOGY

Hypoparathyroidism is the development of decreased PTH leading to a decrease in calcium homeostasis. Primary hypoparathyroidism is the result of parathyroidectomy, destruction of the glands in radiation therapy or accidental excision in thyroidectomy, autoimmune syndromes, and various congenital causes. Secondary disease is due to low PTH levels due to hypercalcemia caused by another etiology. Primary hypoparathyroidism occurs due to defects in the calcium-sensing receptor. Decreases in PTH lead to bone resorption, increased phosphate excretion, and poor absorption of calcium in the diet. Hypocalcemia is the result.

PRESENTATION AND DIAGNOSIS

Hypoparathyroidism presents with symptoms of hypocalcemia. Seizures, personality and mood changes, paresthesias, hoarseness, muscle cramps, and irritability are the result. Positive physical exam signs such as Chvostek sign (facial twitching as a result of facial nerve stimulation) and Trousseau sign (carpal spasm due to blood pressure cuff on arm), and choreoathetosis may occur. Paraplegia, Parkinsonism, dystonia, and other motor defects may also occur due to metastatic calcifications in the basal ganglia. PTH titers are decreased in primary disease with hypocalcemia; secondary hypoparathyroidism may present with low PTH and elevated calcium; pseudohypoparathyroidism presents with elevations in PTH due to hormone insensitivity.

TREATMENT

Treatment of primary disease involves PTH supplements, calcium supplements, and vitamin D supplements. The primary goal is to avoid hypocalcemia and bone resorption.

Table 247 Hypoparathyroidism

	Hypoparathyroidism
Etiology	**Primary**--parathyroidectomy, destruction of the glands in radiation therapy or accidental excision in thyroidectomy, autoimmune syndromes, and various congenital causes. **Secondary**--low PTH levels due to hypercalcemia caused by another etiology.
Presentation	Seizures, personality and mood changes, paresthesias, hoarseness, muscle cramps, and irritability.
Diagnosis	Chvostek and Trousseau signs and choreoathetosis may occur. Paraplegia, Parkinsonism, dystonia, and other motor defects may also occur. PTH titers are decreased in primary disease with hypocalcemia; secondary hypoparathyroidism may present with low PTH and elevated calcium.
Treatment	PTH supplements, calcium supplements, and vitamin D supplements.

PSEUDOHYPOPARATHYROIDISM

ASSESSMENT

Pseudohypoparathyroidism is typically due to genetic defects that lead to hypocalcemia, hyperphosphatemia, increased PTH, and insensitivity to PTH. PHP typically presents early especially with hypocalcemia. It is an exceedingly rare disorder. Patients present with a complex known as Albright hereditary osteodystrophy (AHO), which includes short stature, rounded facies, shortened metacarpals and metatarsals, obesity, dental hypoplasia, and metastatic calcifications. Diagnosis is made by confirmation of hypocalcemia, PTH assays, assessing PTH responsiveness (or lack thereof), and conducting other endocrine function tests. Basal ganglia calcification may also be present on CT.

MANAGEMENT

Treatment of PHP involves IV calcium, vitamin D, calcitriol, and careful management of calcium and phosphate homeostasis. Calcium chloride is the preferred agent.

Table 248 Pseudohypoparathyroidism (PHP)

Pseudohypoparathyroidism (PHP)	
Etiology	Due to genetic defects leading to hypocalcemia, hyperphosphatemia, increased PTH, and insensitivity to PTH.
Presentation	AHO, hypocalcemia.
Diagnosis	Confirmation of hypocalcemia, PTH assays, assessing PTH responsiveness, and conducting other endocrine function tests. Basal ganglia calcification may also be present on CT.
Treatment	Calcium chloride is the preferred agent. IV calcium, vitamin D, calcitriol, and careful management of calcium and phosphate homeostasis.

PARATHYROID TUMORS

The presence of parathyroid cancer when exploring for hyperparathyroidism should elicit a wide excision. Hypercalcemia and nodules in the lung may be other presenting signs of cancer.

ADRENAL

GENERAL CONCEPTS

ANATOMY

The two adrenal glands are located on top of each kidney. They consist of two parts the cortex (which responds to ACTH) and produces the glucocorticoids and mineralocorticoids, and the medulla which produces epinephrine and norepinephrine.

CONGENITAL AND STRUCTURAL

INCIDENTALOMA

Adrenal Gland

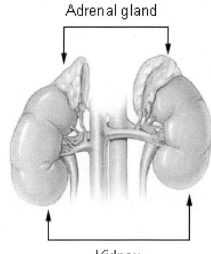

Adrenal gland

Kidney

An incidental adrenal mass may be found on up to 2% of CT scans. Most tend to be nonfunctional. Lesions smaller than 6cm that remains stable and without any clinical findings can be observed. Larger lesions, or those causing clinically-significant symptoms require additional diagnostic testing and surgical intervention. A functional mass due to hyperplasia can be treated with aldactone alone. Adenomas require excision. The workup of a possibly functional mass includes cortisol measurements in the serum and urine, a dexamethasone suppression test (low and high), 24 hour aldosterone level, serum aldosterone level, renin titers, and possible biopsy.

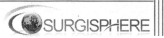

| METABOLIC AND DEGENERATIVE

HYPERCORTISOLISM (CUSHING SYNDROME) ⭐

ETIOLOGY AND PATHOPHYSIOLOGY

Cushing syndrome, also known as hypercortisolism, is the result of excess glucocorticoids commonly due to increased production by the adrenal gland. Neoplasms in the form of an adrenal adenoma may lead to ACTH-independent hypercortisolism, while excess ACTH secretion by a pituitary tumor may lead to the same symptoms. Cushing syndrome is most commonly attributed to excess glucocorticoid administration. It is rare as an endogenous cause. Morbidity and mortality vary depending on the cause. Females are more affected than males.

PRESENTATION AND DIAGNOSIS

Cushing syndrome presents with the typical signs of moon facies, buffalo hump, fat pads in the head and neck, truncal obesity, striae, proximal muscle weakness, bruising, hirsutism, HTN, DM, and symptoms related to other etiologies. A pituitary adenoma that secretes ACTH may present with homonymous hemianopsia due to optic chiasm impingement along with headaches. Peptic ulcers and various endocrinologic abnormalities may also develop over time. Diagnosis is made with excess cortisol production identified by laboratory tests (such as a 24-hour urinary free cortisol [UFC] level), a positive dexamethasone suppression test with elevations in cortisol the morning after administration, and various imaging studies to identify pituitary or adrenal adenomas. Loss of cortisol feedback may lead to ACTH derangements in shock.

TREATMENT

Treatment for Cushing syndrome is a reduction of hypercortisolism through surgical resection in primary disease, whether it involves adrenalectomy or transsphenoidal pituitary resection. Radiation therapy is also used occasionally. Medical intervention is not very successful, but can be attempted using ketoconazole, mitotane, metyrapone, aminoglutethimide, trilostane, and etomidate to decrease cortisol. Glucocorticoid replacement may be necessary. Ectopic production of ACTH should be suspected in the presence of persistent hypercortisolism after resection of a transsphenoid adenoma. Such production may occur in small cell lung cancer.

Table 249 Cushing Syndrome

Cushing Syndrome	
Etiology	Adrenal adenoma, pituitary tumor. Most commonly attributed to excess glucocorticoid administration.
Presentation	Moon facies, buffalo hump, fat pads in the head and neck, truncal obesity, striae, proximal muscle weakness, bruising, hirsutism, HTN, DM.
Diagnosis	Excess cortisol production identified by UFC level, a positive dexamethasone suppression test, and various imaging studies to identify pituitary or adrenal adenomas.
Treatment	Surgical resection in primary disease, radiation therapy. Glucocorticoid replacement may be necessary. Possible chemotherapeutic intervention (see above text).

PSEUDO-CUSHING SYNDROME

ASSESSMENT

Pseudo-Cushing syndrome is a transient excess in cortisol due to increased release of corticotrophin-releasing hormone (CRH). This disorder is commonly due to excess alcohol consumption. Pseudo-Cushing syndrome presents like Cushing syndrome with spontaneous resolution within a matter of weeks or months after avoiding alcohol.

Table 250 PseudoCushing Syndrome

Pseudo-Cushing Syndrome	
Etiology	Excess alcohol consumption
Presentation	Presents like Cushing syndrome with spontaneous resolution within a matter of weeks or months after avoiding alcohol.
Diagnosis	History of alcohol abuse and increased CRH.
Treatment	Spontaneously resolves after avoiding alcohol.

HYPERALDOSTERONISM (CONN SYNDROME)

ETIOLOGY AND PATHOPHYSIOLOGY

Conn syndrome, also known as primary hyperaldosteronism, is the result of increased aldosterone secretion leading to hypernatremia, hypokalemia, and HTN. Increased aldosterone production may also be the result of an adenoma or adrenal hyperplasia. Conn syndrome is rare, and morbidity and mortality are from the HTN and the hypokalemia that can develop.

PRESENTATION AND DIAGNOSIS

Conn syndrome presents with constitutional symptoms, muscle weakness, DI, HTN, CHF, and other symptoms of hypernatremia and hypokalemia. Suppression of the renin-angiotensin axis (RAA) is commonly found. An abnormal 24-hour urine aldosterone test confirms the diagnosis. CT is used to diagnose the extent of adrenal dysfunction due to adenoma or hyperplasia.

TREATMENT

Treatment of Conn syndrome includes symptomatic treatment of HTN and correcting underlying electrolyte disturbances. Sodium restriction is necessary. Diuretics, ACE inhibitors, calcium-channel blockers, and ARBs form the cornerstone of medical therapy. Adrenalectomy is used in cases refractory to medical intervention.

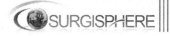

Table 251 Conn Syndrome

Conn Syndrome	
Etiology	Adenoma or adrenal hyperplasia.
Presentation	Muscle weakness, DI, HTN, CHF, and other symptoms of hypernatremia and hypokalemia. Suppression of the RAA.
Diagnosis	Abnormal 24-hour urine aldosterone test, CT.
Treatment	Symptomatic treatment of HTN and correcting underlying electrolyte disturbances. Sodium restriction, diuretics, ACE inhibitors, calcium-channel blockers, and ARBs, adrenalectomy.

HYPOALDOSTERONISM (ADDISON DISEASE)

ETIOLOGY AND PATHOPHYSIOLOGY

Hypoaldosteronism is commonly due to decreased renin production in CRF, leading to defects in potassium handling and subsequent hyperkalemia. Aldosterone is required for proper sodium-potassium exchange by the principal cells of the cortical collecting tubule; defects in aldosterone lead to excess potassium retention. Hyporeninemic hypoaldosteronism is also known as RTA type IV.

PRESENTATION AND DIAGNOSIS

Hypoaldosteronism may lead to arrhythmia from the excessively high potassium levels. Mild acidosis may also be present, along with HTN. Other than these manifestations, hypoaldosteronism is typically subclinical, but presenting signs may include fever, nausea, and vomiting. CRF with hyperkalemia confirms the diagnosis.

TREATMENT

Loop and thiazide diuretics are used to correct the hyperkalemia in hypoaldosteronism. Sodium bicarbonate corrects acidosis, while fludrocortisone serves as an analogue to aldosterone. Resins that bind to potassium are used to remove potassium from the body on an emergent basis.

Table 252 Hypoaldosteronism

Hypoaldosteronism	
Etiology	Decreased renin production in CRF.
Presentation	Arrhythmia, mild acidosis with HTN.
Diagnosis	CRF with hyperkalemia confirms the diagnosis.
Treatment	Loop and thiazide diuretics, sodium bicarbonate, fludrocortisone. Resins that bind to potassium.

ADRENAL INSUFFICIENCY

ETIOLOGY AND PATHOPHYSIOLOGY

Adrenal insufficiency is the acute development of nausea, vomiting, abdominal pain, shock, and subsequent death due to adrenal failure. This leads to the inability to produce cortisol, aldosterone, and various androgens. Prompt diagnosis is essential to avoid death. It may occur in patients who are withdrawn from steroid therapy, as a consequence of septic shock, and in patients who use medications including ketoconazole, phenytoin, rifampin, and mitotane.

PRESENTATION AND DIAGNOSIS

Adrenal insufficiency presents suddenly and can lead to shock as the initial presentation. Inability to regulate temperature, along with nausea and vomiting can also occur. Abdominal pain is common. Diagnosis is made by an abnormal ACTH test that leads to little change in cortisol. Electrolyte abnormalities in adrenal insufficiency include hyperkalemia and hyponatremia. EKG is often done to rule out cardiac manifestations of hyperkalemia.

TREATMENT

Treatment requires glucocorticoid administration. Fluid and electrolyte correction are also necessary. Hypotension is reversed with dopamine or norepinephrine. The glucocorticoid of choice is dexamethasone. Fludrocortisone is a drug sometimes used to correct aldosterone defects. A postop patient with a history ITP and shock should receive hydrocortisone to forestall the adrenal crisis.

Table 253 Adrenal Insufficiency

Adrenal Insufficiency	
Etiology	Adrenal failure. Due to withdrawal from steroid therapy, as a consequence of septic shock and in patients who use certain medications.
Presentation	Presents suddenly and can lead to shock. Inability to regulate temperature, nausea and vomiting can also occur. Abdominal pain is common.
Diagnosis	Abnormal ACTH test that leads to little change in cortisol. EKG.
Treatment	Glucocorticoids administration. Fluid and electrolyte correction, hypotension reversal with dopamine or norepinephrine.

ADRENAL TUMORS

PHEOCHROMOCYTOMA

ASSESSMENT

Pheochromocytomas are catecholamine-secreting tumors that lead to intermittent malignant HTN and cardiac arrhythmia. This highly curable tumor is very rare but is responsible for numerous cases of secondary HTN. Pheochromocytoma may occur in isolation, or with familial syndromes such as MEN 2, MEN 3, neurofibromatosis, and Von-Hippel-Landau (VHL) disease. Presentation is with symptoms of very high BP (such as headache), diaphoresis, chest pain, anxiety, and palpitations. End organ damage may be evident from the excessively high BP. Metanephrine is elevated, along with vanillylmandelic acid

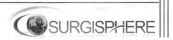

and catecholamines. A contrast-enhancing lesion is often seen on CT scan. Diagnosis includes 24 hour urine collection for VMA, measurement of metanephrine and catecholamine titers, and a possible MIBG scan to localize ectopic tissues.

MANAGEMENT

Pheochromocytoma is treated with alpha blockade using phenoxybenzamine for about a week followed by beta blockade for 24 hours. Preoperative fluid resuscitation is needed prior to surgical resection. A MIBG scan should be conducted when imaging for extra-adrenal pheochromocytoma. These tend to have a higher malignancy potential and tend to be located near the aortic bifurcation. They tend to be on the left side near the origin of the inferior mesenteric artery, in an area known as the organ of Zuckerkandl, a derivation of the neural crest.

Table 254 Pheochromocytoma

Pheochromocytoma	
Etiology	Catecholamine-secreting tumors.
Presentation	Symptoms of very high BP. End organ damage may be evident.
Diagnosis	Metanephrine is elevated, along with vanillylmandelic acid and catecholamines.
Treatment	Alpha blockade using phenoxybenzamine followed by beta blockade. Resection is necessary.

ADRENOCORTICAL CARCINOMA

An adrenocortical carcinoma tends to be unilateral and over 6cm in size when clinically significant. Resection is necessary due to the high potential for metastasis to distant nodes, lung, liver, kidney, and bone.

SOMATOSTATINOMA

A somatostatinoma is associated with MEN I and presents with hyperglycemia, diarrhea, cholelithiasis, and hypochlorhydria. Surgical resection of the primary tumor and all metastatic tumors is necessary.

ENDOCRINE PANCREAS

GENERAL CONCEPTS

ANATOMY

Embedded in the pancreas are the Islets of Langerhans. These Islet contain the alpha cells and the beta cells.

The beta cells produces insulin, which regulates the osmolarity of sugar by storing sugar excesses in the liver and promoting uptake by the body's cells. The alpha cells produce glucagon, which is antagonistic to insulin and releases sugar into the blood stream.

PHYSIOLOGY

INSULIN AND GLUCAGON ✿

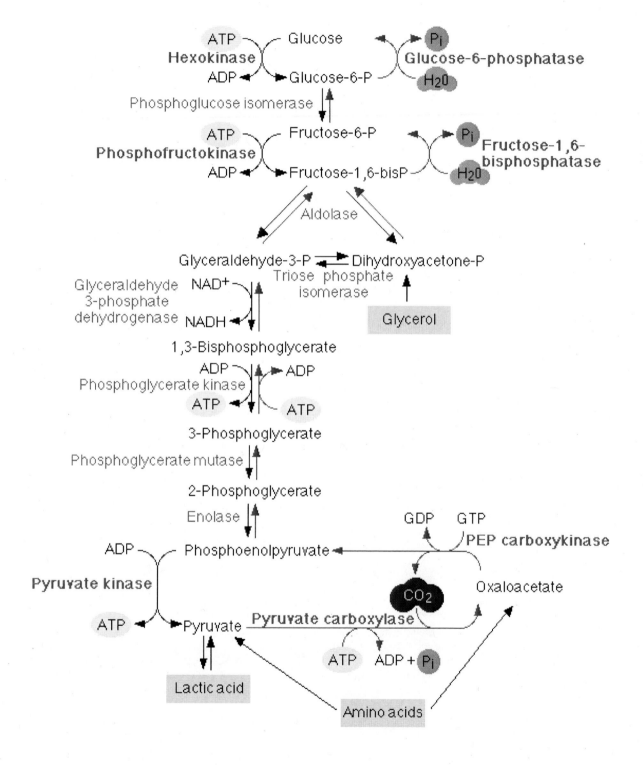

Glucose uptake in the intestines is an active process and requires a sodium gradient. Glucose metabolism in early sepsis is retarded due to decreased utilization. The intermediary between lactate and glucose is pyruvate. **A hormone present in early septic shock is glucagon.**

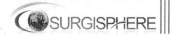

METABOLIC AND DEGENERATIVE

TYPE I DIABETES MELLITUS

Table 255 Type I Diabetes Mellitus

Type I Diabetes Mellitus	
Etiology	Autoimmune destruction of pancreatic beta cells.
Presentation	Polyuria, polydipsia, and polyphagia with symptoms of hyperglycemia, ketoacidosis. Patients tend to be thin and complain of numerous constitutional symptoms. Blurred vision is common.
Diagnosis	Fasting glucose, an abnormal OGTT, and abnormal insulin titers.
Treatment	Insulin and monitoring of glucose levels. Transplant of beta cells can be attempted in some patients. Diet and exercise are the keys to good management.

TYPE II DIABETES MELLITUS

Table 256 Type 2 Diabetes Mellitus

Type 2 Diabetes Mellitus	
Etiology	Multifactorial inheritance with environmental triggers in the form of a poor diet and lack of exercise.
Presentation	Typically asymptomatic. Obesity is a common presentation, and pregnant women may deliver an infant that is LGA. Later complications caused by NIDDM are numerous.
Diagnosis	GCT
Treatment	Reversing deleterious exercise and diet trends. Reducing risk factors. Controlling concurrent diseases. Tight glycemic control. For pregnant women, glyburide. Insulin is the only recommended treatment for women with a history of NIDDM. Medical interventions include sulfonylureas, meglitinides, biguanides, metformin, alpha-glucosidase inhibitors, glitazones, and exenatide. Obese individuals are initially started on metformin. Sulfonylureas are acceptable in persons of normal weight.

DIABETIC KETOACIDOSIS

ETIOLOGY AND PATHOPHYSIOLOGY

DKA is the development of insulin resistance or deficiency that leads to significant hyperglycemia, acidosis, low bicarbonate, and ketonemia. With sufficient time without insulin, breakdown of free fatty acids (FFA) and gluconeogenesis take over to replenish the supply of glucose; beta-oxidation of the FFA produces ketone bodies, which in turn can induce the metabolic acidosis seen in DKA. DKA requires prompt insulin therapy to avoid mortality. It is most likely to occur in IDDM, but can present in NIDDM. Causes include exacerbations of DM, including infection (such as UTI), missing medications, and serious illness or stressors such as MI, CVA, pregnancy, and surgery.

PRESENTATION AND DIAGNOSIS

DKA presents with symptoms of hyperglycemia, constitutional complaints, and general malaise. Dry mucous membranes with decreased skin turgor are evident on physical exam. Reflexes are typically diminished, and respiration is labored. Tachycardia and hypotension can occur, along with tachypnea and hypothermia. A fruity smell of ketones is present on the breath; confusion and coma can rapidly ensue if treatment is not rapidly implemented. Diagnosis is made by hyperglycemia, bicarbonate less than 15, and pH below 7.3. An anion gap metabolic acidosis is present.

TREATMENT

Correct underlying electrolyte abnormalities, especially hypokalemia which can occur quickly. Start with isotonic saline to rehydrate the patient. Rapidly treat underlying infections. Follow NS with ½NS, and replenish potassium. Significantly acidic pH should be corrected with bicarbonate. Insulin is administered to reverse the DKA.

Table 257 Diabetic Ketoacidosis (DKA)

Diabetic Ketosis (DKA)	
Etiology	Exacerbations of DM, including infection, missing medications, and serious illness or stressors such as MI, CVA, pregnancy, and surgery.
Presentation	Hyperglycemia, constitutional complaints, and general malaise. Dry mucous membranes with decreased skin turgor. Reflexes are typically diminished, and respiration is labored. Tachycardia and hypotension can occur, along with tachypnea and hypothermia. A fruity smell of ketones is present on the breath.
Diagnosis	Hyperglycemia, bicarbonate less than 15, and pH below 7.3. An anion gap metabolic acidosis is present.
Treatment	Correct underlying electrolyte abnormalities. Treat underlying infections quickly. Follow NS with ½NS, and replenish potassium. Significantly acidic pH should be corrected with bicarbonate. Insulin is administered to reverse the DKA.

HYPEROSMOLAR HYPERGLYCEMIC NONKETOTIC COMA

ASSESSMENT

Hyperosmolar hyperglycemic nonketotic coma (HHNC) is the development of coma due to dehydration and hyperglycemia. It is commonly secondary to stressors or infection. HHNC occurs more often than DKA and carries a significant risk of mortality. It is most common in elderly individuals, whereas DKA occurs more in middle-aged adults. Symptoms include delirium and other CNS changes, seizures, hemiparesis, paresthesias, and sensory deficits culminating with stupor then coma. Signs and symptoms of dehydration and hyperglycemia are present. As infection is commonly a trigger for HHNC, examination should focus on ruling out easily discernable infections. Electrolyte derangements are commonly present, and glucose is often near 1,000 mg / dL. Some overlap with DKA is possible.

MANAGEMENT

Treatment centers on maintaining the ABCs, correcting the dehydration, and treating the hyperglycemia. Large boluses of NS are given early. Thiamine, dextrose, and naloxone are given if the patient is comatose. Rapid fluid administration is often the key to reversing significant fluid deficits, which can be over 10 L. Insulin therapy can ameliorate symptoms.

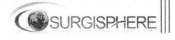

Table 258 Hyperosmolar Hyperglycemic Nonketotic Coma (HHNC)

Hyperosmolar Hyperglycemic Nonketotic Coma (HHNC)	
Etiology	Coma due to dehydration and hyperglycemia. It is commonly secondary to stressors or infection.
Presentation	Delirium and other CNS changes, seizures, hemiparesis, paresthesias, and sensory deficits culminating with stupor then coma. Signs and symptoms of dehydration and hyperglycemia are present.
Diagnosis	Examination should focus on ruling out easily discernable infections. Electrolyte derangements are commonly present, and glucose is often near 1,000 mg / dL. Some overlap with DKA is possible.
Treatment	Maintaining the ABCs, correcting the dehydration, and treating the hyperglycemia. Large boluses of NS are given early. Thiamine, dextrose, and naloxone are given if the patient is comatose. Insulin therapy can ameliorate symptoms.

HYPOGLYCEMIA

ASSESSMENT

Hypoglycemia occurs with a serum glucose titer below 50 mg / dL and can herald systemwide alteration in function. Various stressors, in addition to hyperinsulinemia, can lead to hypoglycemia, and the outcome can be death. Profound mental deficits leading to permanent defects can occur if the hypoglycemia is not reversed in a timely manner. Cardiac defects can also arise, and all of this damage can lead to coma. Hypoglycemia affects older females more than any other group. A history of diabetes is commonly present. C-peptide is elevated with insulinomas and normal or low with exogenous insulin. CT exam may be necessary to identify the precise location of the insulinoma.

MANAGEMENT

Treatment involves admission to the ICU and rapid correction of the glucose deficiency. Glucose should not be infused faster than 4 mg/kg/min. Supportive therapy is required and careful management necessary to help reverse the hypoglycemia and avoid permanent sequelae. A C-peptide level should always be determined in hypoglycemic patients who are suspected of surreptious use of insulin.

Table 259 Hypoglycemia

Hypoglycemia	
Etiology	Various stressors in addition to hyperinsulinemia.
Presentation	Profound mental deficits leading to permanent defects can occur. Cardiac defects can also arise, and all of this damage can lead to coma.
Diagnosis	C-peptide is elevated with insulinomas and normal or low with exogenous insulin. CT exam may be necessary to identify the precise location of the insulinoma.
Treatment	Admission to the ICU and rapid correction of the glucose deficiency. Supportive therapy is required and careful management.

PANCREATIC TUMORS

INSULINOMA

Insulinoma should be confirmed after determining a ratio of insulin to glucose greater than 0.4 by measuring the C-peptide level. Insulinomas can be located anywhere in the pancreas, and typically presents with symptomatic hypoglycemia. Whipple's triad describes the presenting signs, and includes symptomatic hypoglycemia when fasting, a normal blood glucose less than 50 mg/dL, and resolution of symptoms of glucose administration.

MULTIPLE ENDOCRINE NEOPLASIA

MEN 1

ETIOLOGY AND PATHOPHYSIOLOGY OF MEN 1

MEN 1 (Wermer syndrome) leads to tumor formation in the parathyroid gland, endocrine pancreas, and anterior pituitary. The adrenal cortex tumors can also develop, along with lipomas and angiofibromas. The most common effect with MEN 1 is hyperparathyroidism with four gland hyperplasia (95%). Parathyroid effects tend to occur early and presents with a high serum calcium, high parathyroid hormone level, high serum chloride, high urine calcium, and low serum phosphate. Familial hypercalcemic hypocalciuria must be ruled out. The high calcium levels tend to exacerbate ZE syndrome. Gastrinomas may occur in the pancreas, but insulinomas and glucagonomas are all possible (35-75%). Imaging for diagnosis can be done with an octreotide scan. An insulinoma is the second most common tumor and presents with Whipple's triad (fasting glucose less than 45mg/dL, hypoglycemic symptoms, and relief of symptoms with ingestion of glucose). Diagnosis of an insulinoma is made with serum proinsulin, c-peptide levels, the presence of anti-insulin antibodies, and urine sulfonylureas. The anterior pituitary may have a prolactinoma or other pituitary tumor (15-60%). Silent adenomas are typically found in the adrenal gland. MEN 1 is an autosomal dominant disorder found on chromosome 11q13 that leads to defects in the nuclear protein menin. MEN 1 occurs in young adults. The presence of a MEN tumor with a migratory rash should begin a search for a glucagonoma. Glucagonomas typically present with signs and symptoms of diabetes mellitus, glossitis, stomatitis, and a migratory necrolytic erythematous rash. The treatment is octreotide. Both MEN 1 and MEN 2 have hyperparathyroidism. Recall that the therapy for this is total parathyroidectomy with auto reimplantation of a single gland.

MEN 2

ETIOLOGY AND PATHOPHYSIOLOGY OF MEN 2

MEN 2 (also known as MEN 2a, or Sipple syndrome) leads to tumor formation in the thyroid (as medullary carcinoma), pheochromocytoma, and hyperparathyroidism. Hyperplasia of the adrenal medulla may also be present. MEN 2 is an autosomal dominant disorder that affects the RET proto-oncogene. MEN 2 is very rare and occurs very early in life. Medullary thyroid carcinoma occurs 100% of the time by the time the individual reaches the 30s, and is diagnosed by the presence of amyloid within the stroma and parafollicular C cells. Pheochromocytoma occurs in half of all individuals and tends to be located at the aortic bifurcation (organ of Zuckerkandl). 30% of individuals develop parathyroid tumors. Hirschsprung disease is common in infants. Urine catecholamines need to be checked before proceeding with a thyroidectomy in MEN. This is done to rule out a pheochromocytoma. VMA levels should be checked.

MEN 1: PTH (remove first), pancreas (gastrinoma; monitor), anterior pituitary (monitor)
MEN 2: MTC, pheo, PTH
MEN 3: MTC, pheo, neuroma

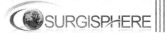

MEN 3

ETIOLOGY AND PATHOPHYSIOLOGY OF MEN 3

MEN 3, previously known as MEN 2b, leads to the development of medullary thyroid carcinoma, pheochromocytoma, and neuromas. A marfanoid habitus is typically found with MEN 3. MEN 3 is also due to a RET proto-oncogene defect (chromosome 10), and is rarer than MEN 2. **A transmembrane tyrosine kinase receptor is encoded by RET.** Overall, death from MEN is due to PUD, distant metastases with cancer effects, hypercalcemia leading to sudden cardiac death through arrhythmia, CHD, CVA, and CHF. MEN 3 presents early in life. Early presentation of medullary thyroid cancer occurs in the teens.

PRESENTATION AND DIAGNOSIS

MEN 1 typically presents with symptoms of hyperparathyroidism in conjunction with Zollinger-Ellison syndrome (ZES). MEN 2 presents with MTC and sometimes also with pheochromocytoma. MEN 3 presents with a marfanoid habitus, neuromas, and MTC. Diagnosis is made by identifying the presence of the tumor through a variety of laboratory tests and imaging studies.

TREATMENT

Treatment options for various neuroendocrinologic disturbances have been described earlier in this chapter. Treatment generally involves subtotal or total removal of the endocrine organ followed by hormone replacement. As MEN subtypes present with several distinct tumors, a careful search for other tumors should take place, and the patient should be closely followed. Treatment of hyperparathyroidism is completed with subtotal parathyroidectomy or **total parathyroidectomy with autoimplantation.** Pancreatic tumors are modified with PPIs and parathyroidectomy, which tends to alleviate the hypercalcemia and symptoms of ZE syndrome. Pituitary tumors are treated with **transsphenoidal resection** for refractory or enlarging tumors. **The first surgery that should be completed is parathyroidectomy.** Medullary thyroid cancer is treated with total thyroidectomy with central node dissection; chemoradiation is not indicated. Pheochromocytoma is treated with adrenalectomy. Malignant tumors are treated with bilateral adrenalectomy.

Table 260 Multiple Endocrine Neoplasm (MEN)

Multiple Endocrine Neoplasm (MEN)	
Etiology	MEN 1--Autosomal dominant disorder found on chromosome 11 that leads to defects in the protein menin. MEN 2—Autosomal dominant disorder that affects RET proto-oncogene. MEN 3—RET proto-oncogene defect.
Presentation	MEN 1--symptoms of hyperparathyroidism in conjunction with ZES. MEN 2--MTC and sometimes also with pheochromocytoma. MEN 3--Marfanoid habitus, neuromas, and MTC.
Diagnosis	Presence of the tumor through a variety of laboratory tests and imaging studies.
Treatment	Generally involves subtotal or total removal of the endocrine organ followed by hormone replacement.

PRACTICE QUESTIONS

 A 34 year old male presents with intermittent but worsening right lower quadrant pain. A CT scan reveals nephrolithiasis, and the patient passes the stone on his own 12 hours later with resolution of his pain. However, an incidental finding on the CT scan indicates a 3cm left adrenal mass. Which of the following is the next best course of action?

A. Monitor with repeat CT scans every 6 months
B. Needle biopsy the mass
C. Open biopsy of the mass
D. Resect the left adrenal gland
E. Start spironolactone

 The best answer is <u>Monitor with repeat CT scans every 6 months</u>. An adrenal mass over six centimeters must be excised en toto in order to avoid the risk for adrenal cortical carcinoma. Masses less than six cm may be monitored with serial CT scans every 6 months as long as it is a non-functioning mass. The laboratory workup for adrenal masses includes checking serum electrolytes, sex hormones, cortisol, renin, catecholamines, steroid levels, and completing a urine VMA. A dexamethasone suppression test is also completed. Any functional adrenal mass should be excised, while bilateral adrenal hyperplasia and aldosterone secreting tumors may be treated with spironolactone.

 A 22 year old male presents with progressive weight gain with an approximately 80 pound increase over the past year, high blood pressure, diabetes, and purple striae around his abdomen. A dexamethasone suppression test is completed. Low dose stimulation leads to a high cortisol level, and high dose stimulation leads to a low cortisol level. What is the next best course in management?

A. Adrenalectomy
B. PET scan
C. Start low dose maintenance steroids
D. Transsphenoidal pituitary resection
E. VATS with mediastinoscopy

 The best answer is <u>Transsphenoidal pituitary resection</u>. This patient has Cushing syndrome with the characteristic weight gain, onset of diabetes, high blood pressure, and purple striae. Other changes may include mental status changes, hirsutism, and a characteristic buffalo hump. Serum cortisol is typically elevated, and a dexamethasone suppression test is completed to identify the location of the secretory tumor. Low dose dexamethasone with low cortisol response means the primary source of the tumor is in the adrenal gland. Low dose dexamethasone with high cortisol response means the primary is either in the pituitary gland or is ectopic. High dose dexamethasone with low cortisol response means the primary is the pituitary. High dose dexamethasone with high cortisol response means the primary is an ectopic source. The treatment for this gentleman is therefore either a transsphenoidal pituitary resection or radiation therapy.

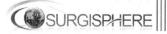

A 42 year old female presents with a blood pressure of 202 / 110. Serum testing yields hypokalemia and hypernatremia. Which of the following is the next best step in management?

A.   Complete a dexamethasone suppression test
B.   Excise the adrenal adenoma
C.   Measure serum renin levels
D.   Start spironolactone
E.   Start steroids

The best answer is <u>Measure serum renin levels</u>. This patient has primary hyperaldosteronism (Conn syndrome) with hypertension, hypokalemia, and hypernatremia. Before a formal diagnosis can be made, serum renin levels are checked as renal hypertension can also lead to elevated aldosterone. If levels are normal, the adrenal glands are evaluated. Unilateral hyperplasia is treated with isolated excision. Bilateral hyperplasia is treated via spironolactone. A dexamethasone suppression test is relevant for Cushing disease. Steroids are reserved for Addison disease.

A 62 year old female who has been treated for rheumatoid arthritis for a number of years presents to your clinic with a symptomatic blood pressure of 72/36. Serum electrolytes yield hyperkalemia and hyponatremia. Cosyntropin is given, which yields a low serum cortisol, and a diagnosis of Addison disease is made. What is the next best step?

A.   Check urine metanephrines and VMA
B.   Complete a dexamethasone suppression test
C.   CT scan of the adrenal glands
D.   Start IV steroids
E.   Start PO steroids

The best answer is <u>Start IV steroids</u>. This patient has Addison disease with acute decompensation. She should be started on IV steroids to forestall further cardiovascular compromise, and transitioned to PO steroids when she stabilizes. She has a characteristic low serum cortisol following stimulation, and a positive ACTH stimulation test. A dexamethasone suppression test is indicated for Cushing syndrome. CT scan of her adrenal glands is more appropriate as part of the workup for Conn syndrome, and checking urine VMA is for pheochromocytoma.

A 51 year old Russian immigrant is consulted by surgery for a 2 cm mass found just left of the aortic bifurcation. The patient presently has a blood pressure of 172/61, intermittent flushing, and episodic hypertension. What is the best test if you suspect metastatic pheochromocytoma?

A.   CT abdomen / pelvis
B.   CT chest / abdomen / pelvis
C.   I-131 metaiodobenzyliquanetine study
D.   MRI abdomen
E.   PET scan

The best answer is <u>I-131 metaiodobenzyliquanetine study</u>. The best test to identify metastatic pheochromocytoma is the I-131 metaiodobenzyliquanetine study. Most metastatic tumors are found at the organ of Zuckerkandl, located just lateral to the aortic bifurcation near the inferior mesenteric artery. The other studies are typically not immediately indicated.

A 51 year old Russian immigrant is consulted by surgery for a 2 cm mass found just left of the aortic bifurcation. The patient presently has a blood pressure of 172/61, intermittent flushing, and episodic hypertension. What is the best preoperative management plan?

A. Phenoxybenzamine and propranolol for 7 days, surgery, fluids
B. Phenoxybenzamine for 7 days, propranolol for 2 days, fluids, surgery
C. Phenoxybenzamine for 7 days, propranolol for 2 days, surgery, fluids
D. Propranolol for 7 days, phenoxybenzamine for 2 days, fluids, surgery
E. Propranolol for 7 days, phenoxybenzamine for 2 days, surgery, fluids

The best answer is <u>Phenoxybenzamine for 7 days, propranolol for 2 days, fluids, surgery</u>. The best preoperative management plan is to start alpha blockade via phenoxybenzamine for a period of 7 days. This should be followed with beta blockade with propranolol. Fluid resuscitation prior to surgery is important given the likelihood of hypotension in the immediate postoperative period. Nipride is the drug of choice if a sudden elevation in blood pressure occurs.

What is the source of the superior anterior pancreaticoduodenal artery?

A. Celiac artery
B. Common hepatic artery
C. Gastroduodenal artery
D. Proper hepatic artery
E. Superior mesenteric artery

The best answer is <u>Gastroduodenal artery</u>. The superior anterior and posterior pancreaticoduodenal arteries are a branch of the gastroduodenal artery. The inferior anterior and posterior pancreaticoduodenal arteries are a branch of the superior mesenteric artery. As the gastroduodenal artery is also removed during a Whipple procedure, the duodenum is also removed due to the loss of its blood supply.

A patient presents with hyponatremia, hyperkalemia, decreased cardiac output, and hypoglycemia. What is the next best step in management?

A. Blood product resuscitation
B. Cortisol stimulation test
C. Intubation and fluid resuscitation
D. IV hydrocortisone
E. Neosynephrine

The best answer is <u>IV hydrocortisone</u>. This patient is suffering from adrenal insufficiency, and requires immediate therapy with 200mg IV hydrocortisone and symptomatic management. There is insufficient time to send off a diagnostic test and wait for the results. Intubation is not required, although crystalloid can be infused immediately. Pressors may be needed with further decompensation. There is no indication for blood transfusion.

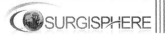

A 36 year old male presents with a blood pressure of 172/110, significant weakness and fatigue, and desire to continually drink fluid and urinate. His serum electrolytes are also noted to be significantly imbalanced, with notable hypokalemia. What is the most likely diagnosis?

A. Addison disease
B. Conn syndrome
C. Cushing disease
D. Diabetes insipidus
E. Renal hypertension

The best answer is <u>Conn syndrome</u>. Conn syndrome, also known as primary hyperaldosteronism, is the result of increased aldosterone secretion leading to hypernatremia, hypokalemia, and HTN. Increased aldosterone production may also be the result of an adenoma or adrenal hyperplasia. Conn syndrome is rare, and morbidity and mortality are from the HTN and the hypokalemia that can develop. Conn syndrome presents with constitutional symptoms, muscle weakness, DI, HTN, CHF, and other symptoms of hypernatremia and hypokalemia. Suppression of the renin-angiotensin axis (RAA) is commonly found. An abnormal 24-hour urine aldosterone test confirms the diagnosis. CT is used to diagnose the extent of adrenal dysfunction due to adenoma or hyperplasia. The primary cause is an adrenal adenoma in 66% of patients, while the majority of the remainder may have an idiopathic bilateral hyperplasia.

Which of the following is not one of the effects of insulin?

A. Fatty acid synthesis stimulation
B. Gluconeogenesis in the liver
C. Glucose absorption by muscle and adipose tissue
D. Increased glycogen synthase activity
E. Muscle protein formation through amino acid incorporation

The best answer is <u>Gluconeogenesis in the liver</u>. Insulin leads to an increase in glycogen synthesis in the liver and muscle, increased fatty acid synthesis, increased fatty acid esterification, decreased proteinolysis, decreased lipolysis, and decreased gluconeogenesis in the liver. Insulin is produced by beta cells of the pancreas.

A patient is diagnosed with MEN I and Zollinger-Ellison syndrome. What is the accepted treatment sequence?

A. Hypophysectomy and pancreatic tumor resection
B. Parathyroidectomy and gastrectomy
C. Parathyroidectomy and pancreatic tumor resection
D. Parathyroidectomy and proton pump inhibitors
E. Parathyroidectomy and truncal vagotomy

 The best answer is <u>Parathyroidectomy and proton pump inhibitors</u>. MEN I includes parathyroid adenomas leading to hypercalcemia, neuroendocrine tumors such as gastrinomas, pituitary tumors, and pancreatic tumors. The therapy is to complete a ¾ gland parathyroidectomy or total parathyroidectomy with reimplantation. If symptomatic ZE syndrome continues, resection of the stomach would then be indicated. Therefore, the initial therapy is to proceed with the parathyroidectomy and use PPIs for symptomatic control. Symptoms of a gastrinoma include diarrhea with hypercalcemia. Recall that hypokalemic, hypochloremic, watery diarrhea with metabolic alkalosis is a sign of a VIPoma.

 A 38 year old female is found to have an isolated hypercalcemia. Upon further diagnostic testing, she is found to have primary hyperparathyroidism. What is the next best step in management?

A. ¾ gland excision
B. Calcium supplementation
C. Parathyroidectomy with reimplantation
D. Radical excision of thyroid lobe
E. Sestamibi scan

 The best answer is <u>Parathyroidectomy with reimplantation</u>. This patient has primary hyperparathyroidism, of which initial presenting symptoms are few but include bone pain, stone formation, and generalized symptoms. In the event of a hypercalcemic crisis, saline and lasix can be used to ameliorate symptoms. Radical thyroid lobe excision is necessary only with parathyroid cancer. While a sestamibi scan is useful in locating parathyroid gland tissue, it is not typically done prior to a parathyroidectomy. Recall that both MEN I and II have hyperparathyroidism. Recall that the superior parathyroids develop from the 4th pouch and the inferior parathyroids from the 3rd pouch. The inferior thyroid artery is the chief blood supply.

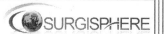

SURGICAL CRITICAL CARE

CHAPTER CONTENTS

SHOCK AND RESUSCITATION

POSTOPERATIVE FEVER

POSTOPERATIVE DAYS 1 AND 2

One of the most common postoperative sequelae is the development of a fever. The most common cause of this fever depends on when the pyrexia occurs. Fevers that occur by postoperative day two include atelectasis. Evidence is accumulating that atelectasis can be minimized or even entirely prevented through the use of incentive spirometry. The mechanism of action is unclear, but it appears as if deep inspiration has a more positive effect in preventing atelectasis rather than inducing a patient to cough. Chances of fever developing on postoperative day one or two increases in patients with ventilator support and in patients who have pain on inspiration due to surgery to the chest wall or ancillary structures.

POSTOPERATIVE DAYS 3 THROUGH 5

The most common cause of postoperative fever between postoperative days three and five is due to urinary tract infection. Prophylactic measures can be taken in patients who are more susceptible than normal for developing UTIs. This population includes patients who have indwelling Foley catheters, and who have a historical predilection for developing UTI.

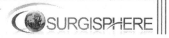

POSTOPERATIVE DAYS 4 THROUGH 6

Deep vein thrombosis is the most common cause of postoperative fever on days four through six. DVT is a serious issue than can lead to sudden death due to a massive pulmonary embolism, and astute surgeons and health care providers take steps to minimize this potentially disastrous outcome. Low-dose heparin given subcutaneously and the use of sequential compressed devices (SCD) have been shown to reduce the incidence of DVT. The best way to reduce the chances of DVT occurring is to have the patient ambulate as soon as possible following surgery. The patient population most at risk of DVT is those who have undergone pelvic procedures, orthopedic surgery, or a general surgery procedure.

POSTOPERATIVE DAYS 5 THROUGH 7

Infections of the surgical wound are most common postoperative days five through seven. Prophylactic antibiotics are an important part of any surgical procedure, even in clean cases.

POSTOPERATIVE DAYS 7 AND BEYOND

Finally, fevers that occur after postoperative day seven are often iatrogenic, often from medications. A mnemonic for remembering the most common causes of postoperative fevers is to recall the five W's, or Wind, Water, Walking, Wound, and Wonder drugs.

Table 261 Fever–Postoperative

Fever-Postoperative	
Days 1-2	Atelectasis—prevent with incentive spirometry.
Days 3-5	UTI-prophylactic measures.
Days 4-6	DVT—prevent with Low-dose heparin and the use of SCD. Have the patient ambulate as soon as possible following surgery.
Days 5-7	Infections of surgical wounds—prevent with prophylactic antibiotics.
Days 7-beyond	Iatrogenic (often from medications).

SYSTEMIC INFLAMMATORY RESPONSE SYNDROME

ASSESSMENT

Systemic inflammatory response syndrome (SIRS) is the presence of fever (not always present in the elderly), tachycardia, narrow pulse pressure, hyperpnea, and hypotension in serious cases. There is no end-organ damage, bacteremia, or significant medical support with SIRS. SIRS should be thought of as a systemwide inflammatory state leading to multiple organ dysfunction syndrome (MODS). The proinflammatory state includes numerous APRs and significant release of various cytokines. The number of organs affected determines mortality. Orders include CBC, ABG, CC1, PT, aPTT, D-dimer, fibrinogen, and LFTs. Pancultures are also collected.

MANAGEMENT

SIRS is treated with admission to the ICU, close observation, and supportive therapy. Fluid repletion is done and monitoring cardiac function through a pulmonary artery catheter (PAC) is often done. SIRS can evolve into sepsis with multiple organ failure, as discussed below.

Table 262 Systemic Inflammatory Response Syndrome (SIRS)

Systemic Inflammatory Response Syndrome (SIRS)	
Presentation	Fever (not always present in the elderly), tachycardia, narrow pulse pressure, hyperpnea, and hypotension in serious cases. There is no end-organ damage, bacteremia, or significant medical support.
Diagnosis	CBC, ABG, CC1, PT, aPTT, D-dimer, fibrinogen, and LFTs. Pancultures are also collected.
Treatment	Admission to the ICU, close observation, and supportive therapy. Fluid repletion, and monitoring cardiac function through a (PAC) is often done.

SEPSIS

ETIOLOGY

The most common cause of sepsis is from gram positive and gram negative bacterial infection migrating to the bloodstream. Most sepsis leading to shock tends to be from gram negative bacteria. The most common source is genitourinary, followed by respiratory and abdomen.

PATHOPHYSIOLOGY

Sepsis leading to shock is the result of progressive SIRS. Diversion of blood flow from the central circulation to the peripheral vessels due to increased heat production from hypermetabolism is the underlying pathophysiologic mechanism. Without fluid repletion at this stage, ischemia of central tissues begins to occur. A diffuse increase in microvascular permeability also occurs secondary to the inflammatory response taking place. Left uncontrolled, the end result is a decrease in urine output from renal hypoperfusion, hypotension from diversion of intravascular volume, and warming of the extremities due to decreased systemic vascular resistance (SVR). Cardiac output increases in an attempt to compensate for the hypotension. Decreased oxygen consumption leads to an increase in mixed venous oxygen content.

PRESENTATION AND DIAGNOSIS

Sepsis meets the criteria for SIRS in addition to a symptomatic bacteremia. Organ dysfunction may also be present. Sepsis typically has an identifiable source of infection and numerous general symptoms are often present. Fever and mental status changes are common. IV lines should be immediately tested and changed, especially central lines. A complete physical exam should be done to identify whether other sources exist. Respiratory alkalosis is often present. Virtually any rampant infection or significant disease process can lead to SIRS and evolve into full-blown sepsis. Laboratory analysis proceeds in a manner similar to that of SIRS. CXR, US, and CT are also often used as necessary. Glucocorticoids in shock lead to insulin resistance. The resulting hyperglycemia is the earliest sign of impending sepsis and may occur up to 24 hours preceding hypotension, low SVR, high CO, and warm extremities. Respiratory alkalosis is, hyperventilation, and altered mental status are other early signs of sepsis. Sepsis is associated with an increase in IL6. Late sepsis will progress with worsening hypotension, a decrease in cardiac output from poor filling pressures (low CVP and BV), increased PVR (compensatory), cold extremities, conversion to lactic acidosis with metabolic acidosis, and hypoventilation.

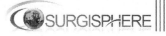

TREATMENT

Supportive therapy and maintaining organ perfusion are essential to decrease morbidity and mortality. Antibiotics as discussed above are essential for most cases of sepsis. Infection by IV lines may be treated with imipenem, meropenem, cefoperazone, cefepime, or vancomycin. Activated protein C (Xigris) used in the treatment of sepsis leads to fibrinolysis.

Table 263 Sepsis

Sepsis	
Etiology	Infection
Presentation	Sepsis meets the criteria for SIRS in addition to a symptomatic bacteremia. Organ dysfunction may also be present. Fever and mental status changes are common. Respiratory alkalosis is often present.
Treatment	IV-lines should be immediately tested and changed, especially central lines. A complete physical exam should be done to identify whether other sources exist. Laboratory analysis proceeds in a manner similar to that of SIRS. CXR, US, and CT are also often used as necessary. Supportive therapy and maintaining organ perfusion are essential to decrease morbidity and mortality. Antibiotics as discussed above are essential for most cases of sepsis. Infection by IV lines may be treated with imipenem, meropenem, cefoperazone, cefepime, or vancomycin.

ANESTHESIA

VENTILATION

Increasing PEEP leads to increased recruitment of alveoli. PEEP also leads to a redistribution of blood flow to the cortex in the kidney.

ANESTHETICS AND ANALGESICS

ANTICHOLINERGICS – NICOTINIC ANTAGONISTS

Table 264 Anticholinergics – Nicotinic Antagonists

DRUG	INDICATIONS	MECHANISM OF ACTION	CONTRAINDICATIONS	NOTES
Succinylcholine	Muscle paralysis Mechanical ventilation	Rapid onset, short duration with decrease in excitatory potential; noncompetitive Initial stage: prolonged depolarization → fasciculations, muscle pain. Second stage: repolarization but blockade of receptors.	Malignant hyperthermia possible with use of Halothane Avoid in patients with increased ICP, burns, DMD, crush injury, MS, and hyperkalemia. May lead to arrhythmia and bradycardia.	Depolarizing NMJ agent Use neostigmine as second stage antidote. No antidote for first stage. Directly competes with acetylcholine.
Cisatracurium		Nicotinic receptor blockade		Cisatracurium is preferred in patients with renal or liver failure due to **Hoffman degradation**.
Vecuronium		Nicotinic receptor blockade	No cardiac effects (pancuronium leads to	Nondepolarizing NMJ agents. Reverse with neostigmine or

			tachycardia)	edrophonium.	
Rocuronium	Facilitate tracheal intubation	Competes for cholinergic receptor at motor end-plates		Nondepolarizing NMJ agents. Reverse with neostigmine or edrophonium.	
Pancuronium			Leads to tachycardia		
Dantrolene	NMS and malignant hyperthermia	Interferes with calcium ion release by sarcoplasmic reticulum	Active hepatic disease, OPD	Calcium channel blocker	
Sildenafil	ED Pulmonary HTN Raynaud phenomenon	PDE-5 blocker that increases cGMP	Vasodilation Priapism MI Arrhythmia and SCD	MI w/ nitrates Do not use if Hx of MI, hypotension, renal or hepatic disease, and retinal disorders	

⚠ Malignant hyperthermia presents as a disorder of calcium metabolism with decreased reuptake by the sarcoplasmic reticulum leading to increased intracellular calcium. An early sign of malignant hyperthermia is an increase in end tidal CO2. The first physical finding is the presence of spasms in the masseter.

⚠ The muscle that is the last to be paralyzed and the first to recover from paralysis is the diaphragm.

SEDATIVES AND HYPNOTICS

Table 265 Sedatives and Hypnotics

DRUG	INDICATIONS	MECHANISM OF ACTION	COMPLICATIONS	NOTES
Midazolam	Preanesthetic		Myocardial depression	Short-acting.
Diazepam	Preanesthetic			Long-acting
Flumazenil	Reversal of sedative effects of benzodiazepines	Competitively inhibits benzodiazepine receptor site	Seizures	Not recommended in cyclic antidepressant poisoning Leads to amnesia, no analgesia

ANESTHETICS – INHALED

Table 266 Inhaled Anesthetics

DRUG	INDICATIONS	COMPLICATIONS	CONTRAINDICATIONS	NOTES
Halothane	Anesthesia	Bradycardia, hepatitis, malignant hyperthermia, arrhythmia, respiratory depression, increased ICP	CV disease, hepatic disease	
Sevoflurane	Anesthesia	Bradycardia, respiratory depression, increased ICP		Rapid onset
Nitrous oxide	Anesthesia	Minimal		Lowest potency, combined with other agents
Desflurane	Anesthesia	Airway irritation, coughing, respiratory depression, increased ICP		Most rapid onset

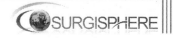

ANESTHETICS – INTRAVENOUS

Table 267 Intravenous Anesthetics

DRUG	INDICATIONS	MECHANISM OF ACTION	COMPLICATIONS	CONTRAINDICATIONS	NOTES
Midazolam	Endoscopy		Respiratory depression, amnesia		Benzodiazepine; reverse w/ flumazenil
Ketamine	Short procedures	Dissociative anesthetic	↑CV, hallucinations, ↑ICP	HTN, stroke.	Amnesia, analgesia, muscle relaxation
Morphine !	GETA	Hyperpolarization and presynaptic inhibition at the mu opioid receptor. Net effect is change in neural activity along various pathways, especially pain pathways.	Substance abuse and dependence, **respiratory depression (brainstem CO2 response), miosis (Edinger-Westphal), CNS depression**, constipation, nausea/vomiting (CTZ)	Emphysema, cor pulmonale	Opioid, good analgesia No tolerance to miosis or constipation. Morphine binds to mu, enkephalins bind to delta, and dynorphins bind to kappa. Codeine is a partial mu agonist.
Fentanyl ⚠	GETA	Lipid soluble, 100X potent compared to morphine	Muscle rigidity at high doses that impedes ventilation		Opioid, good analgesia.. Tolerated in large doses due to lack of histamine response.
Propofol !	Short procedures	Amnestic and sedative, but not analgesic.	Hypotension		No cumulative effects, strict aseptic technique must be maintained.

!　Visceral pain is carried by C-fibers. Nociceptive stimuli are carried via afferent nerves of the spinothalamic tract.

⚠　A risk of general anesthesia in diabetes mellitus is hypoglycemia.

ANESTHETICS – LOCAL

Table 268 Local Anesthetics

DRUG	INDICATIONS	MECHANISM OF ACTION	COMPLICATIONS	NOTES
Lidocaine !	Local anesthesia		Toxicity signs: lightheadedness, dizziness, metallic taste, tinnitus, circumoral paresthesia, numbness, seizure, arrhythmia, cardiac collapse	Greater amounts needed in infected tissue (acidic tissue) Smaller fibers affected first, so pain is lost first, then T, touch, and finally P Give with epinephrine to increase local effects No allergic cross reactivity between esters and amides. Long duration.
Bupivacaine	Local anesthesia	Amides Penetrate in uncharged form, then bind in charged form	CV toxicity	

⚠ Spinal anesthetics are contraindicated when ICP is increased.

ANXIOLYTICS – TYPICAL

Table 269 Typical Anxiolytics

DRUG	INDICATIONS	MECHANISM OF ACTION	COMPLICATIONS	CONTRAINDICATIONS	NOTES
Clonazepam ⚠	Panic disorder Anxiety disorder Absence seizures		CNS depressant.	↑LFTs, glaucoma, pregnancy.	Intermediate-acting
Diazepam ⚠	Anxiety Sedation Withdrawal states	GABA_A receptor agonist that leads to increased frequency of chloride channel opening to decrease synaptic activity	CNS depressant.	Glaucoma, pregnancy, children.	🔍 Longest acting 🔍 Three active metabolites
Midazolam	Sedation Anesthesia		CNS depressant.		Shortest-acting benzodiazepine

BARBITURATES

Table 270 Barbiturates

DRUG	INDICATIONS	MECHANISM OF ACTION	COMPLICATIONS	CONTRAINDICATIONS
Phenobarbital ⚠	Anxiolytic Hypnotic Sedative	Facilitates GABA_A and increase length of chloride channel opening to decrease neuronal firing	Induce tolerance Low therapeutic index Respiratory depression Myocardial suppression	Severe withdrawal

ANALGESICS – NSAIDS

Table 271 NSAIDs

DRUG	INDICATIONS	MECHANISM OF ACTION	COMPLICATIONS	CONTRAINDICATIONS	NOTES
Ibuprofen ⚠	Analgesia Anti-inflammatory Antipyretic	Reversible inhibition of COX-1 and COX-2	Nephrotoxicity, aplastic anemia, PUD	PUD. Renal patients	Block prostaglandin synthesis
Indomethacin ⚠	Analgesia Anti-inflammatory Antipyretic	Reversible inhibition of COX-1 and COX-2	Nephrotoxicity, aplastic anemia, PUD	PUD. Renal patients	Also used to close a PDA
Acetaminophen ⚠	Analgesic Antipyretic	Reversible inhibition of COX in CNS	Hepatic necrosis in OD, glutathione depletion	Hepatitis.	Peripheral inactivation **NOT an anti-inflammatory** Treat OD with N-acetylcysteine
Aspirin ⚠	Analgesic	Irreversible	PUD, Reye	ETOH, **do NOT use in children especially with VZV or influenza**	No effect on PT or PTT Low doses decrease

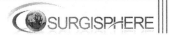

	COX-1 and	syndrome,	**infection**	uric acid secretion
Antipyretic	COx-2	tinnitus, reflex		High doses decrease
Anti-inflammatory	inhibition inhibits prostaglandin formation	acidosis from reflex hypoventilation due to initial hyperventilation (late stage poisoning)		uric acid reabsorption
Antiplatelet aggregation				

FLUID AND ELECTROLYTES

ELECTROLYTE DISTURBANCES

HYPONATREMIA

ETIOLOGY AND PATHOPHYSIOLOGY

Hyponatremia is a plasma sodium less than 135 mEq/L. It is separated into three categories: hypotonic hyponatremia, isotonic hyponatremia, and hypertonic hyponatremia. Hypotonic hyponatremia is divided into hypovolemic hypotonic hyponatremia, isovolemic hypotonic hyponatremia, and hypervolemic hypotonic hyponatremia. Hypovolemic hypotonic hyponatremia is commonly caused by diuretics, salt-wasting syndromes, vomiting, diarrhea, burns, and third-spacing as in pancreatitis or peritonitis. Isovolemic hypotonic hyponatremia is caused by renal failure, secretion of inappropriate antidiuretic hormone (SIADH), deficiencies in glucocorticoids, hypothyroidism, and various medications. Hypervolemic hypotonic hyponatremia is a result of cirrhosis, CHF, and nephrotic syndrome. Isotonic hyponatremia can be attributed to excessive isotonic infusions with glucose or mannitol, and pseudohyponatremia. Hypertonic hyponatremia is caused by hyperglycemia and hypertonic infusions of glucose or mannitol. Glucose increases of more than 100 mL/dL above normal lead to a decrease in sodium concentration by 1.6 mEq/L.

PRESENTATION AND DIAGNOSIS

Moderate hyponatremia presents with confusion, lethargy, anorexia, and myalgia. Severe hyponatremia presents with coma or seizures. Diagnosis is made by examining the osmolarity, carefully assessing the patient for objective signs and symptoms (i.e. tachycardia, dehydration), and measuring serum glucose. Pseudohyponatremia is diagnosed with normal or elevated osmolarity that does not match the calculated osmolarity; common causes include multiple myeloma and hypertriglyceridemia that increase the protein or lipid fraction in the plasma. The sodium deficit can be calculated as follows:

$$Na\ deficit = 0.6 * Wt(kg) * (140 - Na(serum))$$

$$Plasma\ osmolarity = 2 * Na + \frac{Glu}{18} + \frac{BUN}{2.8}$$

TREATMENT

Treatment is to slowly correct the serum sodium, with half corrected in the first 24 hours. A rate no faster than 1 mEq / hr should be used to avoid central pontine myelinolysis (CPM), seizure, and increased intracranial pressure (ICP). Hypovolemic hyponatremia is corrected with 0.9% normal saline (NS); hypervolemic hyponatremia is corrected with sodium and water restriction. ACE-inhibitors may be beneficial in the latter condition. CPM tends to occur in severe hyponatremia, and presents with stupor, confusion, lethargy, and quadriparesis. Some patients recover from CPM over a period of weeks. Conservation of sodium is done through an ADH-independent reabsorption.

Table 272 Hyponatremia

Hyponatremia	
Hypotonic	**Hypovolemic**--diuretics, salt-wasting syndromes, vomiting, diarrhea, burns, and third-spacing **Isovolemic**-- renal failure, SIADH, deficiencies in glucocorticoids, hypothyroidism, & various medications. **Hypervolemic**-- cirrhosis, CHF, and nephrotic syndrome, CPM tends to occur in severe hyponatremia, and presents with stupor, confusion.
Isotonic	Excessive isotonic infusions with glucose or mannitol, and pseudohyponatremia.
Hypertonic	Hyperglycemia and hypertonic infusions of glucose or mannitol.
Presentation	**Moderate** hyponatremia presents with confusion, lethargy, anorexia, & myalgia. **Severe** hyponatremia presents with coma or seizure.
Diagnosis	Examining the osmolarity, carefully assessing the patient for objective signs and symptoms (i.e. tachycardia, dehydration), and measuring serum glucose.
Pseudohyponatremia diagnosis	Normal or elevated osmolarity that does not match the calculated osmolarity; causes include multiple myeloma & hypertriglyceridemia that increase the protein or lipid fraction in the plasma.
Treatment	Correct the serum sodium. Hypovolemic hyponatremia is corrected with 0.9% NS; hypervolemic hyponatremia is corrected with sodium and water restriction. ACE-inhibitors may be beneficial in the latter condition.

HYPERNATREMIA

ETIOLOGY AND PATHOPHYSIOLOGY

Hypernatremia is a serum sodium level greater than 145 mEq/L. It is classified into hypovolemic hypernatremia, isovolemic hypernatremia, and hypervolemic hypernatremia. Hypovolemic hypernatremia is commonly caused by water loss, renal loss through diuretics, GI losses, respiratory losses, or skin losses. Isovolemic hypernatremia is commonly the result of decreased TBW with a decrease in ECF; it may also be due to diabetes insipidus (DI), skin losses, and central defects in osmolarity. Hypervolemic hypernatremia is commonly due to increased TBW with increased sodium, hypertonic fluid or excess salt intake, Conn syndrome, and Cushing syndrome.

PRESENTATION AND DIAGNOSIS

Hypernatremia presents with fatigue, confusion, and lethargy that can progress to seizures and coma.

TREATMENT

Hypovolemic hypernatremia is treated with NS given at 2 mOsm / kg / hr. Isovolemic hypernatremia is treated with 0.45% NaCl (½ NS) with half the water deficit corrected over the first day. No more than 1 mEq / L / hr should be given in an acute setting. Vasopressin is used if the patient has DI. Finally, hypervolemic hypernatremia is treated with ½ NS and loop diuretics to remove excess sodium from the body.

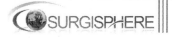

Table 273 Hypernatremia

Hypernatremia	
Hypovolemic	Commonly caused by water loss, renal loss through diuretics, GI losses, respiratory losses, or skin losses.
Isovolemic	Commonly the result of decreased TBW with a decrease in ECF; it may also be due DI, skin losses, & central defects in osmolarity.
Hypervolemic	Commonly due to increased TBW with increased sodium, hypertonic fluid or excess salt intake, Conn syndrome, and Cushing syndrome.
Presentation	Fatigue, confusion, and lethargy that can progress.
Treatment	NS. Vasopressin is used if the patient has DI. Hypervolemic hypernatremia is treated with ½ NS and loop diuretics.

HYPOCHLOREMIA

Hypochloremic alkalosis should be treated with potassium. Vomiting will lead to a hypochloremic metabolic alkalosis.

HYPOKALEMIA

ETIOLOGY AND PATHOPHYSIOLOGY

Hypokalemia is a potassium less than 3.5 mEq / L. Hypokalemia can be attributed to three potential causes, including poor intake (especially in the elderly or in those receiving total parenteral nutrition [TPN]), increased excretion (as in diuretics, mineralocorticoid excess, hyperaldosteronism, osmotic diuresis, excess urine flow, and GI losses from diarrhea or vomiting), and a shift from the extracellular space to the intracellular space (as in acute insulin therapy for hyperglycemia). Other causes include vitamin B12 use, B-blockers, correcting digoxin toxicity with antibody therapy, and alkalosis (each 0.1 pH increase leads to a shift of 0.5 mEq / L of K+).

PRESENTATION AND DIAGNOSIS

Hypokalemia presents with HTN, if the underlying cause is primary hyperaldosteronism or licorice ingestion, while hypotension may suggestion laxative abuse, Bartter syndrome, or bulimia. Hypokalemia may also present with flaccidity, muscle weakness, and loss of deep tendon reflexes (DTRs). Arrhythmia can also occur. Diagnosis is commonly with UA.

TREATMENT

Medical treatment is composed of preventing the potassium loss, replenishing the potassium stores with PO or IV (no more than 10 mEq / hr via peripheral IV due to venous irritation or 40 mEq / hr through central lines in emergent situations), monitoring for hypokalemic toxicity, and avoiding recurrence of symptoms.

Table 274 Hypokalemia

	Hypokalemia
Etiology	Can be attributed to poor intake, increased excretion, and a shift from the extracellular space to the intracellular space. Other causes include vitamin B12 use, B-blockers, correcting digoxin toxicity with antibody therapy, and alkalosis. Hypoaldosteronism.
Presentation	HTN, if the underlying cause is primary hyperaldosteronism or licorice ingestion, while hypotension may suggestion laxative abuse, Bartter syndrome, or bulimia. It may also present with flaccidity, muscle weakness, loss of DTRs, arrhythmia.
Diagnosis	UA
Treatment	Preventing the potassium loss, replenishing the potassium stores with PO or IV, monitoring for hypokalemic toxicity.

HYPERKALEMIA

ETIOLOGY AND PATHOPHYSIOLOGY

Hyperkalemia is the result of either increased intake of potassium, impaired excretion of potassium (the most common cause), or a shift from the intracellular to extracellular space. Decreased excretion is commonly due to potassium-sparing diuretics, ACE-inhibitors, NSAIDs, or type IV RTA. Hyperkalemia is most common in hospitalized patients, in patients who experience rhabdomyolysis, diabetics, and a high risk subset that takes ACE-inhibitors. Mortality occurs with increasing potassium levels, and extremes of age are a positive predictor for mortality. Other implicated drugs include cyclosporine, pentamidine, TMP-SMX, heparin, ketoconazole, and metyrapone. 21-hydroxylase deficiency and 11-beta hydroxylase deficiency are other causes.

PRESENTATION AND DIAGNOSIS

Diagnosis of hyperkalemia is made by renal function tests to identify renal insufficiency, measuring potassium in the urine and plasma along with urine osmolality, and doing an EKG. With elevated potassium, EKG changes (in order) include peaked T waves, PR interval prolongation, QRS widening, disappearance of the P wave, a sine wave pattern, and finally, sinus arrest. Bradycardia may also be present.

TREATMENT

Treatment involves detecting any toxicity caused by the hyperkalemia and treating it. Removing excess sources of potassium is the next step, followed by shifting potassium intracellularly with glucose and insulin administration. Using bicarbonate to repair a metabolic acidosis and using beta-blockers are other effective means of decreasing extracellular potassium. The next step is to increase excretion of potassium with fluorohydrocortisone and stopping any potassium-sparing diuretics and ACE-inhibitors. GI excretion can be increased with potassium-binding resins such as Kayexalate. Dialysis is an option in emergency situations. The last step is to prevent recurrence.

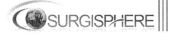

Table 275 Hyperkalemia

Hyperkalemia	
Etiology	Increased intake of potassium, impaired excretion of potassium, or a shift from the intracellular to extracellular space. Decreased excretion is commonly due to potassium-sparing diuretics, ACE-inhibitors, NSAIDs, or type IV RTA. Hyperkalemia is most common in hospitalized patients who experience rhabdomyolysis, diabetes, and a high risk subset that takes ACE-inhibitors. Other implicated drugs include cyclosporine, pentamidine, TMP-SMX, heparin, ketoconazole, and metyrapone, 21-hydroxylase deficiency, and 11-beta hydroxylase.
Presentation	Peaked T waves, PR interval prolongation, QRS widening, disappearance of the P wave, a sine wave pattern, and finally, sinus arrest. Bradycardia may also be present.
Diagnosis	Renal function tests to identify renal insufficiency, and doing an EKG.
Treatment	Detecting and treating any toxicity caused by the hyperkalemia. Removing excess sources of potassium, shifting potassium intracellularly with glucose and insulin administration or using bicarbonate to repair a metabolic acidosis and using beta-blockers. Increase excretion of potassium with fluorohydrocortisone and stopping any potassium-sparing diuretics and ACE-inhibitors. GI excretion can be increased with potassium-binding. Dialysis is an option in emergency situations. Calcium when EKG changes are present

HYPOCALCEMIA

ETIOLOGY AND PATHOPHYSIOLOGY

Hypocalcemia is a serum calcium level less than 8.5 mg / dL. Disarray in normal calcium regulation by vitamin D, parathyroid hormone (PTH), and calcitonin along with derangements in magnesium and phosphorus account for the majority of causes of decreased calcium. Other causes include pancreatitis, sepsis, rhabdomyolysis, tumor lysis syndrome, magnesium deficiency, and exposure to toxins such as fluoride, ethanol, phenytoin, citrate, and cimetidine. Hypoalbuminemia from cirrhosis is another cause of hypocalcemia.

PRESENTATION AND DIAGNOSIS

Presentation of hypocalcemia can be gauged by the presence of circumoral paresthesia, a positive Chvostek sign (facial spasm after tapping on the facial nerve anterior to the tragus), and a positive Trousseau sign (spasm of the wrist after stopping forearm blood flow with a blood pressure cuff). Diagnosis is made by electrolyte panels and EKG findings positive for a prolonged QT interval. Always check albumin levels.

TREATMENT

Treatment of hypocalcemia includes identifying any PTH deficit and replacing with vitamin D or calcitriol along with thiazide diuretics to prevent excess calcium excretion, replenishing any decreases in magnesium, phosphate restriction, oral calcium supplementation, and infusion in emergent situations. Calcium gluconate and calcium chloride are useful as supplements.

Table 276 Hypocalcemia

	Hypocalcemia
Etiology	Disarray in normal calcium regulation by vitamin D, irregularities in PTH and calcitonin along with derangements in magnesium and phosphorus. Other causes include pancreatitis, sepsis, rhabdomyolysis, tumor lysis syndrome, hypoalbuminemia, magnesium deficiency, and exposure to toxins such as fluoride, ethanol, phenytoin, citrate, and cimetidine.
Presentation	Presence of circumoral paresthesia, a positive Chvostek sign, and a positive Trousseau sign.
Diagnosis	Electrolyte panels and EKG findings positive for a prolonged QT interval. Check albumin levels.
Treatment	Identifying any PTH deficit and replacing with vitamin D or calcitriol along with thiazide diuretics, replenishing any decreases in magnesium, phosphate restriction, oral calcium supplementation, and infusion in emergent situations.

HYPERCALCEMIA

ETIOLOGY AND PATHOPHYSIOLOGY

Hypercalcemia is diagnosed with a serum calcium level more than 10.5 mg / dL. Calcium levels are tied to albumin levels, which must be measured in order to determine the amount of free ionized calcium. Hypercalcemia primarily affects the kidneys and CNS leading to fatigue, depression, personality changes, confusion, somnolence, and even coma and death. Nephrolithiasis is the most common renal effect. Positive inotropy and arrhythmias are cardiac effects, while GI effects may lead to constipation and anorexia. The vast majority of cases are due to hyperparathyroidism or malignancy. Most cases of malignancy are due to metastasis of an existing cancer to the bone, while the remainder is due to cancers that secrete parathyroid hormone related peptide (PTHrP). Other conditions include vitamin D excess, granulomatosis, vitamin A excess and renal failure. Some of these specific causes are discussed in more detail below.

PRESENTATION AND DIAGNOSIS

Diagnosis of hypercalcemia includes the presence of the symptoms discussed above. Dehydration is common, and metastatic calcifications in other tissues are common in more severe cases, particularly if phosphorus is also high. PTH levels should be measured and a search for malignancy should be undertaken. A shortened QT interval may be present on EKG. Always check albumin levels.

TREATMENT

Treatment involves volume repletion, mobilization, reducing GI calcium absorption with prednisone and oral phosphate, preventing bone resorption with biphosphonates such as pamidronate, etidronate, risedronate, and alendronate, and administering calcitonin. Dialysis may also be used in more serious cases. A surgical option includes a partial parathyroidectomy. Hypercalcemia with diarrhea should begin a search for MEN syndrome; gastrin levels should be measured.

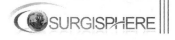

Table 277 Hypercalcemia

	Hypercalcemia
Etiology	Primarily affects the kidneys and CNS leading to fatigue, depression, personality changes, confusion, somnolence, and even coma and death. Nephrolithiasis is the most common renal effect. Positive inotropy and arrhythmias are cardiac effects, while GI effects may lead to constipation and anorexia. The vast majority of cases are due to hyperparathyroidism or malignancy. Most cases of malignancy are due to metastasis of an existing cancer to the bone, while the remainder is due to cancers that secrete PTHrP. Other conditions include vitamin D excess, granulomatosis, vitamin A excess, and renal failure.
Presentation	Presence of the symptoms discussed above. Dehydration is common, and metastatic calcifications in other tissues is common in more severe cases, particularly if phosphorus is also high.
Diagnosis	PTH levels should be measured and a search for malignancy should be undertaken. EKG. Check albumin levels.
Treatment	Volume repletion, mobilization, reducing GI calcium absorption with prednisone and oral phosphate, preventing bone resorption with biphosphonates such as pamidronate, etidronate, risedronate, and alendronate, and administering calcitonin. Dialysis may also be used in more serious cases. A surgical option includes a partial parathyroidectomy. Hypercalcemic coma should be treated with fluid and lasix; dialysis is the first line therapy.

HYPOPHOSPHATEMIA

ETIOLOGY AND PATHOPHYSIOLOGY

Phosphate levels less than 2.5 mg / dL qualify as hypophosphatemia. Poor intake or relatively low intake, increased excretion, and a shift from extracellular to intracellular space are three causes for hypophosphatemia. Alcoholics, patients with eating disorders, Crohn disease, vitamin D deficiency, RTA, antacids that bind to phosphate, hyperparathyroidism, hypokalemia, hypomagnesemia, volume expansion, and acetazolamide are some of the specific causes for hypophosphatemia.

PRESENTATION AND DIAGNOSIS

Presentation of hypophosphatemia includes rhabdomyolysis with muscle weakness, seizures and coma, hemolytic anemia, and platelet dysfunction. Hypophosphatemia is diagnosed by ruling out glucose and insulin infusion, ruling out respiratory alkalosis, and measuring the urine phosphate content. Losses less than 100 mg / d indicate loss due to GI causes or to internal redistribution of phosphate. Losses greater than 100 mg / d indicate possible Fanconi syndrome. High serum calcium points towards primary hyperparathyroidism or malignancy, while low serum calcium points towards secondary hyperparathyroidism, rickets, renal failure, and familial causes.

TREATMENT

Treatment for hypophosphatemia includes oral repletion in minor cases or IV administration if severe. Vitamin D supplementation is also often given. Parathyroidectomy may be indicated with parathyroid causes of hypophosphatemia.

Table 278 Hypophosphatemia

	Hypophosphatemia
Etiology	Poor intake or relatively low intake, increased excretion, and a shift from extracellular to intracellular. Alcoholics, patients with eating disorders, Crohn disease, vitamin D deficiency, RTA, antacids that bind to phosphate, hyperparathyroidism, hypokalemia, hypomagnesemia, volume expansion, and acetazolamide.
Presentation	Rhabdomyolysis with muscle weakness, seizures and coma, hemolytic anemia, and platelet dysfunction.
Diagnosis	Rule out: glucose and insulin infusion, respiratory alkalosis. Measure the urine phosphate content.
Treatment	Oral repletion in minor cases or IV administration if severe. Vitamin D supplementation is also often given. Parathyroidectomy may be indicated with parathyroid causes.

REFEEDING SYNDROME

Refeeding syndrome is due to hypophosphatemia with respiratory weakness exacerbated by feeding a patient. The high carbohydrate load and insulin response leads to decreased availability of phosphate as it is moved intracellularly. This leads to a failure in ATP production. Treatment is to replete phosphate. Hypophosphatemia following refeeding presents as respiratory failure due to the phosphorylation of glucose intermediaries and a drop in available PO4 and subsequent loss of ATP generation.

HYPERPHOSPHATEMIA

ETIOLOGY AND PATHOPHYSIOLOGY

Hyperphosphatemia is diagnosed with a phosphate level greater than 5 mg / dL in the serum. It is commonly due to excessive intake such as with vitamin D intoxication, decreased excretion through renal failure or hypoparathyroidism (including pseudohypoparathyroidism and hypomagnesemia), and a shift from intracellular to extracellular space (as in rhabdomyolysis and tumor lysis syndrome).

PRESENTATION AND DIAGNOSIS

Presentation of hyperphosphatemia includes hypocalcemia and malignant calcification. Most patients are asymptomatic, but muscle cramps, perioral paresthesia, uremic symptoms, and general malaise can all occur.

TREATMENT

Treatment of hyperphosphatemia involves treating renal failure, dietary restriction, phosphate binders such as calcium carbonate, insulin and glucose infusion as a temporary measure, and dialysis in more serious cases.

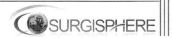

Table 279 Hyperphosphatemia

Hyperphosphatemia	
Etiology	Excessive intake, decreased excretion through renal failure or hypoparathyroidism (including pseudohypoparathyroidism and hypomagnesemia), and a shift from intracellular to extracellular space.
Presentation	Hypocalcemia & malignant calcification. Most patients are asymptomatic, but muscle cramps, perioral paresthesia, uremic symptoms, and general malaise can occur.
Treatment	Treating renal failure, dietary restriction, phosphate binders, insulin and glucose infusion as a temporary measure, and dialysis in more serious cases.

HYPOMAGNESEMIA

ETIOLOGY AND PATHOPHYSIOLOGY

Hypomagnesemia is defined as a magnesium level less than 1.8 mg / dL. It is commonly due to malabsorption or poor dietary intake, excess excretion (due to diarrhea, diuretics, ATN, hypokalemia, hypercalciuria, or endocrine disturbances), and redistribution within the body (hypoalbuminemia, pancreatitis, glucose and insulin administration), and in prolonged exercise.

PRESENTATION AND DIAGNOSIS

Hypomagnesemia presents with weakness, increased reflexes, seizures, hypokalemia, and hypocalcemia. EKG changes include prolonged QT, flattened T waves, and a prolonged PR interval. Atrial fibrillation is a complication, and Torsade de pointes may occur.

TREATMENT

Treatment of hypomagnesemia is by oral magnesium oxide supplements or IV magnesium sulfate (MgSO4). Cardiac dysfunction must be addressed. The remaining suggestions for other electrolyte disturbances also apply for hypomagnesemia.

Table 280 Hypomagnesemia

Hypomagnesemia	
Etiology	Commonly due to malabsorption or poor dietary intake, excess excretion such due to diarrhea, diuretics, ATN, hypokalemia, hypercalciuria, or endocrine disturbances, and redistribution within the body as in hypoalbuminemia, pancreatitis, glucose and insulin administration, and in prolonged exercise.
Presentation	Weakness, increased reflexes, seizures, hypokalemia, and hypocalcemia. Alcoholic patients with hypomagnesemia will present as if they have hypocalcemia; magnesium should be given first.
Diagnosis	EKG changes include prolonged QT, flattened T waves, and a prolonged PR interval. Atrial fibrillation is a complication, and Torsade de pointes may occur.
Treatment	Magnesium oxide supplements or IV magnesium sulfate. Cardiac dysfunction must be addressed. Suggestions for other electrolyte disturbances also apply.

HYPERMAGNESEMIA

ETIOLOGY AND PATHOPHYSIOLOGY

Hypermagnesemia is diagnosed by a serum magnesium titers greater than 2.3 mg / dL. It is typically due to renal failure with decreased excretion, abuse of antacids containing magnesium, tumor lysis syndrome or rhabdomyolysis, redistribution in DKA or pheochromocytoma, and toxicity from lithium.

PRESENTATION AND DIAGNOSIS

Hypermagnesemia presents with decreased DTR, hypotension, paresthesia, coma, and specific EKG changes. EKG changes are opposite of those found with hypomagnesemia.

TREATMENT

Treatment of hypermagnesemia is to treat the EKG changes with IV calcium and use dialysis to regain normal magnesium homeostasis.

Table 281 Hypermagnesemia

Hypermagnesemia	
Etiology	Due to renal failure with decreased excretion, abuse of antacids containing magnesium, tumor lysis syndrome or rhabdomyolysis, redistribution in DKA or pheochromocytoma, and toxicity from lithium.
Presentation	Decreased DTR, hypotension, paresthesia, coma, and specific EKG changes.
Diagnosis	EKG
Treatment	IV calcium and use dialysis to regain normal magnesium homeostasis.

NUTRITION

NUTRITIONAL REQUIREMENTS

Familiarity with nutritional requirements and energy content of various sources of intake are an important component of providing appropriate nutritional care to the surgical patient. The tables and formulas below are an important mainstay in therapy. The major source of protein turnover is skeletal muscle, which becomes significant in prolonged starvation, acute injury, and other deviations from the baseline.

Table 282 Energy Content

Energy Content	
Carbohydrate	3.4 kcal / g
Protein	4 kcal / g
Lipid	9 kcal / g

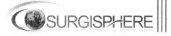

Table 283 Crystalloid Contents

Crystalloid Contents	
Normal saline	154 mEq Na, 154 mEq Cl
Lactated ringers	130 mEq Na, 4 mEq K, 2.7 mEq Ca, 109 mEq Cl, 28 mEq HCO3

The Harris-Benedict equation is used to determine basal energy expenditure. Various modifications are used to determine the estimated caloric needs for patients. The equation varies for men and women. The average caloric need for a 70kg male is about 1700kcal/day. The average caloric need for a 70kg female is slightly less. The metabolic cart can also be used to calculate overall nutritional status and the respiratory quotient. Indirect calorimetry works by calculating CO_2 production. The respiratory quotient is calculated as the ratio between CO_2 produced to O_2 consumed.

$$Male\ BEE = 66 + 13.7 * Wt(kg) + 5 * Ht(cm) - 6.8 * Age$$

$$Female\ BEE = 655 + 9.6 * Wt(kg) + 1.7 * Ht(cm) - 4.7 * Age$$

The respiratory quotient is a unitless number calculated as the **ratio between the amount of carbon dioxide produced and the amount of oxygen consumed.** This value typically correlates to the caloric value for each liter of carbon dioxide produced.

Table 284 Respiratory Quotient

Process	Respiratory Quotient
Carbohydrate oxidation	1
Fat oxidation	0.7
Protein breakdown	0.8
Lipogenesis	> 1.0
Normal	0.8

Table 285 Energy Requirements

Energy Requirements	
Protein requirement	0.9-1.5g/kg/day of protein (normal requirements)
	2-3 g/kg/day of protein (severe burn or sepsis requirements)
	Limit total intake to 40-50g/day in hepatic failure.
Nitrogen balance	Nitrogen:non-protein calories = 1:100-1:200

ENTERAL AND PARENTERAL NUTRITION

Parenteral feeding should be avoided except with specific indications due to the significant morbidity and mortality associated with TPN. Enteral feeding provides the advantage of a decreased risk of sepsis through line infection, induction of the immune system through activation of IgA and stimulation of the small intestine, and maintenance of the gastrointestinal tract. This leads to increased integrity of the GI tract with decreased spontaneous bacterial translocation across the cell wall. The induction of gastrin and other mediators leads to increased insulin release and subsequent anabolic effects. Enteral nutrition, however, has a decreased rate of absorption in the immediate postoperative period. This by itself is not an indication for TPN.

Indications for TPN include malfunction of the gastrointestinal tract, such as in prolonged complete bowel obstruction, the development of high output enterocutaneous fistula, advanced Crohn disease or ulcerative colitis, severe pancreatitis, or congenital or structural anomalies of the GI tract. Patients with severe malnourishment may do well with TPN as an adjunct. Patients with severe burns, head trauma, sepsis, or those receiving high doses of chemoradiation therapy may also benefit from TPN.

Table 286 TPN Composition

TPN Composition	
Protein content	1 g/kg/day (1g nitrogen = 6.25g protein)
Caloric content	4 cal/g x 1g x wt (kg)
Non-protein content	25 cal/kg/day
Water	30-40 mL/kg/day
Total energy	30-60 kcal/kg/day
Amino acids	1-2 g/kg/day
Essential minerals	Acetate/gluconate, calcium, chloride, chromium, copper, iodine, magnesium, manganese, phosphorus, potassium, selenium, sodium, zinc

TPN should be stopped slowly over a period of time to avoid hypoglycemia. The rate of TPN should initially be reduced to 50 ml/hr for several hours, and then stopped. Sudden discontinuation of TPN should be treated with a solution of D10W.

ESSENTIAL AMINO ACIDS

Arginine is an essential amino acid that augments the immune system Glutamine is the amino acid most abundant in circulation Glutamine levels following intestinal surgery are decreased due to an increase in utilization by the intestinal cells.

MALNUTRITION AND OBESITY

OBESITY

ETIOLOGY AND PATHOPHYSIOLOGY

Obesity is an epidemic in the United States, affecting nearly a quarter or more of the population with some estimates indicating nearly half of the population meeting the criteria for excess body fat. It is especially common in American Indians, Hawaiians, Hispanics, and African Americans. Obesity is defined as having a body mass index (BMI) over the 85th percentile or more than 30 kg / m^2, calculated as follows:

$$BMI = \frac{weight\,(kg)}{height\,(m^2)}$$

Obesity appears to be partially related to a genetic inheritance, but changes in society, poor diet, and poor exercise all contribute. Complications of obesity lead to obstructive sleep apnea (OSA), pseudotumor cerebri, liver dysfunction,

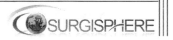

psychosocial impairments, increased cardiovascular disease, HTN, hypertriglyceridemia, arthritis, and numerous other complications. Other causes of obesity include Prader-Willi syndrome, pseudohypoparathyroidism, Down syndrome, Turner syndrome, growth hormone deficiencies, hypothyroidism, and other endocrinologic dysfunction, PCOS, and use of various medications including antidepressants and oral contraceptives.

PRESENTATION AND DIAGNOSIS

Obesity is diagnosed as a BMI over 30 kg / m^2. Numerous concomitant illnesses or diseases may be present.

TREATMENT

Treatment of obesity is a multifaceted response that involves modifications in lifestyle, avoiding additional risk factors (such as smoking or alcohol abuse), and treating any concomitant disorders such as DM, HTN, CVA, and heart disease. The last resort is surgical intervention in the form of bariatric surgery – this is typically used in patients with a BMI exceeding 40 or double their ideal body weight (IBW).

Table 287 Obesity

	Obesity
Etiology	Genetic inheritance, but changes in society, poor diet, and poor exercise all contribute. Other causes of obesity include Prader-Willi syndrome, pseudohypoparathyroidism, Down syndrome, Turner syndrome, growth hormone deficiencies, hypothyroidism, and other endocrinologic dysfunction, PCOS, and use of various medications including antidepressants and oral contraceptives.
Presentation	A BMI over 30 kg / m^2. Numerous concomitant illnesses or diseases may be present.
Treatment	Modifications in lifestyle, avoiding additional risk factors, and treating any concomitant. The last resort is surgical intervention in the form of bariatric surgery.

MALNUTRITION

ETIOLOGY AND PATHOPHYSIOLOGY

Malnutrition may present as kwashiorkor or marasmus, with the former having a telltale sign of significant edema due to protein starvation. Marasmus has both protein and caloric starvation. Deficiencies in multiple vitamins and significantly poor diet are commonly implicated for malnutrition. There are systemwide effects with significant cognitive and physical retardation, and diminished immune activity. Severe malnutrition is rare in the United States; nearly 150 million children worldwide are affected by malnutrition. Chronic illness and multiple food allergies may also lead to malnutrition.

PRESENTATION AND DIAGNOSIS

Malnutrition presents with weight loss, falling off the normal growth curves, and with behavioral changes leading to apathy, anxiety, and deficits in cognition and attention. Iron deficiency presents with constitutional symptoms, anemia, decreased cognition, headache, glossitis, and koilonychia. Vitamin D deficiency presents with hypocalcemia, rickets, and growth retardation. Vitamin A deficiency presents with night blindness, growth retardation, xerophthalmia, and hair changes. Iodine deficiency presents with goiter and physical and mental retardation. Folate and vitamin B12 deficiency have been previously discussed in the form of anemia. Physical exam detects anasarca with kwashiorkor. Cheilosis, angular stomatitis, fatty hepatomegaly, and skin hyperpigmentation with peeling are present. Thin and brittle hair is commonly found. Albumin is not recommended for acute monitoring as changes tend to occur over time from the high half-life. Pre-albumin has a shorter half-life.

TREATMENT

Treatment involves identifying the particular dietary inadequacies and having a full replacement of missing proteins, calories, vitamins, and minerals. Up to 150 kcal / kg / d may be necessary to regain the weight deficit. Severe cases require admission to a medical facility.

Table 288 Malnutrition

Malnutrition	
Etiology	Deficiencies in multiple vitamins, and significantly poor diet are commonly implicated for malnutrition. Chronic illness and multiple food allergies may also lead to malnutrition.
Presentation	Weight loss, falling off the normal growth curves, and behavioral changes leading to apathy, anxiety, and deficits in cognition and attention. Iron deficiency presents with constitutional symptoms, anemia, decreased cognition, headache, glossitis, and koilonychia. Vitamin D deficiency presents with hypocalcemia, rickets, and growth retardation. Vitamin A deficiency presents with night blindness, growth retardation, xerophthalmia, and hair changes. Iodine deficiency presents with goiter and physical and mental retardation.
Treatment	Identifying the particular dietary inadequacies and having a full replacement of missing proteins, calories, vitamins, and minerals.

VITAMIN DEFICITS

VITAMIN A DEFICIENCY

ETIOLOGY

Retinol deficiency is primarily due to poor diet and excessive rice consumption, and secondarily due to malabsorption syndromes and malnutrition syndromes.

PRESENTATION

Vitamin A deficiency presents with growth retardation, night blindness, xerophthalmia, keratomalacia, follicular hyperkeratosis, and Bitot spots with foamy patches in the conjunctiva. Treat with vitamin A administration.

VITAMIN C DEFICIENCY

ETIOLOGY

Vitamin C deficiency is due to poor diet, pregnancy, thyrotoxicosis, inflammatory disease, after surgery, burns, and diarrhea.

PRESENTATION

Scurvy presents with splinter hemorrhages in the nail bed, swollen and friable gums, loss of teeth, breakdown of old scars, poor healing, spontaneous hemorrhage, petechiae, and hyperkeratotic hair follicles. Treat with ascorbic acid administration.

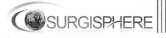

VITAMIN D DEFICIENCY

ETIOLOGY

Vitamin D deficiency is primarily due to poor sunlight exposure or poor intake of calcium or phosphorus. Secondary causes include hypoparathyroidism, hereditary diseases, and poor absorption.

PRESENTATION

The effect of vitamin D deficiency is rickets in children and osteomalacia in adults. Treatment is adequate intake of calcium, phosphorus, and vitamin D supplements.

VITAMIN E DEFICIENCY

ETIOLOGY

Tocopherol deficiency is a natural state in infants but may present later in life with poor intake, malabsorption syndromes, or genetic causes.

PRESENTATION

Vitamin E deficiency presents with hemolytic anemia, reticulocytosis, hyperbilirubinemia, abetalipoproteinemia, neuropathy such as spinocerebellar ataxia and loss of DTRs, and retinopathy. Treatment is repleting vitamin E stores.

VITAMIN K DEFICIENCY

ETIOLOGY

Vitamin K is a lipid soluble vitamin that is essential for the formation of clotting factors. It is produced by colonic bacteria. Terminal ileum disease prevents normal vitamin K production and absorption. It presents as hemorrhagic disease of newborns (HDN) in infants; in adults, it presents as a bleeding diathesis. Other causes include parenchymal liver disease such as cirrhosis, in which case vitamin K supplements have little effect (fresh frozen plasma [FFP] is required), malabsorption syndromes, biliary disease, cholestyramine, coumadin, and various other medications (INH, rifampin, barbiturates, and others), lupus anticoagulant, DIC, polycythemia vera, cystic fibrosis, and leukemia. Vitamin K is responsible for forming coagulation factor II (prothrombin), factor VII (proconvertin), factor IX (Christmas factor), and factor X (Stuart factor). Protein C, protein S, and several bone matrix proteins reliant on glutamic acid residue conversion by vitamin K are also modified by vitamin K. Loss of bacteria that synthesize vitamin K in the gut and malabsorption syndromes can lead to deficiency. Coumadin therapy may exacerbate vitamin K changes.

PRESENTATION

Vitamin K deficiency, if severe enough, presents as complaints of significant hemorrhage following mild trauma. Ecchymoses, petechiae, hematomas, and oozing of blood are common. GI bleeds, hematuria, menorrhagia, epistaxis, and mucosal bleeds occur frequently. PT and aPTT are elevated. Des-gamma-carboxy prothrombin (DCP) is present in the absence of vitamin K. Phylloquinone is given as therapy.

TREATMENT

Treatment for vitamin K deficiency involves correcting the cause of the underlying deficit and providing vitamin K supplements. FFP is necessary in severe disease. Subcutaneous injections of phylloquinone (vitamin K 1) can be given; menadione (vitamin K 3) can be given orally in malabsorption syndromes. Phytonadione can also be directly injected in severe disease. Green leafy vegetables and oils provide a good source of vitamin K.

Table 289 Vitamin K Deficiency

Vitamin K Deficiency	
Etiology	Terminal ileum disease. Other causes include parenchymal liver disease, malabsorption syndromes, biliary disease, cholestyramine, coumadin, and various other medications, lupus anticoagulant, DIC, polycythemia vera, cystic fibrosis, & leukemia.
Presentation	Significant hemorrhage following mild trauma. Ecchymoses, petechiae, hematomas, and oozing of blood. GI bleeds, hematuria, menorrhagia, epistaxis, and mucosal bleeds.
Diagnosis	PT and aPTT are elevated. DCP is present in the absence of vitamin K.
Treatment	Correct the cause of the underlying deficit and providing vitamin K supplements. FFP is necessary in severe disease.

VITAMIN B1 DEFICIENCY

ETIOLOGY

Primary thiamine deficiency is due to decreased intake especially in a high-rice diet. Secondary deficiency is due to hyperthyroidism, pregnancy, fever, malabsorption syndromes, diarrhea, and liver disease. Alcoholism impairs utilization.

PRESENTATION

Thiamine deficiency presents as dry beriberi with peripheral neurologic symptoms including distal extremity paresthesias, cramps, and pain, CNS symptoms including Wernicke-Korsakoff syndrome (Korsakoff syndrome occurs first with mental confusion and confabulations, Wernicke encephalopathy happens last and consists of nystagmus, ophthalmoplegia, and coma), and cardiovascular symptoms including high output cardiac failure with tachycardia, diaphoresis, warm skin, and lactic acidosis. Shock can occur and death ensues rapidly if treatment is not started in time. Treatment is with thiamine administration and magnesium sulfate given to reduce peripheral resistance to thiamine. Electrolyte replacement may also be necessary.

VITAMIN B2 DEFICIENCY

ETIOLOGY

Riboflavin deficiency is due to decreased intake of milk and animal products; secondary deficiency is due to malabsorption syndromes, diarrhea, liver disease, and alcoholism.

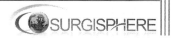

PRESENTATION

Riboflavin deficiency presents with pallor, mucosal ulceration such as angular stomatitis and cheilosis, and linear fissures in the skin commonly infected by *Candida*. A red tongue is present, and cutaneous lesions leading to erythema and acanthosis may occur. Keratitis may lead to lacrimation and photophobia. Riboflavin is treated with repletion.

NICOTINIC ACID DEFICIENCY

ETIOLOGY

Niacin deficiency is due to excessive maize corn consumption, amino acid imbalances, malabsorption syndromes, cirrhosis, and alcoholism. Pellagra ensues.

PRESENTATION

Pellagra presents with a photosensitive rash, red stomatitis, glossitis, bloody diarrhea, and CNS changes. Desquamation, keratosis, edema of the tongue and other mucous membranes, GI discomfort, confabulations, cogwheel rigidity, and psychiatric changes may occur. Tryptophan deficiency may present in a similar manner. Deficiency is treated with niacinamide along with replenishment of other lacking vitamins.

VITAMIN B6 DEFICIENCY

ETIOLOGY

Pyridoxine deficiency is rarely a primary deficiency; secondary causes include the same as those for other vitamins, plus oral contraceptive use, use of hydralazine, cycloserine, or penicillamine, and increase metabolic activity.

PRESENTATION

Seborrheic dermatosis, cheilosis, glossitis, peripheral neuropathy, lymphopenia, seizures, and anemia develop with worsening deficiency. Treatment is to cease offending medications and provide pyridoxine supplements.

BIOTIN DEFICIENCY

ETIOLOGY

Biotin deficiency occurs in raw egg consumption or long term total parenteral nutrition (TPN).

PRESENTATION

Biotin deficiency presents with alopecia, keratoconjunctivitis, immunologic deficiencies, and retardation of development. Treatment is to provide supplements.

Table 290 Vitamin Deficiency

Vitamin	Etiology	Presentation	Treatment
Vitamin Deficiency			
A	Primarily due to poor diet and excessive rice consumption, and secondarily due to malabsorption syndromes and malnutrition syndromes.	Growth retardation, night blindness, xerophthalmia, keratomalacia, follicular hyperkeratosis, and Bitot spots with foamy patches in the conjunctiva.	Vitamin A administration.
B1	Decreased intake, especially in a high-rice diet. Secondary deficiency is due to hyperthyroidism, pregnancy, fever, malabsorption syndromes, diarrhea, and liver disease. Alcoholism impairs utilization.	Dry beriberi with peripheral neurologic symptoms including distal extremity paresthesias, cramps, and pain, CNS symptoms including Wernicke-Korsakoff syndrome, and cardiovascular symptoms including high output cardiac failure with tachycardia, diaphoresis, warm skin, and lactic acidosis. Shock can occur and death ensues rapidly if treatment is not started in time.	Thiamine administration and magnesium sulfate given to reduce peripheral resistance to thiamine. Electrolyte replacement may also be necessary.
B2	Riboflavin deficiency is due to decreased intake of milk and animal products; secondary deficiency is due to malabsorption syndromes, diarrhea, liver disease, and alcoholism.	Pallor, mucosal ulceration such as angular stomatitis and cheilosis, and linear fissures in the skin commonly infected by *Candida*. A red tongue is present, and cutaneous lesions leading to erythema and acanthosis may occur. Keratitis may lead to lacrimation and photophobia.	Repletion
B6	Pyridoxine deficiency is rarely a primary deficiency; secondary causes include the same as those for other vitamins, plus oral contraceptive use, use of hydralazine, cycloserine, or penicillamine, and increase metabolic activity.	Seborrheic dermatosis, cheilosis, glossitis, peripheral neuropathy, lymphopenia, seizures, and anemia develop with worsening deficiency.	Cease offending medications and provide pyridoxine supplements. **Administration** of B6 can **minimize** effects of **homocystinuria**.
Biotin	Occurs in raw egg consumption or long term TPN.	Alopecia, keratoconjunctivitis, immunologic deficiencies, and retardation of development.	Provide supplements
C	Due to poor diet, pregnancy, thyrotoxicosis, inflammatory disease, after surgery, burns, and diarrhea.	Splinter hemorrhages in the nail bed, swollen and friable gums, loss of teeth, breakdown of old scars, poor healing, spontaneous hemorrhage, petechiae, and hyperkeratotic hair follicles	Ascorbic acid administration.
D	Primarily due to poor sunlight exposure or poor intake of calcium or phosphorus. Secondary causes include hypoparathyroidism, hereditary diseases, and poor absorption.	Rickets in children and osteomalacia in adults.	Adequate intake of calcium, phosphorus, and vitamin D supplements
E	A natural state in infants but may present later in life with poor intake, malabsorption syndromes, or genetic causes.	Hemolytic anemia, reticulocytosis, hyperbilirubinemia, abetalipoproteinemia, neuropathy such as spinocerebellar ataxia and loss of DTRs, and retinopathy.	Repleting vitamin E stores.

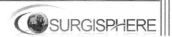

K	Loss of bacteria that synthesize vitamin K in the gut and malabsorption syndromes can lead to deficiency. Coumadin therapy may exacerbate vitamin K changes.	May present as HDN with cutaneous, GI or intrathoracic bleeds, or as hemorrhage later in life. Bruising, mucosal bleeding, hematuria, menorrhagia, and oozing from wounds occurs. PT and aPTT are increased.	Phylloquinone is given as therapy.
Niacin	Niacin deficiency is due to excessive maize corn consumption, amino acid imbalances, malabsorption syndromes, cirrhosis, and alcoholism. Pellagra ensues.	Pellagra presents with a photosensitive rash, red stomatitis, glossitis, bloody diarrhea, and CNS changes. Desquamation, keratosis, edema of the tongue and other mucous membranes, GI discomfort, confabulations, cogwheel rigidity, and psychiatric changes may occur. Tryptophan deficiency may present in a similar manner.	Niacinamide along with replenishment of other lacking vitamins.

A vitamin deficiency that occurs following a Whipple procedure is iron.

VITAMIN TOXICITY

VITAMIN A TOXICITY

Excessive vitamin A causes thickening of hair and increased hair loss throughout the body. As the toxicity worsens, pseudotumor cerebri, headache, and weakness may develop. Hepatosplenomegaly is also seen.

VITAMIN D TOXICITY

Vitamin D toxicity leads to anorexia, nausea, vomiting, polyuria, polydipsia, pruritus, azotemia, proteinuria, metastatic calcifications from hypercalcemia, and anxiety. Consider acidifying the urine and using corticosteroids for treatment.

VITAMIN E TOXICITY

Tocopherol toxicity has few toxic effects other than decreasing the effectiveness of vitamin K, which with coumadin therapy, may lead to spontaneous hemorrhage.

VITAMIN K TOXICITY

Vitamin K toxicity is rare, but very high doses of its precursor, menadione, may lead to hemolytic anemia and kernicterus.

VITAMIN B6 TOXICITY

Excessive vitamin B6 consumption may lead to sensory ataxia and decreased lower extremity proprioception.

Table 291 Vitamin Toxicity

Vitamin	Presentation
A	Thickening of hair and increased hair loss throughout the body. As the toxicity worsens, pseudotumor cerebri, headache, and weakness may develop. Hepatosplenomegaly is also seen.
B6	May lead to sensory ataxia and decreased lower extremity proprioception.
D	Anorexia, nausea, vomiting, polyuria, polydipsia, pruritus, azotemia, proteinuria, metastatic calcifications from hypercalcemia, and anxiety. Consider acidifying the urine and using corticosteroids for treatment.
E	Few toxic effects other than decreasing the effectiveness of vitamin K, which with coumadin therapy, may lead to spontaneous hemorrhage.
K	Rare, but very high doses of its precursor, menadione, may lead to hemolytic anemia and kernicterus.

PRACTICE QUESTIONS

 Due to a defect in the sarcoplasmic reticulum, a patient develops malignant hyperthermia following administration of succinylcholine during induction of anesthesia. Which of the following is the best therapy?

A. Dantrolene, insulin, and bicarbonate
B. Nipride drip, bicarbonate
C. Nitroglycerin, diazepam
D. Dantrolene
E. Hydralazine, plasmapheresis

 The best answer is <u>Dantrolene, insulin, and bicarbonate</u>. The best treatment for malignant hyperthermia caused by succinylcholine or lidocaine is to stop the anesthesia, give dantrolene, followed by insulin and bicarbonate to mitigate the hyperkalemia and acidosis that will follow. This will forestall any further damage and also avoid arrhythmias from the hyperkalemia. Succinylcholine is a competitive agonist that competes with acetylcholine.

 A patient who is undergoing a bedside wound debridement suddenly experiences perioral numbness and tinnitus in his ear, followed by seizures and cardiac arrest. What is the most likely etiology?

A. Lidocaine toxicity
B. Pulmonary embolism
C. Massive cardiovascular accident
D. Toxic hypokalemia
E. Toxic hypercalcemia

 The best answer is <u>Lidocaine toxicity</u>. This patient likely received an overdose of lidocaine leading to perioral paresthesias and tinnitus in his ear. Seizures may follow with sufficient medication, followed by ventricular fibrillation and cardiac arrest. No more than 4-5mg per kg should be used if lidocaine is given without epinephrine. Up to 7mg per kg can be used with epinephrine.

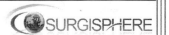

An ICU patient who has significant respiratory compromise is intubated using succinylcholine. During intubation, the patient becomes asystolic. What is the immediate treatment required?

   A. Calcium gluconate, insulin, and epinephrine
   B. Vasopressin
   C. IV KCl with epinephrine
   D. Cardioversion
   E. Etomidate

 The best answer is <u>Calcium gluconate, insulin, and epinephrine</u>. This patient likely developed hyperkalemia due to succinylcholine administration, leading to arrhythmia that degenerated into asystole. Treatment includes bringing the potassium levels down with calcium gluconate, insulin, bicarbonate, and glucose, and treatment with epinephrine. As a result of this complication, succinylcholine is contraindicated in any high potassium state such as burn injury, renal disease, crush injuries to the muscles, and skeletal muscle disorders such as myasthenia gravis.

 Which of the following paralytic agents is best used in a patient with liver and kidney failure?

   A. Atracurium
   B. Propofol
   C. Etomidate
   D. Succinylcholine
   E. Ketamine

 The best answer is <u>Atracurium</u>. The drug of choice for muscle paralysis in patients with combined liver and kidney failure is atracurium as it undergoes breakdown by Hoffman elimination. Propofol is an anesthetic agent that leads to amnesia and sedation, with a side effect of hypotension. Etomidate may lead to adrenal insufficiency. Succinylcholine can lead to arrhythmias and is contraindicated in kidney failure. Ketamine is a smooth muscle relaxant and dissociative amnesic agent used to induce anesthesia. Halothane can cause arrhythmias.

 Which of the following is a contraindication to spinal anesthesia?

   A. Liver surgery
   B. Kidney surgery
   C. Vasculopathy
   D. INR of 1.5
   E. Hypertension

The best answer is <u>Liver surgery</u>. Contraindications to spinal anesthesia include coagulopathy with an INR greater than 1.5, sepsis, increased intracranial pressure, and hepatic surgery.

An 84 year old male who has a myocardial infarction is transferred to the ICU. A Swan-Ganz catheter is floated and a significant elevation in PCWP is noted. What is the underlying cause?

A. Increased EDV, increased SVR, and decreased CO
B. Increased EDV
C. Increased SVR
D. Decreased CO
E. Increased EDV and increased SVR

 The best answer is <u>Increased EDV, increased SVR, and decreased CO</u>. This patient has an increase in end diastolic volume due to cardiac hypocontractility, leading to an increase in systemic vascular resistance. The hypocontractility directly leads to a drop in cardiac output.

 A 76 year old male who has a myocardial infarction is brought to the ICU in cardiogenic shock. Which of the following is the best initial course of therapy?

A. Dobutamine
B. Norepinephrine
C. Milrinone
D. Vasopressin
E. Epinephrine

 The best answer is <u>Dobutamine</u>. The best initial vasopressor is dobutamine due to its improvement in cardiac contractility without significantly increasing myocardial oxygen consumption. The result is a mitigation in ischemic damage due to failure to increase oxygenation. Hypertrophic subaortic stenosis should be treated with ACE inhibitors, beta blockers, and a possible balloon pump placement to decrease myocardial oxygen demand. Pressors that increase oxygen demand should be avoided in hypertrophic subaortic stenosis.

 An ICU patient who has been improving over a period of days cannot be weaned from his ventilator. His tube feeds were recently started and is thought to be the cause of his difficulty. Which of the following is the most likely reason for failure to extubate?

A. Overfeeding
B. Hypoglycemia
C. Starvation
D. Refeeding syndrome
E. TPN toxicity

 The best answer is <u>Overfeeding</u>. Overfeeding leads to increased carbon dioxide production, leading to greater demands on the lungs to remove this from the body. The increased carbon dioxide production is the result of increased nutrient metabolism. Overworking the lungs leads to continued dependence on the ventilator. The treatment is to reduce carbon dioxide production by changing the composition of the tube feeds and re-evaluating intake.

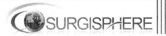

Which of the following is the fastest anesthetic agent that also leads to the most rapid clearing?

A. Propofol
B. Ketamine
C. Midazolam
D. Diazepam
E. Lorazepam

The best answer is Propofol. Propofol is a rapid anesthetic agent with rapid onset and rapid clearing. It is cleared quickly through hepatic metabolism. It is therefore contraindicated in patients with significant hepatic disease.

The ratio of carbon dioxide production to oxygen production for carbohydrates is:

A. 1
B. 0.7
C. 0.5
D. 1.2
E. 1.5

The best answer is 1. The respiratory quotient for carbohydrates is 1. That for fats is 0.7.

Which of the following is the best description of normal nutritional needs for an adult?

A. 25 kcal / kg / day
B. 70 kcal / kg / day
C. 10 kcal / kg / day
D. 50 kcal / kg / hour
E. 20 kcal / kg / hour

The best answer is 25 kcal / kg / day. The best estimate for normal nutritional needs for an adult is 25 kcal / kg / day, or approximately 1750 kcal / day for a 70kg adult. A neonate requires nearly 5 times this amount, at 120 kcal / kg / day. Injuries or increased metabolic stress can double the nutritional needs for an adult to 35-40 kcal / kg / day.

Which of the following is not an indication for TPN?

A. Crohn disease exacerbation

B. Short gut syndrome

C. Pancreatitis

D. Small bowel fistula

E. Small bowel obstruction

 The best answer is <u>Crohn disease exacerbation</u>. The presence of short gut syndrome, pancreatitis, enterocutaneous fistula, small bowel obstruction, or being NPO for more than a week are all indications for TPN. Being NPO for over a week leads to the body breaking down skeletal muscle protein as its chief energy source, leading to significant muscle weakening before the body is able to switch over to lipolysis. Normal TPN should have a glucose concentration of 60%, lipid concentration of 30%, and protein concentration of 10%. Glucose generates 3.4 cals / gm and is given at 5 gm / kg / hr. Lipids generate 9 cals / gm. Protein should be given at 1 gm / kg. The ratio of nitrogen intake to caloric intake should be 1:100; 6.25 grams of protein has 1 gram of nitrogen in it.

TRANSPLANT SURGERY AND IMMUNOLOGY

CHAPTER CONTENTS

IMMUNOLOGY

GENERAL CONCEPTS

PHARMACOLOGY

Table 292 Transplant Medications

DRUG	INDICATIONS	MECHANISM OF ACTION	COMPLICATIONS	CONTRAINDICATIONS	NOTES
Prednisone	Immunosuppression	Suppresses cytokine production and decreases TNF-α action. Bind to intracellular receptors that affect DNA binding proteins and increase gene transcription; decreases MHC upregulation and IFN-gamma production. Inhibits IL-1 expression in macrophages	Dependency. Addisonian crisis if sharp cessation. Hyperglycemia	Use with care in active DM. Use with care in hepatic disease	Improve graft survival
FK506	Maintenance of immunosuppression. Drug of choice	Inhibits IL-2 expression in T-cells by NF-AT inhibition	Similar to cyclosporin but more neurotoxic		Tacrolimus
Mycophenolate	Immunosuppression	Noncompetitive inhibitor of B and T cell proliferation through purine synthesis inhibition (IMP dehydrogenase inhibitor). Works on lymphocytes due to missing salvage pathway for GMP			Cellcept
Cyclosporin	Maintenance of	Inhibits IL-2 expression through	Nephrotoxicity		Also

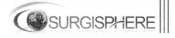

immunosuppression	calcineurin inhibition leading to T-cell inhibition	Fibrosis HTN Hyperkalemia Gingival hyperplasia		increases TGF-B Bile excretion
OKT3	Immunosuppression Acute rejection	Monoclonal antibody to T-cells via CD3 receptor Give with methylprednisone	Cytokine release syndrome: hypotension, pulmonary edema, cardiac depression	Risk of aseptic meningitis
Azathioprine	Antiproliferative and immunosuppressant	Converted to 6-MP by liver to inhibit DNA synthesis (DNA precursor alkylation and chromosomal breakage)	Intestinal sloughing, liver toxicity	Affects all rapidly dividing cells
ALG	Induction agent	Polyclonal antilymphocyte globulin Induction agents shut down T-cell response	Thrombocytopenia, rash, fevers, chills	
Rapamycin	Maintenance of immunosuppression	Impairs IL-2 signal transduction leading to arrest prior to S-phase		Sirolimus

ANTIBODY CLASSES

Table 293 Antibody Classes

TYPE	FEATURES	NOTES	DIFFERENCES
IgG	Monomeric 65%	Most abundant immunoglobulin found throughout the body. Freely crosses the placenta and provides for maternal-fetal immunity during early neonatal period. Binds to wide variety of infective organisms, activates complement (classic pathway) and through opsonization. IgG1 is the most common subtype (IgG1 – 4). IgG2 does not bind to macrophages but is a common antibody to carbohydrates (celiac sprue). IgG3 does not play a role in rheumatoid factor antigen but strongly binds to complement compared to the other IgGs. IgG4 does not fix complement (C1q) or bind to macrophages. Most versatile is IgG1 followed by IgG3. IgG has higher affinity than IgM. May lead to ITP.	**IgG can cross placenta; the others cannot.** Fixes complement, but IgM is more potent. No passive transfer reaction capability. Longest half-life. Long-lasting immunity.
IgM	Monomeric or Pentameric 10%	Primary response to antigen that often signifies early disease. Converted to IgG to give long-lasting immunity. Antigen receptor that is also located on B cell surface. Forms pentamers. High avidity and is the first immunoglobulin to be expressed. IgM has higher avidity than IgG.	Does not cross placenta. Strongly fixes complement. Early antibody response.
IgA	Monomeric or dimeric 20%	IgA1 is readily broken down by bacterial IgA protease. IgA2 is not. Forms dimers. **Secreted on mucus membranes** to play a role in protecting mucosal surfaces. Secretory component added during excretion from epithelial cells. **Also found in breast milk, saliva, tears, GI tract, and lungs.**	Protective barrier on mucosal surfaces. Dimers.
IgD	Monomeric 1%	Found on the surface of B cells and in lesser amounts in serum. Low in concentration with an unclear role to date. Coexpressed with IgM in naïve B cells. Deficiency does not appear to hinder immune function.	Mostly intravascular (like IgM).
IgE	Monomeric 1%	Type I hypersensitivity reaction (anaphylaxis) with a gate-keeper-like function. Induces degranulation from mast cells, basophils, and eosinophils. Very high elevations typically signify parasitic infections. Heat-labile (only one). Does not activate complement.	Passive transfer reaction capability.

- Allotype – amino acid substitutions in constant region due to random change between individuals of a species; used for paternity testing.

- Idiotype – Variations in the variable region within a particular class of immunoglobulins; permits recognition of wide range of epitopes.
- Isotype – Specific classes of immunoglobulins including IgG, IgM, IgA, IgD, and IgE.
- The constant region is an example of an isotype; the variable region is an example of idiotype.

MHC DOMAINS

Table 294 MHC Domains

TYPES	FUNCTION	NOTES
MHC-I	Antigen processing (A, B, C). Binds to CD8 (cytotoxic T-cells → cell-mediated pathway).	Host cell infected by bacteria, virus, or transformed. Found on all nucleated cells and platelets within the body. Transmembrane alpha chain and beta-2-microglobulin. Interacts with cytotoxic T-cells (CD8+ cells) which induce apoptosis, after pairing with antibodies and inducing humoral response. Proteins are generated in cytoplasm. Loading occurs in rough endoplasmic reticulum. Primarily responsible for graft rejection.
MHC-II	Peptide loading (**DM, DP, DQA, DQB, DRA, DRB**) Binds to CD4 (helper T-cells → cell-mediated or humoral pathway).	Macrophage or phagocytic host with bacteria, viruses, or particulate matter. Found on macrophages, dendritic cells, activated T-cells, B-cells. Alpha and beta chain with proteins digested in lysosomes, with presentation to CD4+ helper T-cells (may induce a humoral or cell-mediated immune response). Mediate organ-rejection following transplantation. Loading occurs in lysosome.
MHC-III	Complement, cytokines.	C2, C4, TNF-alpha, and TNF-beta function.

- Human leukocyte antigen genes code for the major histocompatibility complex, and these genes are associated with various diseases (discussed further down) based on linkage disequilibrium (non-Mendelian inheritance).
- The antigen-presenting cells (APCs) are macrophages, dendritic cells, activated T-cells, and B-cells.
- MHC matching (crossmatch) is determined by lymphocytotoxicity assay and the MLC assay. Class I is tested with the lymphocytotoxicity assay; class II is tested by PCR.
- A negative crossmatch improves outcome with kidney, pancreas, and heart transplantation. Crossmatch status has no effect on morbidity with liver transplantation.

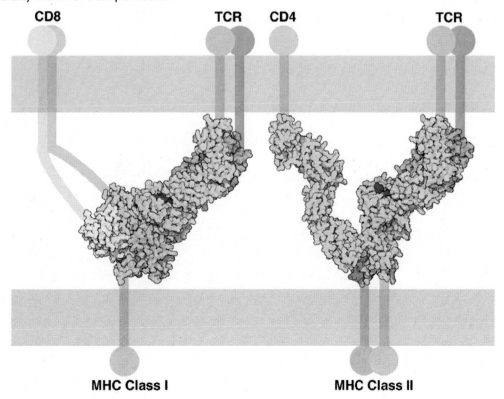

MHC Class I   MHC Class II

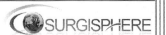

CELLS OF THE IMMUNE SYSTEM

IMMUNE CELLS

Table 295 Immune Cells

Cell Type	Surface Proteins	Function	Notes
Macrophage	CD14, MHC II	Phagocytosis, antigen presentation to helper T cell (MHC II), cell-mediated immunity. Form granulomas (histiocytosis X, TB, chronic granulomatous disease, sarcoidosis, rheumatic fever (Aschoff bodies), gummas in syphilis. Role in atherosclerosis (progressive plaque formation). Reservoir of HIV in HIV/AIDS. **Produce TNF**, important mediator in gram-negative sepsis.	Liver – Kupffer cells. Skin – Langerhans cells. Bone – Osteoclasts. Brain – Microglia. Spleen – Sinusoidal.
B-cell	CD19, CD20 IgM	Humoral immune system activation. Overall half-life of 3 weeks. Plasma B-cells – secrete large amounts of antibody and form a clonal population. Memory B-cells – long-lasting humoral immunity with ability to rapidly form a clonal population when reactivated.	
Tc-cell	CD3, CD8 TCR	Destruction of infected cells after activation by macrophages or other APCs. Deficiency may lead to candidiasis and Pneumocystis carinii infections. Calcium-dependent release of perforin or calcium-independent apoptosis of target cells.	Cytotoxic T-cells.
TH1-cell	CD3, CD4, CD28 TCR	Activate cell-mediated response through secretion of IFN-gamma and IL2.	Induced by IL12.
TH2-cell	CD3, CD4, CD28 TCR	Activate humoral response through secretion of IL4, IL5, and IL10.	Induced by IL4.
Regulatory T-cells	CD4, CD25	Suppress immune system activation and help avoid autoimmune diseases.	
NK cell	CD16, MHC I	Major role in killing cancerous cells.	
Dendritic cells	CD80, CD86	Strong T-cell activators through antigen-presentation (MHC II). Role in allergies and autoimmune disease.	
Somatic cells	MHC I	Includes all nucleated cells and platelets	All cells in body except RBCs.

P-selectin modulates endothelial cell adherence. E-selection mediates lymphocyte adhesion to the endothelium.

CYTOKINES AND GROWTH FACTORS

INTERLEUKINS AND GROWTH FACTORS

Table 296 Interleukins

TYPE	FEATURES	NOTES
IL-1	Secreted by macrophages and activates acute phase reaction. Catabolic.	Increases body temperature (resets hypothalamus temperature regulation) and increases adhesion factor expression by cells (promotes extravasation of immune mediators). IL-1 receptor antagonist is used for the treatment of RA. **Pyrogen**.
IL-2	Secreted by T-cells and stimulates T-cell response.	Used as adjunctive therapy in cancer, especially malignant melanoma and **renal cell carcinoma**. Activates regulatory T-cells to moderate reaction to self (NK cells → lymphokine-activated killer cells). Stimulates B-cells.
IL-6	**Secreted by macrophage** and activates acute phase reaction.	Very high levels following trauma, burns, and tissue damage. Stimulates osteoblasts to stimulate osteoclasts (almost all pathways are indirect like this). Estrogen inhibits IL-6 and so can theoretically be used for the treatment of osteoporosis. Induces fever. Works through gp130. **Pyrogen**.

GROWTH FACTORS AND ACUTE PHASE REACTANTS

Table 297 Growth Factors and Acute Phase Reactants

TYPE	FEATURES	NOTES
IFN-alpha	Inhibit viral protein synthesis.	Activate NK cells. Induces MHC I and II.
IFN-beta	Inhibit viral protein synthesis.	Activate NK cells. Induces MHC I and II.
IFN-gamma	Increase MHC I and MHC II expression by cells to increase antigen-processing.	Activate cell-mediated pathway and NK cells. Inhibits humoral pathway. Used in hairy cell leukemia.
TNF-alpha	Major role in inflammation and acute phase response. Released by WBCs during infection / inflammation and endothelium due to damage. Stimulates CRH, suppresses appetite, resets thermostat, and increases APRs by liver. Strong chemotaxis for neutrophils. Induces IL-1 production and increases insulin resistance. Catabolic.	Also known as cachexin. Synthetic forms used for the treatment of autoimmune disorders but increased risk of TB or activation of latent infection (CMV, EBV, VZV). Tumor lysis.
PDGF	Platelet derived growth factor is released by platelet alpha granules and attracts neutrophils, fibroblasts, and macrophages.	Stimulates ECM production.
TGF-B	Transforming growth factor beta stimulates collagen synthesis and inhibits ECM degradation. Attracts macrophages and fibroblasts.	Stimulates fibrosis.
EGF	Epidermal growth factor is an autocrine mediator that stimulates epithelialization.	
VEGF	VEGF is stimulated by hypoxemia, which induces angiogenesis.	Required for angiogenesis. Produced by cancer cells.

⚠ Granulocytes include neutrophils, eosinophils, and basophils.

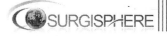

- The acute phase response leads to antibody production, a cytotoxic response, phagocytosis, complement activation, leukocytosis, fever, increased antigen processing, decreased viral or bacterial replication, and developing of adaptive immune response.
- Active immunity – from attenuated live viruses (best), killed vaccinations, or actual infection with long-lasting immunity and numerous B-cells.
- Passive immunity – mother to baby (IgG), serum transfer (i.e. rabies Rx) with rapid onset but short duration.
- Glucocorticoids have the greatest catabolic effect.

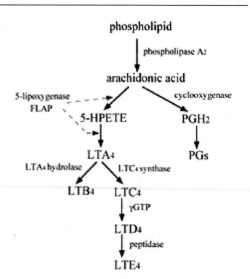

COMPLEMENT

Table 298 Complement

Type	Function	Notes
C1	Binds to antigen-antibody complex. C1q induces classical complement pathway with target cell death.	Opsonization; inhibited by C1EI.
C2	Binds to antigen-antibody complex / activated.	Opsonization.
C3	Broken down into C3a and C3b / activated by C2/C4 or C3b,Bb.	Opsonization.
C3a	Weak neutrophil chemotaxis, anaphylaxis reaction / inflammation.	Anaphylaxis.
C3b	Combines with C2b, C3a and C4b to form C5 convertase (classic pathway) or combines with C3b, Bb, C3a to form C5 convertase.	Opsonization.
Bb	Alternative pathway.	
C4	Binds to antigen-antibody complex / activated.	Opsonization.
C5	Broken down into C5a and C5b.	
C5a	Strong neutrophil chemotactic agent.	Anaphylaxis and neutrophil chemotaxis (strong).
C5b	Membrane attack complex.	Important in *Neisseria* infection.
C6	Membrane attack complex.	Important in *Neisseria* infection.
C7	Membrane attack complex.	Important in *Neisseria* infection.
C8	Membrane attack complex.	Important in *Neisseria* infection.
C9	Membrane attack complex.	Important in *Neisseria* infection.
DAF	Found on surface of cells to prevent complement-deposition and activation.	Decay-accelerating factor.
C1EI	Inactivates complement to prevent complement activation and cell destruction.	C1 esterase inhibitor.

- The alternative pathway provides a means of activating the immune system without antibodies.
- C3b is critical in both classic and alternative pathways.
- The classic pathway is activated by IgM or IgG.
- Toxins, IgA, and spontaneous activation occurs in the alternative pathway.

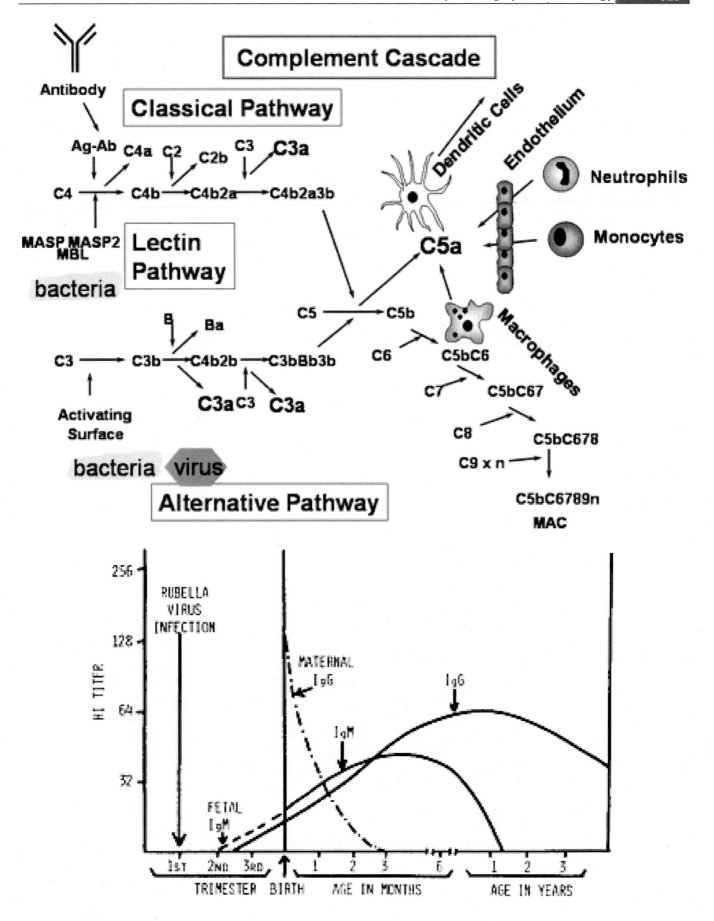

HYPERSENSITIVITY REACTIONS

Table 299 Hypersensitivity Reactions

TYPE	FEATURES	NOTES	DISEASES
Type I	IgE mediated response that leads to activation of mast cells and granulocytes following initial sensitization. Net result is a degranulation of histamine, proteoglycans such as heparin, serine proteases, prostaglandin D2 (vasodilation), cytokines, and leukotriene C4.	Rapid response with immediate reaction that presents with anaphylaxis, hives, wheals, flares, urticaria, and intense pruritus.	Occurs in allergic reactions (bee stings, peanut allergies, drug allergies).
Type II	IgG and IgM mediated response that leads to direct antibody-mediated cell toxicity with cell destruction; either direct phagocytosis or complement-mediated cell death.	Direct antibody-mediated destruction of self and with activation of membrane attack complex through complement pathways (classic pathway).	Autoimmune hemolytic anemia, erythroblastosis fetalis (Rh disease), Goodpasture, rheumatic fever, Graves', bullous pemphigoid.
Type III	Indirect IgG and IgM mediated response that leads to antibody-antigen complexes. These complexes deposit in various tissues leading to inflammation and cellular destruction.	Activation of immune system with neutrophils and macrophages leading to cell damage.	Serum sickness occurs with horse serum components in some vaccines or serum transfers leading to tissue damage. Arthus reaction occurs with local antigen injection leading to complex deposition within skin and local urticaria; occurs in fungal infections of the lung Other diseases include PAN, SLE, PSGN, RA.
Type IV	Delayed T-cell mediated cytotoxicity leading to direct T-cell mediated cellular destruction.	T-cell effects.	TB test, contact dermatitis.

TRANSPLANT REJECTION

Table 300 Transplant Rejection

TYPE	FINDINGS	TREATMENT
Hyperacute	Type II reaction with preformed IgM or IgG antibodies from prior sensitization leading to antibody-mediated destruction. Occurs over minutes to hours and uses preformed antibodies. Avoid by satisfactory preoperative crossmatch. Vascular rejection is a subset of hyperacute rejection and is due to undetectable antibodies. Initial graft function with deterioration at POD3. Treated with plasmapheresis and IVIG.	Remove transplant.
Acute	Type IV reaction with cytotoxic T-cell-mediated destruction. Occurs over 1-3 weeks and is treated with OKT3. Prevent with cyclosporin or tacrolimus and prednisone. Occurs in 20-40% of recipients.	OKT3
Chronic	Type II and III reaction with antibody-antigen deposition and direct antibody cytotoxicity. Occurs over months to years. No cure. Leads to gradual loss of blood supply.	Remove transplant.
Graft-vs.-host disease	Type IV reaction with cytotoxic T-cell-mediated destruction.	Remove transplant.

ADOPTIVE IMMUNOTHERAPY

Adoptive immunotherapy is when donor immune cells are transferred to the recipient to permit destruction of a tumor. Formation of NK cells (and subsequent conversion to LAK cells) occurs via IL-2. Bulky cancers tend to be affected the most.

This therapy may have potential in the treatment against lymphoma, leukemia, melanoma, sarcoma, and breast cancer. Immune chimera is a transplant patient with immune cells from the donor.

FINDINGS IN DISEASE

- Positive cross-match for donor requires search for new donor.
- Lymphocyte proliferation assay is used to assess lymphocyte function.
- Lymphoproliferation following transplant may be attributable to EBV infection.
- Inclusion bodies in pneumonia following transplant may be attributable to CMV infection.

AUTOANTIBODIES

Table 301 Sepsis

TYPE	DISEASE	NOTES
c-ANCA	Wegener's granulomatosis	Cytoplasmic
Centromere	CREST	
Mitochondrial	Primary biliary cirrhosis	AMA
nAChR	Myasthenia gravis	
Neutrophil	Vasculitis	
pANCA	Polyarteritis nodosa	Perinuclear
Scl-70	Scleroderma	Topoisomerase
Smooth muscle	Autoimmune hepatitis	
Thyroid peroxidase	Hashimoto thyroiditis	
TSH-R	Graves disease	
VGCC	Lambert-Eaton syndrome	

ORGAN TRANSPLANTATION

HEART TRANSPLANT

Indications for a heart transplant are end stage cardiac failure with an expected survival of less than six months. Patients must have no other terminal diseases, such as cancer or serious infection. Heart transplant is commonly done for HCM, RCM, DCM, infectious cardiomyopathy, postpartum cardiomyopathy, and terminal valve disease. A size-matched organ is used. Complications include infection, stroke, or rejection in the early postoperative course and chronic rejection leading to CAD in the late postoperative course. Patient survival is 80% after the first year and about 70% after 5 years. Cause of death after 10 years is from silent myocardial infarction due to progressive atherosclerosis (graft vs. host disease). There are no pain symptoms associated with the MI due to denervation of the transplanted heart. Overall, the most common post-transplant infection for any organ is CMV, which is treated with ganciclovir.

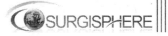

LUNG TRANSPLANT

Lung transplant is performed in patients with irreversible pulmonary disease including interstitial pulmonary fibrosis, pulmonary hypertension, alpha-1-antitrypsin deficiency, cystic fibrosis, and emphysema. Lung cancer is a contraindication for transplant. Elderly patients are also typically rejected as candidates. Rejection is diagnosed by the presence of infiltrates on CXR and confirmed by biopsy. The presence of such infiltrates is an indication for immunosuppression. Development of infiltrates following a course of immunosuppression is likely due to CMV infection and therefore an indication for ganciclovir. Breakdown of the anastomosis will occur in 5% of patients. Posterolateral thoracotomy is used for single lung transplantation, and a transverse thoracotomy used for double lung transplantation. Patients have a 75% 1 year survival and a 50% survival at 3 years.

HEART-LUNG TRANSPLANT

A heart-lung transplant is indicated in cases of Eisenmenger physiology leading to irreversible cardiopulmonary disease, pulmonary hypertension that accompanies severe cardiac disease, and with congenital defects. Complications are similar to those of heart and lung transplant. Fibrosis of the lung can occur; one year survival is about 60%.

LIVER TRANSPLANT

INDICATIONS

Liver transplantation is the final option in progressive, irreversible hepatic failure. Indications include cirrhosis, primary sclerosing cholangitis, fulminant hepatitis, HCC, and hepatic vein thrombosis with less than a 1 year survival. It has a 5-year survival approaching 90%. A donor liver must be matched with ABO groups and be similar in size. No HLA or Rh matching is necessary. Recipients must be free of malignancy or serious infection.

SIDE EFFECTS

Liver transplantation requires the use of immunosuppressive drugs including OKT3, tacrolimus, and cyclophosphamide. Failure to maintain immunosuppression may lead to acute rejection, which presents with onset of fever, RUQ pain, and elevations in several LFTs. Acute rejection is treated with the steroid methylprednisone, which is the first line agent. Antibodies to lymphocytes may also be used to control the immune reaction. Cyclophosphamide can lead to hemorrhagic cystitis in up to 10% of patients due to production of the fixative acrolein. Adequate hydration and use of N-acetylcysteine can mitigate this risk. Early postoperative complications include hemorrhage and bleeding disorders, thrombosis, biliary stricture or leaks, and occasionally, acute rejection. Late postoperative complications include biliary tree stenosis, hepatitis, chronic rejection, and toxicity from cyclosporin. Biliary stricture may be a result of ischemia.

Table 302 Liver Transplant

Liver Transplant	
Indications	Final option due to irreversible hepatic failure due to sclerosis, cirrhosis, HCC, hepatic vein thrombosis, fulminant hepatitis.
Side effects	Rejection due to failure of immunosuppression.
Liver dialysis	Experimental therapy. Temporary substitute until transplantation.

LIVER DIALYSIS

The use of liver dialysis is gaining popularity in certain centers. This experimental therapy seeks to utilize the same theory as renal dialysis – to remove toxins and dangerous substances that can amplify liver damage. Liver dialysis is a temporary substitute in individuals with full hepatic failure awaiting liver transplant.

KIDNEY TRANSPLANT

ESRD is the chief indication for kidney transplant. Patients are free of infection and cancer, and a wide range of ages is acceptable for the recipient. The graft is placed in the iliac fossa, and is extraperitoneal. The early postoperative course may be complicated by acute rejection, excess diuresis, urinary leak, hemorrhage, thrombosis, graft rupture, and perigraft lymphocele formation. Acute rejection presents with decreased urine output, hypertension, fever, proteinuria, and rising BUN/Cr. Late complications include ureteral or renal artery stenosis, chronic rejection, and cancer. One year survival for the graft is 80% for cadaveric transplant and 95% for living-related transplant. HLA matching has a strong benefit for the recipient.

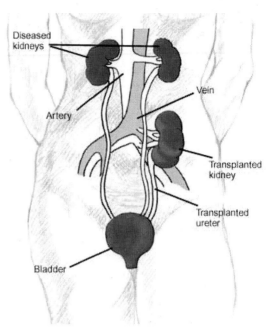

PANCREAS TRANSPLANT

The chief indication for pancreas transplant is type I DM. Complications include rejection, thrombosis, and leakage at the anastomosis. In a pancreas transplant, the donor duodenum is transplanted together into the intraperitoneal pelvis. The duodenum is attached to the bladder, permitting monitoring of the donor pancreas through urinary amylase levels. A pancreas transplant has a 95% 1 year survival.

INTESTINAL TRANSPLANT

Transplant of the intestines is done for short gut syndrome, Crohn disease, and necrotizing enterocolitis. At least 100cm of small bowel is necessary. Complications are numerous and survival is limited to 50-80% after 1 year.

PRACTICE QUESTIONS

 Which of the following immunoglobulins is found in breast milk in significant amounts?

    A. IgA
    B. IgD
    C. IgE
    D. IgG
    E. IgM

The best answer is IgA. IgA is found in breast milk. It is also secreted in the saliva and intestine.

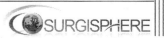

A 12 year old child has his spleen removed for hereditary spherocytosis. However, due to an administrative error, he does not receive antibiotics following the splenectomy, and soon develops overwhelming post-splenectomy sepsis. Which of the following immunologic mediators is responsible for this decompensation?

A. IgA
B. IgD
C. IgE
D. IgG
E. IgM

The best answer is IgM. IgM is responsible for mediating the immune function of the spleen, and alterations in the immune system following splenectomy prevent production of antibodies targeted against encapsulated organisms. The end result is serious infection that can lead to sepsis and death.

A kidney transplant patient three days out from his surgery develops an elevated white blood cell count and low-grade fevers. The donor kidney was CMV positive, and the recipient CMV negative. Which of the following is the next best step in management?

A. Continue to observe
B. Increase antirejection drugs
C. IV gancyclovir
D. PO valcyclovir
E. Vancomycin, zosyn, and diflucan

The best answer is IV gancyclovir. This patient should be treated for a presumed CMV infection with IV ganciclovir. PO medications at this stage are not indicated unless he has severe renal failure or other contraindications.

Which of the following immune cells produces IL-2?

A. Helper T-cell
B. Macrophage
C. Memory B-cell
D. Natural killer cell
E. Neutrophil

The best answer is Helper T-cell. Helper T-cells produce IL-2 to induce activation of the immune system. T-cell function is tested by delayed hypersensitivity skin testing. CD-8 cytotoxic cells are activated by IL-2. IL-1 is released by macrophages and leads to fever through central activation. Adhesion molecules used by neutrophils include P-selectins (found in platelets and endothelial cells), E-selection (endothelium), and L-selection (lymphocytes). TNF is secreted by macrophages and activated T-cells and leads to increased antigen presentation by MHC I and II sites.

Which of the following is the next step in management following a kidney transplant where the transplanted organ turns blue in vivo regardless of a good vascular anastomosis?

A. OKT3
B. Pulse corticosteroids
C. Sirolimus
D. Tacrolimus
E. Transplant nephrectomy

The best answer is <u>Transplant nephrectomy</u>. This patient has hyperacute rejection, which requires removal of the transplanted organ. This type of rejection is mediated by preformed antibodies in the host against the graft and is the result of an undetected failed crossmatch. Hyperacute rejection is likely with a positive T-cell crossmatch. Treatment with tacrolimus (which inhibits calcineurin and IL2) will have no effect, along with Sirolimus (inhibition of dendritic cells and cytokine release), and OKT3 (CD3 lymphocyte inhibition). Anti-thymocyte globulin is used in acute rejection only, along with pulse steroids. Chronic rejection is mediated by natural killer cells and long-term T cell activation, leading to atherosclerosis and eventual graft failure. The presence of a post-transplant lymphoproliferative disorder is likely mediated by EBV and may require chemotherapy if decreasing immunosuppression does not work. The most common cancer in transplant patients is squamous cell cancer of the skin.

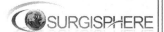

GYNECOLOGY

CHAPTER CONTENTS

BREAST

BREAST DISEASES

FIBROADENOMA

Fibroadenomas are the most common breast tumor found in women less than 35 years of age. It presents as a freely movable mass under the skin.

FIBROCYSTIC DISEASE

Fibrocystic disease in breast is most likely to develop into cancer if it is due to atypical ductal hyperplasia. Fibrocystic changes lead to multicentric ductal discharges.

BENIGN BREAST PAIN

Breast pain may be reduced with the use of bromocryptine to inhibit the release of prolactin. A male adolescent with gynecomastia only requires reassurance.

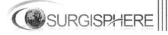

BREAST CANCER

EPIDEMIOLOGY

Breast cancer is most commonly the result of an invasive ductal adenocarcinoma; the remaining causes are generally attributable to lobular carcinoma. It is the second most common cause of death in women, and <u>1 in 7 women</u> will eventually develop breast cancer, and there are nearly a million cases a year throughout the world with nearly 50,000 deaths in the US. Risk factors include early age of menarche, late age of menopause, late first pregnancy or nulliparity, use of oral contraceptives, hormone replacement therapy (HRT), high fat intake, alcohol abuse, smoking, exposure to radiation, and a positive history. Breast feeding appears to be somewhat protective. Klinefelter disease is a positive risk factor for breast cancer in men.

ETIOLOGY

BRCA-1 is associated with breast cancer (85% by age 70), ovarian cancer (44%), colon cancer, and prostate cancer in men. BRCA-1 accounts for 40% of familial breast cancer. Chromosome 17 tumor suppressor gene. BRCA is a nuclear oncogene. BRCA-2 is associated with breast cancer, ovarian cancer (27%), and male breast cancer (10%). Genetic testing is recommended in families that develop breast cancer before the age of 45. Chromosome 13 tumor suppressor gene. Approximately 10% of breast cancer is due to germline mutations. 75% of patients with breast cancer have an elevation in CA 15-3.

RISK FACTORS

Risk factors for the development of breast cancer include early onset of menarche, late menopause, first gestation at a late age, a positive family history in first degree relatives, a history of prior breast cancer, the presence of lobular carcinoma in situ, atypical hyperplasia in fibrocystic disease, and living in Western society. Of moderate risk is the presence of atypical ductal or lobular hyperplasia. The highest association of tumor developing into breast cancer is the presence of atypical ductal hyperplasia. An excisional biopsy is required for diagnosis. Radiation is a significant risk factor for breast cancer; smoking is not.

PRESENTATION

Breast cancer may be entirely asymptomatic, but more commonly, a unilateral bloody nipple discharge or a palpable new mass are present. Retraction of the skin or nipple in a peau d'orange sign may be present. Nipple ulceration can occur. Erythema or edema of the skin overlying the breast may be present, along with axillary and supraclavicular lymphadenopathy. Bone pain, hepatomegaly, and pleural effusion may be present in later stages. Breast cancer should be differentiated from the nonmalignant lesions of fibrocystic breast disease, which varies according to the point in the menstrual cycle and is clearly nonmalignant on biopsy. An early sign of malignancy is enlargement of the cell.

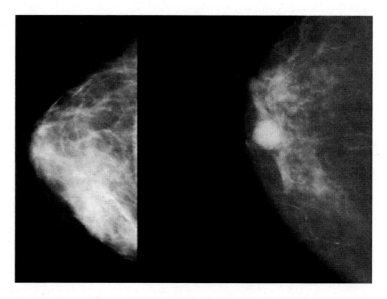

DIAGNOSIS

Diagnosis of breast cancer is made by focused history, physical exam, mammogram, FNA, and open-excisional biopsy. Physical exam is approximately 55% sensitive in detecting existing cancer. The presence of a palpable mass requires ultrasound or a fine needle aspiration. The presence of a cystic mass is followed by aspiration and repeat ultrasound in six weeks. The presence of a solid mass requires a core biopsy; benign findings are excised without margins, while malignant findings require advanced therapy. Mammogram can visualize the majority of breast cancers, especially in women over 35 years of age. They should be done every two years after the age of 40, and annually after the age of 50. Mammograms have a 10% false negative and a 10% false positive rate; as a result, mammograms have been shown to reduce the specific mortality for breast cancer, but not the overall mortality. Bone scans, liver ultrasound, and CXR are used in women with late stage disease. Lesions that cannot be palpated need to be biopsied using stereotactic methods, which is a less morbid and less expensive approach compared to excisional biopsy. Excisional biopsy following needle localization is also used, which can be therapeutic in select patients. If no sentinel lymph nodes are identified, an axillary lymph node dissection is required. Radio-guided breast biopsy is indicated for open biopsy to confirm the diagnosis of atypical hyperplasia. The greatest decrease in breast cancer death has been attributed to mammography for early detection.

DUCTAL CARCINOMA IN-SITU

Fibrocystic disease with proliferative changes is at risk of developing into DCIS. It presents with transformed cells that do not penetrate the basement membrane. 50% of cases will develop into infiltrating ductal carcinoma. The standard therapy is lumpectomy with 5mm margins followed by radiotherapy. Radiotherapy has been shown to decrease the recurrence of DCIS and mitigate the risk of carcinogenesis. Mastectomy with 1cm margins followed by radiotherapy is required for high grade lesions larger than 2.5cm in size, or in multicentric disease. The comedo form presents with necrotic cellular debris and microcalcifications. It is associated with a higher cancer risk due to the higher rate of mitosis. Lymph node dissection is not required unless the lesion is larger than 2.5cm, the comedo form is present, there is microinvasion, or there is multicentric disease. Concurrent DCIS and invasive cancer is at significant risk for local recurrence.

LOBULAR CARCINOMA IN-SITU

The presence of LCIS at the margin of breast excision requires no further therapy. Tamoxifen reduces the risk of invasive ductal cancer by 49%. LCIS is a disease of the breast lobules and acini. The average age of onset is 45 years. LCIS typically presents as incidental findings on a biopsy, with no palpable masses on physical exam or findings on a mammogram. 1/3 of cases develop into breast cancer within 20 years, with equal risk of cancer in either breast. LCIS is a bilateral disease. Close followup is required and possibly tamoxifen and/or prophylactic bilateral mastectomy with a strong family history.

INTRADUCTAL PAPILLOMA

Bloody nipple discharge but a normal mammogram is likely intraductal papilloma and requires excision of the ducts. Intraductal papilloma is the most common cause of spontaneous bloody discharge from the nipple. Total excision is required. There is little risk of cancer.

PAGET'S DISEASE

Paget's disease of the nipple is a variant of ductal carcinoma. It leads to eczematous changes in the nipple. Prognosis is determined by the extent of underlying disease.

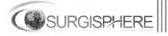

CYSTOSARCOMA PHYLLODES

Phyllodes tumor of the breast is managed by a wide local excision as nearly a quarter of them are malignant. These tumors do not spread via the lymphatics so no nodal dissection is required. This is the most common non-epithelial tumor of the breast. Therapy includes wide excision with clear margins. Recurrent disease is treated with mastectomy. This tumor is responsive to chemotherapy. Due to hematogenous spread, lymph node sampling is not required with phyllodes tumor.

INFLAMMATORY CANCER

Inflammatory breast cancer may invade the dermal lymphatics and so requires lymph node dissection. Inflammatory breast cancer typically presents with tumor, dolor, rubor, calor, and orange-peel skin. Inflammatory breast cancer sometimes mimics mastitis, but is differentiated by its lack of response to antibiotics. Therapy includes neoadjuvant chemotherapy followed by radiotherapy and a modified radical mastectomy.

INFILTRATING DUCTAL CARCINOMA

The presence of an infiltrating ductal carcinoma is the most common form of breast cancer. Local excision is required with margins greater than 2mm. Sentinel lymph node mapping is completed and radiotherapy may be required. Selected patients receive a modified radical mastectomy with sentinel lymph node mapping in lieu of radiotherapy. Only unilateral therapy is required. The mechanism of angiogenesis is local proliferation and migration of cells. This may be mediated by VEGF, a paracrine angiogenesis factor. Angiosarcoma of the breast is treated with mastectomy and postoperative chemoradiation if it is high grade. Large, bulky tumors are relatively insensitive to radiation due to tumor hypoxia. Cancer cells use glutamine as their primary energy source.

 Glutamine is the fuel source for cancer cells.

SURGICAL ANATOMY

Damage to the long thoracic nerve can cause winged scapula due to denervation of the serratus anterior. Damage to the thoracodorsal nerve innervating the latissimus dorsi presents with difficulty doing pull ups. Damage to the intercostobrachial nerve is common and occasionally intentional, and typically presents with loss of sensation to the proximal medial portion of the arm and sometimes to the upper lateral thorax. Level I lymph nodes are lateral to the border of the pectoralis minor. Level II lymph nodes are under the pectoralis minor. Level III lymph nodes are medial to the pectoralis minor. Level III nodes are not resected in a modified radical mastectomy.

STAGING

Locally advanced breast cancer is typically treated with neoadjuvant chemotherapy for tumors larger than 5 cm, invasion of lymph nodes, inflammatory cancers, and stage 3 cancers. A post-menopausal female with ER+ stage IIa breast cancer requires tamoxifen and chemotherapy. A contraindication to segmental mastectomy is the presence of multicentric disease.

Table 303 T Status in Breast Cancer Staging

T Status	Criteria
T1	< 2 cm
T2	2-5 cm
T3	> 5 cm
T4	Involvement of the skin or chest wall

Table 304 N Status in Breast Cancer Staging

N Status	Criteria
N0	Lack of nodes
N1	Presence of lymph nodes
N2	Fixed lymph nodes
N3	Internal mammary nodes

Table 305 M Status in Breast Cancer Staging

M status	Criteria
M0	No metastasis
M1	Presence of supraclavicular nodes

CHEMOTHERAPY

Tamoxifen is a selective estrogen receptor modifier that functions by competitively blocking the binding of estrogen to nuclear receptors. Estrogen receptor is a marker for tumor differentiation. It can be used for up to five years and is limited by its increased risk of DVT and endometrial carcinogenesis due to its partial estrogen agonist ability. There is a 50% annual recurrence reduction. Tamoxifen should be used on patients who are ER+/PR+. Taxol is another drug used in breast cancer patients, and functions by inhibiting mitosis. Anastrozole (Arimadex) is more effective than tamoxifen in ER+ patients and has a concomitant decrease in the incidence of DVT and endometrial carcinogenesis (ATAC trial). Anastrozole is an aromatase inhibitor that blocks estrogen synthase. Herceptin is a monoclonal antibody to the Her-2/neu growth factor receptor. It is used in patients who overexpress this receptor and in those with positive lymph node or metastatic disease.

Table 306 Tamoxifen

DRUG	INDICATIONS	MECHANISM OF ACTION	COMPLICATIONS	NOTES
Tamoxifen	Breast CA	SERM	Retroperitoneal fibrosis (rare)	Estrogen is used to determine sensitivity of breast CA to tamoxifen Can also be used for gynecomastia The STAR trial compared the effectiveness of tamoxifen with raloxifene; tamoxifen is used for breast cancer, raloxifene for osteoporosis

REPRODUCTIVE SYSTEM

CONGENITAL AND STRUCTURAL

ECTOPIC PREGNANCY

A young woman who presents with sudden lower back pain and goes into shock has likely experienced a ruptured ectopic pregnancy. This is always on the differential of acute appendicitis.

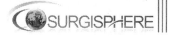

INFLAMMATORY AND INFECTIOUS

PELVIC INFLAMMATORY DISEASE

Table 307 Pelvic Inflammatory Disease (PID)

Pelvic Inflammatory Disease (PID)	
Etiology	Causes of PID include *Chlamydia trachomatis*, CMV, *Gardnerella vaginalis*, *Haemophilus influenza*, *E. coli*, *Peptococcus spp.*, *Streptococcus agalactiae*, *Bacteroides fragilis*, and *Neisseria gonorrhea*.
Presentation	Dull, aching pain that is worsened with intercourse or exercise. Vaginal discharge, bleeding, fever, and various constitutional symptoms are present. Cervical motion tenderness, adnexal tenderness, and purulent discharge are present on exam. WBCs are increased.
Treatment	Cefoxitin and doxycycline. Clindamycin or metronidazole may be added for more complicated cases. Clindamycin and gentamicin are alternative treatments. Ofloxacin with clindamycin or metronidazole can also be used, and is more suitable for outpatient treatment. This latter regimen works well against both gonococcal and chlamydial causes.

Cervical motion tenderness plus vaginal discharge and adnexal tenderness requires admission to the hospital and treatment with IV antibiotics.

ENDOMETRIOSIS

A bluish genital mass and dysmenorrhea is endometriosis and may respond to hormonal therapy.

CANCER

ENDOMETRIAL CANCER

ETIOLOGY AND PATHOPHYSIOLOGY

Endometrial cancer may occur in women with increased time of fertility, HRT, tamoxifen therapy for prior breast cancer, obesity, nulliparity, DM, and HTN, along with a positive family history. Endometrial cancer arises from the superior portion of the uterus and may be focal with a friable mass, diffuse, or a polyp. Nearly 1 in 100 women may develop endometrial cancer. Prognosis is generally favorable with early diagnosis and treatment.

PRESENTATION AND DIAGNOSIS

Diagnosis of endometrial cancer is made with a biopsy through endocervical curettage. Ultrasound is commonly used to analyze the anatomy of the female pelvis; transabdominal sonography (TAS) and transvaginal sonography (TVS) are often used; the latter is preferred over CT for diagnosis, but not for staging.

TREATMENT

Surgery is preferred for endometrial cancer, along with radiation therapy and chemotherapy. A total abdominal hysterectomy with bilateral salpingo-oophorectomy (TAHBSO) is preferred. Progesterone is often given as an adjuvant, along with cisplatin, doxorubicin, cyclophosphamide, paclitaxel, and carboplatin. The latter agents function by alkylating the DNA leading to strand breakage and misreading. Tamoxifen increases the risk of endometrial cancer and should not be used for more than five years. Tamoxifen also increases the risk of thrombosis.

Table 308 Endometrial Cancer

Endometrial Cancer	
Etiology	May occur in women with increased time of fertility, HRT, tamoxifen therapy for prior breast cancer, obesity, nulliparity, DM, and HTN, along with a positive family history.
Presentation	Peri-or postmenopausal vaginal bleeding. Progression leads to enlarged uterus and softening of the cervix.
Diagnosis	Biopsy through endocervical curettage. Ultrasound is commonly used to analyze the anatomy of the female pelvis; TAS and TVS are often used; the latter is preferred over CT for diagnosis, but not for staging.
Treatment	Surgery, radiation therapy and chemotherapy. A TAHBSO is preferred. Progesterone is often given as an adjuvant, along with cisplatin, doxorubicin, cyclophosphamide, paclitaxel, and carboplatin.

OVARIAN CANCER

ETIOLOGY AND PATHOPHYSIOLOGY

Ovarian cancer can occur at any age and affects nearly 1 out of 100 women. It is also the most common cause of death due to genital cancer. Causes include epithelial ovarian cancer including serous or mucinous cystadenocarcinoma, endometroid carcinoma, undifferentiated carcinoma, and clear cell carcinoma. Germ cell tumors such as dysgerminomas and endometrial sinus tumors may occur. Teratomas, embryonal carcinomas, polyembryona, and choriocarcinoma are other rarer causes of ovarian cancer. Risk factors include the use of fertility drugs such as clomiphene, HRT, and nulliparity. Inheritance of BRCA 1 or BRCA 2 is another risk factor, along with HNPCC.

PRESENTATION AND DIAGNOSIS

Endometrial carcinoma presents with a pelvic mass or adnexal mass, lymphadenopathy, ascites, and hydrothorax. Constitutional symptoms are common, along with frequent urination, abnormal uterine bleeding (AUB) or dysfunctional uterine bleeding (DUB), constipation, and referred pain to the back. Diagnosis relies on a careful history and physical exam, followed by CA-125 titers, US using TVS, and various other imaging studies.

TREATMENT

Treatment of ovarian cancer includes laparoscopic debulking, chemotherapy, and possible TAHBSO, if future pregnancy is not desired. The presence of ovarian cancer with peritoneal metastasis requires a total abdominal hysterectomy with bilateral salpingooopherectomy, omentectomy, and selective node sampling. The site of first metastasis tends to be the peritoneum. Ovarian cancer is the most likely cancer to lead to ascites and carcinomatosis.

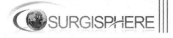

Table 309 Ovarian Cancer

Ovarian Cancer	
Etiology	Serous or mucinous cystadenocarcinoma, endometroid carcinoma, undifferentiated carcinoma, and clear cell carcinoma. Germ cell tumors such as dysgerminomas and endometrial sinus tumors may occur. Teratomas, embryonal carcinomas, polyembryona, and choriocarcinoma are other rarer causes of ovarian cancer.
Presentation	Pelvic mass or adnexal mass, lymphadenopathy, ascites, and hydrothorax. Constitutional symptoms are common, along with frequent urination, AUB or DUB, constipation, and referred pain to the back.
Diagnosis	A careful history and physical exam, followed by CA-125 titers, US using TVS, and various other imaging studies.
Treatment	Laparoscopic debulking, chemotherapy, and possible TAHBSO, if future pregnancy is not desired.

CERVICAL CANCER

ETIOLOGY AND PATHOPHYSIOLOGY

Cervical cancer is the first cancer that is preventable with a vaccination against human papilloma virus 16 and 18. Cervical cancer begins with infection by HPV, a sexually-transmitted disease (STD). Premalignant lesions followed by invasive disease occur. Risk factors for cervical cancer include those that increase risk of contracting HPV, such as early intercourse, frequent intercourse, and low SES. Exophytic cervical cancer which arises from the exocervix is the most common form, and leads to bulky and friable tumors. Nodular cervical cancer forms nodules within the endocervix. Infiltrative cervical cancer leads to hardening of the cervix. Ulcerative cervical cancer leads to sloughing and ulceration of the cervical tissue with purulent drainage. Most types of cervical cancer are squamous cell carcinomas (SCC), but the incidence of adenocarcinoma has been rising in the form of mucinous adenocarcinoma, papillary adenocarcinoma, and clear-cell adenocarcinoma. Cervical cancer occurs more frequently than endometrial cancer and ovarian cancer. It is the most common genital malignancy worldwide. Prognosis is good with early detection.

PRESENTATION AND DIAGNOSIS

Cervical cancer may be entirely asymptomatic, but abnormal vaginal bleeding, abnormal discharge, and local pain with dyspareunia may be present. A Pap smear is required and should be performed in all women at risk. A minority of Pap smears is positive for high-grade squamous intraepithelial lesion (HSIL); about 20% are positive for low-grade squamous intraepithelial lesion (LSIL); nearly 80% agree with negative results on colposcopy. Infrequently, a negative Pap smear may miss an invasive carcinoma. With a positive Pap smear, a reflex HPV test can be done to determine the risk of developing cervical cancer. These tests may lead to colposcopy, in which the cervix is visualized and a cone biopsy is taken for further investigation of any putative lesions. Methods for taking a cone biopsy include cold-knife conization, laser excision, and loop electrosurgical excision procedure (LEEP). Uterine cervical cancer spreads to the obturator lymph node group.

TREATMENT

Treatment for cervical dysplasia depends on the type of intraepithelial lesion encountered. LSIL is typically monitored on a regular basis with repeated Pap smears. HSIL with sufficient risk factors may lead to LEEP, laser conization, laser vaporization (not preferred since no histologic analysis can be done), and cold-knife conization. With microinvasive disease or recurrent HSIL, a hysterectomy is typically performed. Radiation therapy and use of cisplatin chemotherapy is often done with a hysterectomy.

Table 310 Cervical Cancer

Cervical Cancer	
Etiology	Infection by HPV
Presentation	May be entirely asymptomatic, but abnormal vaginal bleeding, abnormal discharge, and local pain with dyspareunia may be present.
Diagnosis	Pap smear, colposcopy, cone biopsy
Treatment	**LSIL**- typically monitored on a regular basis with repeated Pap smears. **HSIL**- with sufficient risk factors may lead to LEEP, laser conization, and cold-knife conization. **Microinvasive disease or recurrent HSIL**-, a hysterectomy is typically performed. Radiation therapy and use of cisplatin chemotherapy is often done with a hysterectomy.

PRACTICE QUESTIONS

 A 52 year old female who has a screening mammography is found to have a radial scar. What is the next best step in management?

    A.   Bilateral modified radical mastectomy
    B.   Core biopsy
    C.   Excisional biopsy
    D.   Radiation therapy
    E.   Unilateral modified radical mastectomy

 The best answer is <u>Excisional biopsy</u>. Patients with a radial scar on mammography should receive an excisional biopsy for definitive diagnosis and putative treatment. Core biopsy is indicated for other limited lesions. Signs of breast cancer on mammography include radial scars, stellate lesions, calcifications, and asymmetry.

 A 57 year old female is diagnosed with a 2 cm mass with pathology that indicates ductal carcinoma in-situ. What is the best course of therapy?

    A.   Chemoradiation then modified radical mastectomy
    B.   Lumpectomy, sentinel lymph node biopsy
    C.   Lumpectomy, sentinel lymph node biopsy, then radiation therapy
    D.   Modified radical mastectomy then chemoradiation
    E.   Tamoxifen, then radiation, then modified radical mastectomy

 The best answer is <u>Lumpectomy, sentinel lymph node biopsy, then radiation therapy</u>. The appropriate treatment for any DCIS mass greater than 1 cm is to proceed with a lumpectomy and sentinel lymph node biopsy, followed by radiation. Tamoxifen has been shown to decrease recurrence by nearly half and is often given with radiation. A modified radical mastectomy is not indicated unless it is an infiltrating cancer.

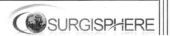

What is the appropriate therapy for a patient who is diagnosed with atypical ductal hyperplasia?

A. Chemoradiation
B. Core biopsy
C. Full axillary lymph node dissection
D. Modified radical mastectomy
E. Needle localized excisional biopsy

The best answer is <u>Needle localized excisional biopsy</u>. Atypical ductal hyperplasia is treated with needle localization the day of surgery, followed by an excision biopsy.

Which of the following best describes the effects of tamoxifen on cancer reduction in LCIS?

A. Tamoxifen decreases cancer risk by 10%
B. Tamoxifen decreases cancer risk by 25%
C. Tamoxifen decreases cancer risk by 50%
D. Tamoxifen decreases cancer risk by 75%
E. Tamoxifen plays no role in LCIS therapy

The best answer is <u>Tamoxifen decreases cancer risk by 50%</u>. Tamoxifen decreases cancer risk by 50% in patients with LCIS.

A 62 year old female undergoes a sentinel lymph node biopsy with 3/3 lymph nodes positive for cancer. What is the next best step?

A. Chemoradiation
B. Full axillary lymph node dissection
C. Modified radical mastectomy
D. Modified radical mastectomy followed by chemoradiation
E. Radical mastectomy

The best answer is <u>Full axillary lymph node dissection</u>. The appropriate treatment plan for a positive sentinel lymph node biopsy is to complete a full axillary lymph node dissection. A modified radical mastectomy is reserved only when the primary is not known. A full axillary lymph node dissection should be completed if a sentinel lymph node cannot be identified. Chemoradiation is necessary for this patient (tamoxifen). Contraindications to a segmental mastectomy include pregnancy in the first two trimesters, multicentric disease, or extensive disease that may preclude tumor-free margins. Indications for radiation therapy include more than four positive lymph nodes or extensive existing lymph node disease, more than 5 cm of chest wall involvement, positive margins, or the presence of inflammatory cancer. Chemotherapy may be started after the first trimester.

A 49 year old female who recently underwent an axillary lymph node dissection for breast cancer develops purple nodules on her arm. What is the best diagnosis?

A. Angioedema
B. Cystic hygroma
C. Hodgkin lymphoma
D. Staphylococcus infection
E. Stewart-Treves syndrome

The best answer is <u>Stewart-Treves syndrome</u>. This patient has Stewart-Treves syndrome, or lymphangiosarcoma. This disorder presents as swelling and edema of the arm following a lymph node dissection. Purple nodules are common. It progresses to an ulcer with crusting, and finally to an extensive necrosis involving the skin and subcutaneous tissue. It metastasizes quickly. It was previously a relatively common complication of the massive lymphedema of the arm which followed removal of axillary (arm pit) lymph nodes and lymphatic channels as part of the classical Halstedian radical mastectomy, as a treatment for breast cancer. The classical radical mastectomy was abandoned in most areas of the world in the late 1960's to early 1970's, being replaced by the much more conservative modified radical mastectomy and, more recently, by segmental breast tissue excision and radiation therapy. Because of this change in clinical practice lymphedema is now a rarity following breast cancer treatment - and post-mastectomy lymphangiosarcoma is now vanishingly rare. When it occurs following mastectomy it is known as Stewart-Treves Syndrome.

A 62 year old female is seen in clinic regarding changes to her right breast. On exam, the breast appears grossly warm and erythematous, tender to touch, and edematous. A punch skin biopsy shows dermal lymphatic invasion and a diagnosis of inflammatory breast cancer is made. What is the next step in management?

A. Chemoradiation followed by modified radical mastectomy
B. Chemotherapy followed by modified radical mastectomy and radiation
C. Modified radical mastectomy
D. Modified radical mastectomy followed by chemoradiation
E. Radiation followed by modified radical mastectomy and chemotherapy

The best answer is <u>Chemotherapy followed by modified radical mastectomy and radiation</u>. Inflammatory breast cancer is best treated with neoadjuvant chemotherapy followed by modified radical mastectomy and postoperative radiation therapy.

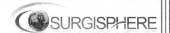

A 71 year old female presents with a nontender mass that is mobile. A diagnosis of Phyllodes tumor is made. What is the next best step?

A. Chemoradiation followed by modified radical mastectomy
B. Core biopsy
C. Modified radical mastectomy with axillary lymph node dissection
D. Modified radical mastectomy with chemoradiation
E. Segmental mastectomy

The best answer is <u>Segmental mastectomy</u>. This patient has Phyllodes tumor, which is treated by a segmental mastectomy without a lymph node dissection or chemotherapy.

What is the most likely diagnosis in a 32 year old woman who has intermittent bloody discharge from her nipple?

A. Ductal carcinoma in-situ
B. Fibroadenoma
C. Intraductal papilloma
D. Invasive ductal carcinoma
E. Paget disease

The best answer is <u>Intraductal papilloma</u>. Intraductal papilloma is the most common cause of spontaneous bloody discharge from the nipple. Total excision is required. There is little risk of cancer. Bloody nipple discharge but a normal mammogram is likely intraductal papilloma and requires excision of the ducts. Paget's disease of the nipple is a variant of ductal carcinoma. It leads to eczematous changes in the nipple. While the other diseases may lead to bloody discharge from the nipple, the most common cause in a 32 year old female is likely to be intraductal papilloma. Carcinoma must be ruled out, as it can lead to bloody discharge in 5% of cases. A circum-areolar biopsy with duct exploration is the course of action that should be followed.

Which of the following is the most common site for metastasis in breast cancer?

A. Bone
B. Brain
C. Liver
D. Lung
E. Pleura

The best answer is <u>Bone</u>. The most common site of metastasis in breast cancer is the bone, which occurs in about half of all patients. 20% of patients can have metastasis to the lung. The next most common sites include the pleura and liver.

A 21 year old female is seen by her breast surgeon for evaluation of a small, mobile lump in her breast. What is the most likely diagnosis?

A. DCIS
B. Fibroadenoma
C. Fibrocystic lesion
D. Intraductal papilloma
E. Lymphoma

 The best answer is <u>Fibroadenoma</u>. The most common tumor that affects women under the age of 35 is a fibroadenoma. This mobile lesion within breast tissue can be removed using local anesthesia, and is typically not removed until maturity of the patient in order to ensure multicentric disease is not present. Up to 15% of patients with fibroadenoma develop multicentric disease.

 Approximately what percentage of women with breast cancer have inheritance via BRCA1 or BRCA2?

A. 1%
B. 5%
C. 10%
D. 25%
E. 75%

 The best answer is <u>5%</u>. Less than 5% of all breast cancers are due to BRCA1 or BRCA2 mutations. However, women under the age of 25 who develop breast cancer are 25% likely to have an inherited form of breast cancer.

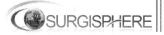

UROLOGY

CHAPTER CONTENTS

GENERAL CONCEPTS

ANATOMY

The left gonadal vein travels to the left renal vein, which enters the portal circulation. The right gonadal vein goes directly to the IVC. The presence of a left-sided varicocele may be a late sign of renal cell carcinoma.

Left **varicocele** = left RCC

PHYSIOLOGY

Aldosterone increases potassium secretion and sodium reabsorption in the distal tubule. Aldosterone increases sodium reabsorption in exchange for hydrogen and potassium; this function occurs on the sodium/hydrogen transporter. Creatinine clearance is less accurate than urea clearance when calculating GFR. Renin is secreted by the juxtaglomerular cells

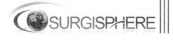

KIDNEY, URETERS, AND BLADDER

CONGENITAL AND STRUCTURAL

ADULT POLYCYSTIC KIDNEY DISEASE

ETIOLOGY AND PATHOPHYSIOLOGY

Adult polycystic kidney disease (APKD) is an autosomal dominant (AD) disorder, and one of the most common inherited disorders. APKD is the etiology responsible for 10% of all patients on dialysis. APKD leads to ESRD through progressive cystic dilation of the renal tubules. Other manifestations of APKD include hepatic cysts, aneurysms, and abnormalities of the cardiac valves. APKD leads to mortality through renal failure, intracranial aneurysms (ICAs) and subarachnoid hemorrhages. Symptoms increase with age.

PRESENTATION AND DIAGNOSIS

APKD presents with progressive decreases in renal function leading to ESRD. HTN heralds renal failure, and stroke can occur. UA is positive for hematuria. One of the most common symptoms is flank pain. Flank masses are obvious on physical exam, and hepatomegaly with nodular enlargement is also present. Family history is typically positive in this hereditary disorder. The preferred initial imaging study is US, followed by the more sensitive CT scan. Magnetic resonance angiography (MRA) is used to diagnose ICAs.

TREATMENT

Treatment involves careful observation and control of symptoms. Dialysis is eventually required, along with medical management with ACE-inhibitors. Renal transplant is eventually required. Cysts in the kidney and liver may become infected and require treatment through surgery and antibiotics.

Table 311 Adult Polycystic Kidney Disease (APKD)

Adult Polycystic Kidney Disease (APKD)	
Etiology	AD disorder which leads to ESRD through progressive cystic dilation of the renal tubules.
Presentation	Progressive decreases in renal function leading to ESRD. HTN heralds renal failure, and stroke can occur. Flank pain and flank masses are obvious on physical exam, and hepatomegaly with nodular enlargement is also present. Family history is typically positive. The preferred initial imaging study is US, followed by the more sensitive CT scan. MRA is used to diagnose ICAs.
Diagnosis	UA is positive for hematuria. The preferred initial imaging study is US, followed by the more sensitive CT scan. MRA is used to diagnose ICAs.
Treatment	Careful observation and control of symptoms. Dialysis is eventually required, along with medical management with ACE-inhibitors. Renal transplant is eventually required. Cysts in the kidney and liver may become infected and require treatment through surgery and antibiotics.

BLADDER DYSFUNCTION

INCONTINENCE

ETIOLOGY AND PATHOPHYSIOLOGY

Improper relaxation of the sphincter, or increased activity of the detrusor muscle lead to abnormalities in the micturition reflex and subsequent involuntary voiding or dysfunction. Common causes include stress incontinence from increased intraabdominal pressure with weakness of the pelvic floor, urge incontinence from increased activity of the detrusor muscle without proper neuronal control, overflow incontinence from poor detrusor muscle activity, continuous incontinence commonly from fistula formation, congenital malformations, traumatic damage to nerves or structures, and enuresis. Multiparous women may suffer from stress incontinence, along with men who have had invasive prostate surgery.

PRESENTATION AND DIAGNOSIS

Incontinence presents with frequency, certain patterns, identifiable precipitants, dysuria, incomplete emptying, and urge. A full neurologic exam is often done along with a pelvic exam. A Q-Tip test is used to identify excessive movement of the bladder or urethra, indicating poor support against pelvic pressure. Stress testing is also done to identify weaknesses in the pelvic muscles. Leaking when completing the Valsalva maneuver is diagnostic for stress incontinence.

TREATMENT

Treatment for incontinence is determined by the particular etiology. Overactivity of the detrusor is treated with behavioral modification therapy (BMT), bladder training, relaxing the bladder with various medications, and creating an artificial sphincter in more serious cases. Stress incontinence is treated by increasing sphincter tone, weight reduction, and Kegel exercises to strengthen the pubococcygeus muscles. Concomitant conditions should be treated, including cough and other causes of increased intraabdominal pressure. Outlet obstruction leading to overflow incontinence can be reversed with prazosin to decrease the sphincter tone, or the use of a catheter. Urinary retention is treated with the use of a parasympathomimetic; it is especially likely to occur following an APR.

Table 312 Incontinence

Incontinence	
Etiology	**Stress incontinence-** from increased intraabdominal pressure with weakness of the pelvic floor **Urge incontinence-** from increased activity of the detrusor muscle without proper neuronal control **Overflow incontinence-** from poor detrusor muscle activity, **Continuous incontinence-** commonly from fistula formation, congenital malformations, traumatic damage to nerves or structures, and enuresis.
Presentation	Frequency, certain patterns, identifiable precipitants, dysuria, incomplete emptying, and urge
Diagnosis	A full neurologic & pelvic exam. A Q-Tip test is used to identify excessive movement of the bladder or urethra, indicating poor support against pelvic pressure. Stress testing is also done to identify weaknesses in the pelvic muscles.
Treatment	**Overactivity of the detrusor** is treated with BMT, bladder training, relaxing the bladder with various medications, and creating an artificial sphincter in more serious cases. **Stress incontinence** is treated by increasing sphincter tone, weight reduction, and Kegel exercises. Concomitant conditions should be treated. **Overflow incontinence-** can be reversed with prazosin to decrease sphincter tone, or the use of a catheter.

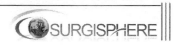

METABOLIC AND DEGENERATIVE

ACUTE TUBULAR NECROSIS

ETIOLOGY

ATN is often secondary to medications that have a toxic effect on the kidneys, and include drugs such as aminoglycosides, amphotericin, cisplatin, and lithium; however, nearly an equally common cause is complications following surgery. General causes for ATN include hypotension, toxic injury, and deposition of muscle fibers in rhabdomyolysis or diagnostic contrast agents that may lead to renal injury. The prodromal phase is without any signs or symptoms immediately following injury; the oliguric or anuric phase occurs following the damage; and the postoliguric phase takes place during resolution where excessive diuresis of accumulated fluid occurs. More severe courses of ATN have a more dismal prognosis. The typical length of renal failure is a few weeks.

DIAGNOSIS

ATN is diagnosed by the presence of brown urine and epithelial casts from tubular cells. There is significant hypernatriuria with a fractional excretion of sodium (FENA) greater than 1%. Complications of ATN include electrolyte abnormalities, volume overload with hyponatremia, uremic syndrome, and infections from indwelling catheters used during treatment. ATN can be avoided by maintaining good CO, IV hydration, and monitoring renal function tests during administration of renotoxic substances. Intrinsic renal failure typically has proteinuria and sedimentation via RBCs, RBC casts, WBC casts, and epithelial casts in the urine. ATN is characterized by epithelial cell casts and granular casts in the urine. Sedimentation with RBC casts, hematuria, proteinuria, and urine with low SG is more indicative of glomerulonephritis. Serology can further identify the cause of ARF: antibodies to the glomerular basement membrane (GBM) occur in Goodpasture syndrome; antibodies to neutrophils (ANCA) occur in polyarteritis nodosa (PAN) and Wegener syndrome; finally, antibodies to nuclei (ANA) occur in SLE.

TREATMENT

ATN typically progresses to severe renal failure followed by a falling BUN to creatinine ratio, an increase in urine output, and hypercalcemic diuresis. Treatment in the early stages of ATN include IV hydration with diuretics to maintain urine flow, restricting protein and potassium intake, and matching renal output with oral input. Slow correction of metabolic acidosis should be done, and any concurrent infections treated quickly. Fever in ATN or ARF should begin with a CXR, pancultures of the sputum, blood, and urine, and the use of antibiotic therapy tailored to the offending organism. Calculating FENA is a sensitive measure of detecting ATN.

Table 313 Acute Tubular Necrosis (ATN)

Acute Tubular Necrosis (ATN)	
Etiology	Often secondary to medications that have a toxic effect on the kidneys, complications following surgery. General causes include hypotension, toxic injury, and deposition of muscle fibers in rhabdomyolysis or diagnostic contrast agents.
Phases	**Prodromal** is without any signs or symptoms immediately following injury. **Oliguric or anuric** occurs following damage; **Postoliguric** takes place during resolution.
Diagnosis	Presence of brown urine and epithelial casts from tubular cells. There is significant hypernatriuria with a FENA greater than 1%. Intrinsic renal failure typically has proteinuria and sedimentation via RBCs, RBC casts, WBC casts, and epithelial casts in the urine. ATN is characterized by epithelial cell casts and granular casts in the urine. Serology can further identify the cause of ARF: antibodies to the GBM.
Treatment	Treatment in the early stages of ATN includes IV hydration with diuretics, restricting protein and potassium intake, and matching renal output with oral input. Slow correction of metabolic acidosis should be done, and any concurrent infections treated quickly. Fever in ATN or ARF should begin with a CXR, pancultures of the sputum, blood, and urine, and the use of antibiotic therapy tailored to the offending organism.

$$FE_{Na} = \frac{U_{Na} \times P_{Cr}}{U_{Cr} \times P_{Na}} \times 100$$

NEPHROLITHIASIS

ETIOLOGY AND PATHOPHYSIOLOGY

The formation of renal calculi is a relatively common renal disorder, affecting some 2% of the population annually. Two pathologic processes can lead to nephrolithiasis. The first is increased urine content of calcium, oxalate, and uric acid leading to supersaturation and spontaneous crystallization. The majority of kidney stones are due to calcium excess. Another cause is renal dysfunction or damage leading to a predisposition to crystallization. Nephrolithiasis is more common in males, and tends to occur in young adults or middle-aged adults. Calcium oxalate stones account for 70% of all stones; 10% are calcium phosphate, 10% contain magnesium, phosphate, and aluminum (struvite stones), and the minority contain uric acid or cystine. Calcium stones form with vitamin D excess, familial causes, and excess resorption or calcium as in hyperparathyroidism or multiple myeloma. Oxalate stones form with enteric causes leading to fat malabsorption or with familial causes. Low citrate can also lead to excess calcium absorption. Uric acid stones form in gout, hematologic conditions, and Crohn disease. Cystine stones are common in various genetic disorders. Infection by *Proteus*, *Staphylococcus*, *Pseudomonas*, and *Klebsiella* can cause struvite stones.

PRESENTATION AND DIAGNOSIS

Nephrolithiasis presents with symptoms only with significant obstruction of the ureters. Renal colic occurs with undulating cramps and severe pain, nausea and vomiting, and pain that migrate from the flank towards the scrotal or labial region as the stone moves. Staghorn calculi tend to remain within the kidney and present with renal failure. A UA is done and typically shows hematuria. A predisposition towards calculus formation is indicated with positive blood tests for electrolyte abnormalities. Diagnosis is made by plain films (positive for calcium-containing stones, which are 85% of all stones), sonograms (for renal stones), intravenous pyelogram (IVP), and helical CT.

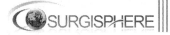

TREATMENT

Treatment for nephrolithiasis includes pain management (including morphine sulfate), increased water intake to promote stone passage, antiemetics (metoclopramide, prochlorperazine), NSAIDs (ibuprofen), and observation. Failure to pass a stone or significant renal stones is treated with extracorporeal shock-wave lithotripsy (EWSL), ureteroscopy, stent placement, and percutaneous nephrostolithotomy.

Table 314 Nephrolithiasis

Nephrolithiasis	
Etiology	Increased urine content of calcium, oxalate, and uric acid, and renal dysfunction or damage leading to a predisposition to crystallization.
Presentation	Symptoms only with significant obstruction of the ureters. Renal colic occurs with undulating cramps and severe pain, nausea and vomiting, and pain that migrates from the flank towards the scrotal or labial region as the stone moves. Staghorn calculi tend to remain within the kidney and present with renal failure. A UA is done and typically shows hematuria. A predisposition towards calculus formation is indicated with positive blood tests for electrolyte abnormalities. Diagnosis is made by plain films, sonograms, IVP), and helical CT.
Diagnosis	A UA is done and typically shows hematuria. A predisposition towards calculus formation is indicated with positive blood tests for electrolyte abnormalities. Diagnosis is made by plain films, sonograms, IVP, and helical CT.
Treatment	Pain management, increased water intake, antiemetics, NSAIDs, and observation. Failure to pass a stone or significant renal stones is treated with EWSL, ureteroscopy, stent placement, and percutaneous nephrostolithotomy.

RENAL FAILURE

PRERENAL FAILURE

Prerenal failure is due to decreased renal perfusion. Common causes that lead to decreased renal perfusion include decreased blood volume through hemorrhage, use of diuretics, third spacing of fluids in pancreatitis or following abdominal surgery, dehydration, CHF, nephrotic syndrome, septic shock, renal artery stenosis (RAS), and Addison disease. Prerenal failure is characterized by BUN that is 20 times greater than creatinine. The use of ACE-inhibitors and NSAIDs can exacerbate prerenal failure. Overall, a FENA less than 1 indicates prerenal failure. Urine sodium tends to be less than 20 mEq / L; intrinsic renal failure has a urine sodium over 30 mEq / L. Prerenal failure produces concentrated urine (UOsm > 400 mOsm / L).

INTRINSIC RENAL FAILURE

Intrinsic renal failure is a consequence of direct renal failure, most likely a result of acute tubular necrosis (ATN). Allergic interstitial nephritis (AIN) with drug-induced immune reactions can occur and lead to ATN. Pigment deposition in myoglobinuria or hemoglobinuria, protein deposition in multiple myeloma (MM), crystal deposition by way of oxalate crystals or urate crystals, vascular disorders leading to thromboembolic phenomenon or vasculitis, IV contrast, NSAIDs, glomerular failure are other causes of intrinsic renal failure leading to ARF.

Table 315 Other Causes of Intrinsic Renal Failure

Other Causes of Intrinsic Renal Failure	
Pigments	Excessive release of hemoglobin from hemolysis and myoglobin from rhabdomyolysis. ATN results due to precipitation of these heavy proteins within the tubules and glomeruli and the direct renal damage they cause.
Proteins	Multiple myeloma produces excessive amounts of Bence-Jones protein, which can coalesce within the glomeruli and tubules and cause ATN. The pathophysiology of damage is similar to that of pigment deposition.
Crystals	Deposition of oxalate crystals in ethylene glycol administration and primary disease, and the deposition of urate crystals in gout and following apoptosis of cancer cells can lead to damage to the renal parenchyma.
Toxins	Most common **causes** are acetaminophen and aspirin poisoning. The effect of these and other NSAIDs is a direct toxic effect leading to necrosis of the renal parenchyma, inhibition of afferent arteriole dilation with subsequent renal ischemia, and interstitial nephritis. **Signs** and **symptoms** of renal failure develop with hematuria, proteinuria, and pyuria. Other toxins include aminoglycosides, cephalosporins, amphotericin B, IV contrast, anticancer drugs, radiation, heavy metal poisoning, and cyclosporine. **Management** involves IV fluids, diuretics, dopamine, and avoidance of protein.

POSTRENAL FAILURE

Postrenal failure is commonly a result of outflow obstruction from the kidney. Common causes include benign prostatic hypertrophy (BPH), bilateral obstruction of the ureters (as in cancer), stricture formation, and bladder obstruction. Postrenal failure presents with hydronephrosis and postobstructive diuresis once the blockage is removed.

Table 316 Renal Failure

Renal Failure	
Acute ARF	Increasing BUN to creatinine ratio with oliguria. The buildup of toxic solutes can occur, along with electrolyte imbalances, volume overload, and multisystemic failure.
Prerenal causes	Due to decreased renal perfusion. Causes include decreased blood volume through hemorrhage, use of diuretics, third spacing of fluids in pancreatitis or following abdominal surgery, dehydration, CHF, nephrotic syndrome, septic shock, RAS, and Addison disease.
Intrinsic causes	Direct renal failure, most likely a result of ATN. AIN with drug-induced immune reactions can occur and lead to ATN. Pigment deposition in myoglobinuria or hemoglobinuria, protein deposition in MM, crystal deposition by way of oxalate crystals or urate crystals, vascular disorders leading to thromboembolic phenomenon or vasculitis, IV contrast, NSAIDs. Glomerular failure is other causes of intrinsic renal failure leading to ARF.
Postrenal causes	Result of outflow obstruction from the kidney. Causes include benign BPH, bilateral obstruction of the ureters, stricture formation, and bladder obstruction. Presents with hydronephrosis, and postobstructive diuresis, once the blockage is removed.

UREMIC SYNDROME

ETIOLOGY AND PATHOPHYSIOLOGY

Uremic syndrome is the development of pruritus, nausea, vomiting, anorexia, polydipsia, proteinuria, tubular casts, purpura, wasting, and pallor associated with CRF. Complications of uremic syndrome include pericarditis, anemia, coagulopathy, GI disruption, and CNS changes. Renal osteodystrophy and peripheral neuropathies are other features of uremic syndrome.

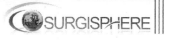

PRESENTATION AND DIAGNOSIS

Uremia presents with seizures, myopathies, clonus, asterixis, HTN, IHD, valvular heart disease, pulmonary edema and effusions, normochromic normocytic anemia, increased bleeding time, reduction in WBCs, GI bleeds, hypertriglyceridemia, and other systemic manifestations. Uremia manifests its hematologic effects by causing a dysfunction of the platelets.

TREATMENT

Uremia is treated by treating the underlying etiology causing CRF and ESRD.

Table 317 Uremic Syndrome

Uremic Syndrome	
Etiology	Development of pruritus, nausea, vomiting, anorexia, polydipsia, proteinuria, tubular casts, purpura, wasting, and pallor associated with CRF. Complications include pericarditis, anemia, coagulopathy, GI disruption, and CNS changes, renal osteodystrophy and peripheral neuropathies.
Presentation	Seizures, myopathies, clonus, asterixis, HTN, IHD, valvular heart disease, pulmonary edema and effusions, normochromic normocytic anemias, increased bleeding time, reduction in WBCs, GI bleeds, and hypertriglyceridemia.
Treatment	Uremia is treated by treating the underlying etiology causing CRF and ESRD.

END-STAGE RENAL DISEASE

ETIOLOGY AND PATHOPHYSIOLOGY

Chronic renal failure (CRF) is progressive decreases in renal function that leads to end stage renal disease (ESRD). CRF is typically secondary to DM leading to diffuse or nodular glomerulosclerosis, HTN, chronic glomerulonephritis, tubulointerstitial disease, APKD, and idiopathic causes. In CRF, progressive loss of nephrons leads to artificially high GFR in the remaining nephrons. This predisposes them to additional insult and injury, leading to a rapidly increasing downward spiral. Renal endocrine function decreases with this continuing injury, leading to a decrease in erythropoietin (EPO) formation and decreased vitamin D.

PRESENTATION AND DIAGNOSIS

CRF is initially asymptomatic as the existing nephrons compensate for the ongoing renal injury. When GFR drops to less than half below baseline, there is initially decreased urine concentration with sodium loss and dehydration. Later symptoms lead to volume overload through renal failure-induced hypernatremia. Potassium excretion decreases, anion gap metabolic acidosis develops, hypocalcemia and hyperphosphatemia occur. The calcium imbalance can lead to bone resorption and ectopic calcification. Creatinine also increases due to decreased renal clearance, along with BUN. CRF presents with signs and symptoms of renal failure, including uremic syndrome, nephrotic syndrome, and ESRD.

TREATMENT

Treatment of CRF centers around maintaining existing renal function through medical management and dialysis until a renal transplant becomes inevitable. Protein restriction is required to minimize renal nitrogen load, along with sodium and phosphate restriction.

Table 318 End Stage Renal Disease (ESRD)

End Stage Renal Disease (ESRD)	
Etiology	CRF is typically secondary to DM leading to diffuse or nodular glomerulosclerosis, HTN, chronic glomerulonephritis, tubulointerstitial disease, APKD, and idiopathic causes.
Presentation	Initially asymptomatic. When GFR drops to less than half below baseline, there is initially decreased urine concentration with sodium loss and dehydration. Later symptoms lead to volume overload through renal failure-induced hypernatremia. Potassium excretion decreases, anion gap metabolic acidosis develops, hypocalcemia and hyperphosphatemia occur. Creatinine also increases, along with BUN. CRF presents with signs and symptoms of renal failure, including uremic syndrome, nephrotic syndrome, and ESRD.
Treatment	Maintaining existing renal function through medical management and dialysis until renal transplant becomes inevitable. Protein restriction is required to minimize renal nitrogen load, along with sodium and phosphate restriction.

INFLAMMATORY AND INFECTIOUS

ACUTE PYELONEPHRITIS

Table 319 Acute Pyelonephritis

Acute Pyelonephritis	
Etiology	The result of a bacterial infection typically emanating from a superiorly progressing UTI.
Presentation	Presents with worsening symptoms of a lower UTI followed by flank pain radiating to the back or pubic region, fever, and numerous constitutional symptoms. CVA tenderness is common.
Treatment	Supportive care and antibiotics tailored to the infecting organism. Surgery to correct anatomic defects and repair renal damage is sometimes done.

PERINEPHRIC ABSCESS

Table 320 Perinephric Abscess

Perinephric Abscess	
Presentation	Constitutional symptoms including fever and abdominal pain, dysuria, and occasionally, a flank mass apparent on exam
Diagnosis	Elevation in WBCs is noted and anemia is common. ESR is elevated. Blood cultures are not specific nor sensitive. Urinalysis typically indicates pyuria, proteinuria, hematuria, and positive cultures. Ultrasound and CT are preferred.
Treatment	Percutaneous drainage, with open drainage used in certain cases. Penicillins, aminoglycosides, and directed antibiotic treatment following sensitivity reports from culture are used. In intractable cases, nephrectomy.

URINARY TRACT INFECTION

ETIOLOGY AND PATHOPHYSIOLOGY

Urinary tract infection (UTI) may present as a lower tract infection (cystitis) or upper tract infection (pyelonephritis, discussed previously). UTI with the formation of calculi, infected cysts, abscess formation, in diabetes, in pregnancy, in

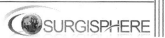

immunocompromised patients, or with certain pathogens is referred to as complicated UTI. The majority of UTIs are caused by *E. coli*, but *S. saprophyticus, Proteus spp., Klebsiella spp., Enterococcus faecalis*, and various yeast also contribute. Risk factors for the development of UTI include frequent intercourse, the presence of anatomic or structural defects, and indwelling catheters. There are over 7 million cases of UTI every year.

PRESENTATION

Hesitancy, dysuria, urgency, polyuria, incomplete voiding, fever, incontinence, and other symptoms are typical of UTI. Acute cystitis presents with these symptoms along with hematuria and low back pain. Constitutional symptoms may also be present. As discussed previously, pyelonephritis presents with the triad of CVA tenderness, fever, and nausea and vomiting. Stone formation, abscess formation, fistulas, or renal failure all may be a part of a complicated UTI.

DIAGNOSIS

Laboratory diagnosis includes urinary glucose, protein, blood, nitrite, and leukocyte esterase titers to determine the relative risk of a UTI. Microscopic inspection for RBCs, WBCs, casts, and any obvious bacteria is also done. Elevated leukocytes is virtually diagnostic of a UTI. WBC casts may be found in pyelonephritis. Nitrite is elevated with bacterial infection. A low grade proteinuria is typically present with UTI. Complicated UTIs also receive ultrasound imaging.

TREATMENT

Therapy for three days is the standard of care. Regimens include TMP-SMX and fluoroquinolones. Cystitis is sometimes treated for up to a week and phenazopyridine may be used to decrease symptoms of dysuria. As discussed previously, mild pyelonephritis is treated with fluoroquinolones and / or TMP-SMX, while more serious infection is treated with ceftriaxone or gentamicin, then TMP-SMX. Complicated UTIs with calculi typically require surgical intervention for removal of the staghorn calculus. Abscess formation requires surgical drainage and treatment with penicillins and aminoglycosides. Cranberry juice decreases the recurrence of UTI.

Table 321 Genitourinary Infection

	Genitourinary Infection
Etiology	*E. coli*, but *S. saprophyticus, Proteus spp., Klebsiella spp., Enterococcus faecalis*, and various yeast also contribute. Risk factors include intercourse, anatomic or structural defects, and indwelling catheters.
Presentation	Hesitancy, dysuria, urgency, polyuria, incomplete voiding, fever, incontinence. Pyelonephritis presents with CVA tenderness, fever, and nausea and vomiting. Stone formation, abscess formation, fistulas, or renal failure all may be a part of a complicated UTI.
Diagnosis	Run urinary glucose, protein, blood, nitrite, and leukocyte esterase titers to determine the relative risk of a UTI. Microscopic inspection for RBCs, WBCs, casts, and any obvious bacteria is also done. Elevated leukocytes are virtually diagnostic of a UTI. WBC casts in pyelonephritis. Nitrite is elevated with bacterial infection.
Treatment	Therapy for three days is the standard of care. Regimens include TMP-SMX and fluoroquinolones. Cystitis is sometimes treated for up to a week and phenazopyridine may be used to decrease symptoms of dysuria. Mild pyelonephritis is treated with fluoroquinolones and / or TMP-SMX, while more serious infection is treated with ceftriaxone or gentamicin, then TMP-SMX. Complicated UTIs with calculi typically require surgical intervention for removal of the staghorn calculus. Abscess formation requires surgical drainage and treatment with penicillins and aminoglycosides. Cranberry juice decreases the recurrence of UTI.

SYPHILIS

Table 322 Syphilis

Syphilis	
Etiology	Infection by *Treponema pallidum*
Presentation	A nontender chancre on the penis or vulva in the form of a solitary, raised papule 3-4 centimeters in diameter. Secondary syphilis occurs thereafter with a diffuse maculopapular rash and generalized lymphadenopathy. The disease continues to be nontender. Syphilis typically leads to a latent phase for as much as 25 years before evolving into tertiary syphilis. Slow progression of tertiary syphilis affects multiple systems with the development of gummas, especially throughout the skeleton and liver. Constitutional symptoms and jaundice are common. Cardiac manifestations may lead to the formation of an aneurysm; neurosyphilis may lead to degradation of CNS function
Diagnosis	Confirmed with the RPR test, VDRL test, FTA-ABS, and other immunoassays. Plain films and CTs are done in tertiary disease.
Treatment	Penicillin G, doxycycline, tetracycline, and erythromycin.

GONORRHEA

Table 323 Gonorrhea

Gonorrhea	
Etiology	Gonorrhea is a sexually transmitted disease that is caused by *Neisseria gonorrhea*
Presentation	Males: Dysuria and yellow discharge are sometimes present. Females: Might have dysuria, vaginal discharge, symptoms of pelvic inflammatory disease
Diagnosis	Gram stain of discharge grown on a Thayer-Martin medium
Treatment	Cephalosporins or fluoroquinolones. Pregnant women should not be administered quinolones and tetracycline

HIV AND AIDS

EPIDEMIOLOGY

Some authorities estimate that nearly one million persons are infected with HIV in the United States with at least 40,000 new cases annually and tens of thousands of deaths due to AIDS every year. The US Public Health Services (PHS) estimates that about 3 out of 10,000 persons have HIV – the exact number is difficult to calculate as HIV requires mandatory reporting in only half the states. However, AIDS is a mandatory reportable illness and in 2001, nearly 1/3 of a million persons had confirmed AIDS. The number of deaths due to AIDS has declined tremendously over the past ten years. Morbidity and mortality from HIV / AIDS is due to various opportunistic infections that assail the body due to a weakness in host defenses. All persons of all races and ages can be affected by HIV / AIDS. However, six times as many men as women are infected with HIV, and sexually-active adults are the most commonly affected population. African-Americans and Hispanics are more affected than Caucasians. Nearly ten years (or more) may elapse between HIV infection and the development of AIDS.

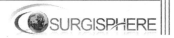

ETIOLOGY

HIV infection is due to one of several subtypes of human immunodeficiency virus. The major viruses are HIV-1 and HIV-2, of which the former is significantly more common in the United States. Infection by HIV leads to acquired immunodeficiency syndrome (AIDS). Infection by numerous opportunistic infections can occur with sufficient breakdown in the immune system, along with several primary diseases.

PATHOPHYSIOLOGY

AIDS is defined as the progression of HIV disease such that CD4 cell counts are less than 200. Early stage HIV has CD4 counts more than 500, intermediate stage with CD4 counts more than 200, and advanced disease with the diagnosis of AIDS. Virus-mediated destruction of CD4 cells leads to the immunodeficiency and a predisposition to numerous infections.

PRESENTATION OF ACUTE INFECTION

HIV infection in the acute stage presents as a flu-like illness, known as an acute retroviral syndrome that commonly occurs 1-6 weeks after infection and similar to infection by EBV leading to infectious mononucleosis. HIV is usually entirely asymptomatic for up to 10 years, then a pre-AIDS complex develops for several years as immunity begins to wane.

PRESENTATION OF THE PRE-AIDS COMPLEX

As disease progresses and CD4 counts drop, a generalized lymphadenopathy develops. Oral thrush and hairy leukoplakia may be present. Past infections with HSV or VZV may recur. Anemia and thrombocytopenia are common. Primary CNS changes or CNS changes secondary to various infections are common, with infection by toxoplasmosis, cryptococcus, CMV, HTLV, TB, syphilis, progressive multifocal leukoencephalopathy (PML), and lymphoma. Aseptic meningitis may occur along with peripheral neuropathies. Kaposi sarcoma (KS) may develop with a CD count more than 200. Other CNS infections are more common with CD4 counts dropping below 200. The pre-AIDS complex that occurs a few years before full-blown AIDS presents with persistent generalized lymphadenopathy (PGL), nodal enlargement, purpura, cotton-wool spots in the retina with hemorrhages and microaneurysms, hairy leukoplakia, fungal infections throughout the body, molluscum contagiosum, psoriasis, seborrheic dermatitis, and numerous constitutional symptoms. HIV-related encephalopathy and dementia (discussed previously) may develop with numerous CNS effects.

PRESENTATION OF AIDS

With the development of AIDS, serious opportunistic infections develop and lead to a rapid decline in health. Pneumocystis carinii pneumonia (PCP) may present with abrupt onset of constitutional symptoms, cough, DOE, tachypnea, and a CD4 count below 250. Candidiasis, pneumonia, CMV, TB, and HSV infections are common. Toxoplasmosis may occur leading to CNS lesions and changes in consciousness, focal neurologic findings, and mental status changes. *Bartonella* infection may lead to bacteremia, angiomatosis, and peliosis with hepatosplenomegaly and splenic or osseous damage. Mycobacterium avium complex (MAC) may develop, leading to anemia, lung disease, lymphadenopathy, and numerous constitutional symptoms. *Cryptococcus* meningitis and *Cryptococcus* pneumonia can occur followed by dissemination throughout the body. Coccidiomycosis may lead to a pleural friction rub, hepatosplenomegaly, tachycardia, increased DTRs, tenosynovitis, erythema nodosum, toxic erythema, and meningitis – this infection is rapidly fatal if severe. Histoplasmosis presents with septicemia and neurologic manifestations. Cryptosporidiosis can lead to watery diarrhea, a malabsorption syndrome, and biliary disease. Other common diseases include *Salmonella septicemia, shigella, campylobacter,* isosporiasis (like cryptosporidiosis), *Microsporidia* (also like cryptosporidiosis), PML (JC papovavirus leading to demyelination and subsequent dementia and encephalopathy), malignancy with Kaposi sarcoma (HHV8), Burkitt lymphoma (abdominal mass with jaw involvement and elevated uric acid), and CNS lymphoma.

DIAGNOSIS

Diagnosis of HIV infection is confirmed by history, physical exam, and viral cultures for various opportunistic infections. ELISA is done first and confirmed with Western blot. PCR, HIV RNA assays, p24 antigen tests, and HIV cultures are other diagnostic tests. Note that ELISA may be negative in the acute phase of disease. CD4 cell counts, viral load, CBC, CC1, and serologic testing for intercurrent infection should be done on a routine basis for all HIV positive patients. Specific testing for various opportunistic infections should be carried out with a sufficient clinical suspicion or with plummeting CD4 counts. AIDS is diagnosed with any CD4 count less than 200 or with infection by an opportunistic disease – reporting is required in all states.

TREATMENT

Treatment for various infections in HIV has been discussed elsewhere. Briefly, antifungals are used for oral thrush, oral hairy leukoplakia is treated with ACV, HSV and VZV with ACV, FCV, and VCV or foscarnet, anemia with recombinant epoetin therapy, and general supportive care. Vaccinations for pneumonia (23 valent), HAV, HBV, tetanus booster, influenza, and VZIG are done. Antiretroviral therapy is given to all patients with acute infection, within 6 months of seroconversion, in those with symptomatic infection, and with CD4 counts dropping below 350. All patients with AIDS should receive antiretroviral therapy. Treatment is complex, but involves efavirenz, indinavir, nelfinavir, ritonavir, saquinavir, stavudine, didanosine, lamivudine, zidovudine, and didanosine. PCP prophylaxis is started in all with CD4 counts below 200 and is best done with TMO-SMX, dapsone with pyrimethamine and leucovorin, pentamidine, or atovaquone. Toxoplasmosis encephalitis is treated with TMO-SMX or the agents listed for PCP. TB is treated as necessary. MAC is treated with azithromycin, clarithromycin, or rifabutin.

TRAUMA

BLADDER RUPTURE

A patient with an extraperitoneal rupture of the bladder can have a foley placed and be observed. An intraperitoneal bladder rupture requires operative management with closure of the rupture in two layers. A foley catheter is placed and retained for at least 10 days.

CANCER

RENAL CELL CARCINOMA

Resection of a single pulmonary metastasis from renal cell cancer increases survival. Suprahepatic IVC resections are not contraindicated.

MALE REPRODUCTIVE ORGANS

CONGENITAL AND STRUCTURAL

PHIMOSIS

The presence of phimosis prior to an elective case should be treated with the creation of a dorsal slit.

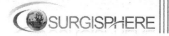

HYPOSPADIAS

Incomplete distal urethral development.

PEYRONES DISEASE

Penile shaft induration. Treatment includes remodeling of the penis and possible prosthetic implantation.

METABOLIC AND DEGENERATIVE

BENIGN PROSTATIC HYPERPLASIA

ETIOLOGY AND PATHOPHYSIOLOGY

Benign prostatic hyperplasia (BPH) usually begins in many males after the age of 40, which can lead to urinary tract outflow obstruction. Frequency of urination increases as the detrusor muscle undergoes hypertrophy to overcome the afterload and expel urine. Incomplete emptying of the bladder may result, and a predisposition to UTIs.

PRESENTATION AND DIAGNOSIS

Presentation of BPH includes hesitancy, frequency, incomplete urination, and urine leaking. Nighttime urinary symptoms may also be present, and hematuria may sometimes occur. Constitutional symptoms may also occur in severe cases. Diagnosis is made by DRE, PSA to screen for prostate cancer, and imaging studies.

TREATMENT

BPH is treated with the alpha-blocker terazosin, prazosin, or doxazosin to relax the prostate, and finasteride or dutasteride to decrease the mass of the prostate. Transurethral resection of the prostate (TURP) is a common surgical intervention to relieve pressure. Incision of the prostate (TUIP) may also be undertaken. Finally, microwave therapy (TUMT) may also be used. Cranberry juice is recommended to avoid UTIs, along with avoiding liquids several hours before sleeping to avoid nighttime symptoms.

Table 324 Benign Prostate Hypertrophy (BPH)

Benign Prostate Hypertrophy (BPH)	
Etiology	Detrusor muscle undergoes hypertrophy.
Presentation	Includes hesitancy, frequency, incomplete urination, and urine leaking. Nighttime urinary symptoms may also be present, and hematuria may sometimes occur. Constitutional symptoms may also occur in severe cases.
Diagnosis	DRE, PSA to screen for prostate cancer, and imaging studies.
Treatment	Alpha-blocker terazosin, prazosin, or doxazosin to relax the prostate, and finasteride or dutasteride to decrease the mass of the prostate. TURP is a common surgical intervention to relieve pressure. TUIP or TUMT may also be used. Cranberry juice is recommended to avoid UTIs, along with avoiding liquids several hours before sleeping to avoid nighttime symptoms.

FOURNIER GANGRENE

Treatment involves debridement and antibiotics. A suprapubic catheter with diverting colostomy may be required to permit satisfactory healing.

CANCER

PROSTATE CANCER

ETIOLOGY AND PATHOPHYSIOLOGY

Prostate cancer is a common but difficult to detect cancer. This slow growing tumor is sometimes detected with elevated prostate-specific antigen (PSA), and the majority of tumors are adenocarcinomas. Most cancer occurs in the peripheral zone (PZ), with the remainder in the transitional zone (TZ). The tumors in the PZ are more aggressive and invasive than those in the TZ. It is the second most common cause of cancer-related death in men, with nearly 30,000 deaths annually from 220,000 cases. Incidence is highest in African American males with exponentially increasing risk with age. A high fat diet and a positive family history are also positive risk factors.

PRESENTATION AND DIAGNOSIS

Prostate cancer is typically asymptomatic until a positive exam through digital rectal exam (DRE) is conducted and hard nodules found, or an elevated PSA found in a screening test. Urinary tract obstructions, through impingement of the outflow tract, are sometimes present. As metastasis to the bone is common, bone pain may be a presenting sign. PSA is a better marker for following up in patients with established prostate cancer, but some clinicians use it as a screening test. Beware that PSA may be negative in a patient with prostate cancer. Biopsy through transrectal ultrasound (TRUS) is the preferred method of diagnosis and prognosis. Imaging studies are also commonly used.

TREATMENT

Treatment of prostate cancer centers on symptomatic management and resection. Radiation therapy is commonly used along with radical prostatectomy. As more men die with prostate cancer than from prostate cancer, simply waiting in an older patient may also be the best course of action.

Table 325 Prostate Cancer

Prostate Cancer	
Etiology	Adenocarcinoma
Presentation	Asymptomatic until a positive DRE is conducted and hard nodules found, or an elevated PSA found in a screening test. Urinary tract obstructions are sometimes present. As metastasis to the bone is common, bone pain may be a presenting sign
Diagnosis	PSA, DRE, biopsy, imaging studies
Treatment	Symptomatic management and resection. Radiation therapy is commonly used along with radical prostatectomy. As more men die with prostate cancer than from prostate cancer, simply waiting in an older patient may also be the best course of action.

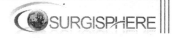

SQUAMOUS CELL CARCINOMA OF THE PENIS

The presence of squamous cell carcinoma of the penis should be treated with a partial penectomy if lymph nodes are negative. If inguinal lymph nodes are positive, six weeks of antibiotics and a lymph node dissection should be performed.

TESTICULAR CANCER

The aggressiveness of non-seminomatous germ cell tumors can be predicted by alpha fetoprotein and beta hCG levels. Initial treatment is a radical inguinal orchiectomy with a high ligation of the spermatic cord.

PRACTICE QUESTIONS

 Which of the following vessels comes from the aorta, runs posterior to the inferior vena cava, posterior to another vascular structure, and inserts into the anterior portion of the renal pelvis?

- A.   Left renal artery
- B.   Left renal vein
- C.   Right renal artery
- D.   Right renal vein
- E.   Ureter

 The best answer is <u>Right renal artery</u>. The right renal artery is a branch of the aorta, travels posterior to the inferior vena cava and posterior to the right renal vein, and turns anterior to insert into the renal pelvis.

 A 76 year old male is diagnosed with a malignant testicular tumor while undergoing an inguinal hernia repair. Blood tests reveal an increase in beta-hCG. Which of the following is the most likely cause of this tumor?

- A.   Choriocarcinoma and seminomas
- B.   Leydig tumor
- C.   Non-seminomatous germ cell tumor
- D.   Sarcoidosis
- E.   Seminoma

The best answer is <u>Choriocarcinoma and seminomas</u>. Germ cell tumors can be divided into seminomatous and non-seminomatous tumors. Seminomas tend to be malignant and approximately 10% of them have an elevation in hCG. Non-seminomatous germ cell tumors such as choriocarcinoma almost always secrete hCG, and AFP about half the time. Yolk sac tumors tend to secrete aFP. Teratomas tend not to secrete any of these markers.

What is the drainage of the left testicular vein?

A. Inferior vena cava
B. Left hypogastric vein
C. Left inferior epigastric vein
D. Left internal iliac vein
E. Left renal vein

The best answer is <u>Left renal vein</u>. The left testicular vein drains into the left renal vein. The right testicular vein drains directly into the inferior vena cava. The left testicular vein anatomy is important in that a left sided renal tumor migrating through the renal vein may present as left testicular venous congestion and subsequent edema.

 A 46 year old male presents with a testicular mass. He complains of having blood with his ejaculate and has pain in his left scrotum. A localized tumor is found during surgical exploration and is diagnosed as a seminoma. All lymph nodes are negative. What is the next best step in management?

A. Orchiectomy and monitor AFP
B. Orchiectomy and monitor B-hCG
C. Orchiectomy with chemoradiation
D. Orchiectomy with radiation therapy
E. Orchiectomy with retroperitoneal lymph node dissection

The best answer is <u>Orchiectomy with radiation therapy</u>. This patient has a non-metastatic seminoma, for which the treatment is to proceed with an orchiectomy followed by radiation therapy. Chemotherapy is necessary if metastatic disease is present. Seminoma spreads to the retroperitoneal lymph nodes and para-aortic nodes. Seminoma does not produce AFP, but it can produce B-hCG. AFP can be followed by non-seminomatous tumors. Non-seminomas are treated with orchiectomy, retroperitoneal node dissection, and chemotherapy with cisplatin if metastasis is present. Non-seminomas are resistant to radiation.

 A 66 year old male presents with a left sided varicocele. He is also found to have some erythrocytosis, and a palpable left flank mass is evident. He is diagnosed with renal cell carcinoma. Where is the most common site of metastasis?

A. Brain
B. Liver
C. Lung
D. Pancreas
E. Prostate

The best answer is <u>Lung</u>. Renal cell carcinoma is most likely to metastasize to the lung and bones. A paraneoplastic syndrome can occur due to excess production of erythropoietin, leading to erythropoiesis. Hematuria, flank pain, and a palpable flank mass are common presenting signs; if a left-sided tumor is present, a left varicocele can occur due to the left testicular vein draining into the left renal vein. A right-sided tumor may present with signs of inferior vena cava obstruction. Renal cell cancer can lead to a syndrome with liver failure, hypertension, and hypercalcemia. Treatment is radical nephrectomy.

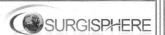

ORTHOPEDIC SURGERY

CHAPTER CONTENTS

GENERAL CONCEPTS

BIOMECHANICS

Alkaline phosphatase is the active enzyme in osteoblasts.

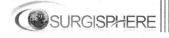

HEAD, NECK, AND SPINE

LUMBAR DISC HERNIATION

ASSESSMENT

Herniation of a lumbar vertebral disc either between L4-L5 or L5-S1 is a common cause of lower back pain. Prolapse of the nucleus pulposus through the annulus fibrosis leads to symptoms of decreased ROM, pain, paresthesia, and decreased reflexes. The specific losses depend on the spinal nerves that are affected. L4 impingement leads to weakened knee reflexes and weakness of the tibialis anterior. L5 effects lead to weakness in the extensor hallucis longus and diminished sensation over the lateral leg. Pinching of S1 leads to a decreased ankle jerk reflex and diminished sensation over the lateral foot.

MANAGEMENT

Treatment of lumbar disc herniation is to alleviate pain with NSAIDs. Surgery is used only with significant neurologic symptoms or pain.

Table 326 Lumbar Disc Herniation

Lumbar Disc Herniation	
Etiology	Herniation of lumbar vertebral disc.
Presentation	Decreased ROM, pain, paresthesia, and decreased reflexes
Diagnosis	**L4 impingement** leads to weakened knee reflexes and weakness of the tibialis anterior. **L5** effects lead to weakness in the extensor hallucis longus and diminished sensation over the lateral leg. **Pinching of S1** leads to a decreased ankle jerk reflex and diminished sensation over the lateral foot.
Treatment	NSAIDs, surgery.

CAUDA EQUINA SYNDROME

ASSESSMENT

Saddle anesthesia, incontinence, sciatica, and loss of motor or sensory function in the lower extremities are the most common effects of lumbar and sacral root compression in cauda equina syndrome (CES). CES is commonly secondary to spinal stenosis, disk herniations, and tumor expansion.

MANAGEMENT

Treatment of CES involves resting on a hard surface at night and adequate pain control. Laminectomy may become necessary to alleviate severe pain and neurologic symptoms.

Table 327 Cauda Equina Syndrome (CES)

Cauda Equina Syndrome (CES)	
Etiology	Sacral and lumbar root compression, secondary to spinal stenosis, disk herniations, and tumor expansion.
Presentation	Saddle anesthesia, incontinence, sciatica, and loss of motor or sensory function in the lower extremities.
Treatment	Resting on a hard surface at night and adequate pain control. Laminectomy.

UPPER EXTREMITIES

SHOULDER AND ARM

A fracture of the mid-humeral shaft should prompt an exploration for radial nerve injury. Volkmann's ischemic contracture may be due to a supracondylar humerus fracture. A patient with a humerus fracture and no radial pulse should have the fracture reduced first. Drop wrist may be due to a distal humerus fracture. Displaced supracondylar fractures of the humerus should be reduced and distal pulses verified. This is the overall management of any extremity fracture.

HAND AND WRIST

CARPAL TUNNEL SYNDROME

ASSESSMENT

Carpal tunnel syndrome is an acquired disorder in which compression of the median nerve occurs as it passes under the flexor retinaculum. Compression of the nerve occurs in a classic repetitive stress injury (RSI) or following direct trauma to the region. Pregnant women are especially at risk due to the generalized edema of pregnancy. Presentation is with distal weakness, thenar atrophy, and tingling in the fingers. Phalen's sign is positive in which paresthesia occurs in the distal extremity following 90 degree wrist flexion ("prayer hand"); Tinel's sign is positive in which tapping on the region of the median nerve at the wrist elicits pain and tingling that radiates distally to the phalanges.

MANAGEMENT

Treatment is straightforward. RICE, or rest, icing, compression, and elevation are done to decrease inflammation. Steroids may be used on a temporary basis to alleviate symptoms. Surgery is the treatment of choice and is a relatively straightforward process in which the flexor retinaculum is incised and the carpal tunnel decompressed.

Table 328 Carpal Tunnel Syndrome (CTS)

Carpal Tunnel Syndrome (CTS)	
Etiology	Compression of the median nerve occurs due to RSI or following direct trauma to the region.
Presentation	Distal weakness, thenar atrophy, and tingling in the fingers.
Diagnosis	Positive Phalen's and Tinel's signs.
Treatment	Rest, icing, compression, and elevation. Steroids may be used temporarily, surgery.

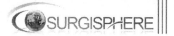

TENOSYNOVITIS

Tenosynovitis is commonly due to penetrating trauma leading to bacterial infection. It presents with fusiform swelling and tenderness with pain on passive motion. The extremity is typically flexed. Management includes antibiotics and possible incision and drainage. Failure to diagnose and treat can result in amputation of the affected region.

LOWER EXTREMITIES

PELVIS

PELVIC FRACTURE

A fracture of the pelvis may occur following high speed motor vehicle accidents. Bleeding can occur into the pelvis and lead to shock. Management includes placement of an external fixation device followed by possible angiography with coil embolization if bleeding does not remit. Surgical intervention is the last resort due to difficulty with visualization and achieving control. Groin pain following a particularly strong kick may be due to a tear of the sartorius muscle.

URETHRAL TRANSECTION

Blood at the urethral meatus should be explored by means of a retrograde urethrogram.

HIP AND THIGH

FEMORAL FRACTURE

Early open reduction and internal fixation should be the therapy of choice in patients with femoral shaft fractures in the setting of multiple traumas. Stabilization with a splint or rod fixation is done early to permit early mobilization of the patient. Arteriography is required with any disruption in distal pulses. Children with open fractures require aggressive debridement to avoid infection. Secondary closure over a week is the preferred therapy.

KNEE AND LEG

KNEE DISLOCATION

Dislocation of the knee posterior requires an angiogram to ensure that the popliteal artery is intact. Disruption leading to thrombosis and possible distal embolization may occur in up to half of all affected patients.

TIBIA AND FIBULA FRACTURE

The initial treatment in a patient with an open tibia and fibula is immediate irrigation and debridement in the operating room. The presentation of a shortened leg and adduction following trauma is likely due to a posterior hip dislocation. The common peroneal nerve must be preserved in the context of a fibulectomy. An arteriogram must be performed to assess for arterial injury following popliteal dislocation. A positive Lachman test indicates injury to the ACL.

AMPUTATION

Lower extremity amputation is the best course of action in patients with significant distal infection that is refractory to maximum medical management. Most patients with wet gangrene of the lower extremity are started on a trial of piperacillin/tazobactam and vancomycin with aggressive surgical debridement. Failure to resolve typically results in a below knee amputation (BKA). Another indication for amputation is the presence of rest pain and dry gangrene without the possibility of bypass to distal arteries. Malignant tumors limited to the lower extremity and significant unsalvageable trauma to the extremity are other indications for amputation. A below knee amputation is the preferred operation in most patients due to the possibility of returning to a functional status via prosthesis and being able to continue to bear weight on the affected limb. However, a BKA may be revised to an above knee amputation (AKA) if it does not heal. Failure of an AKA to heal portends very high mortality. Amputation of the foot is possible in a procedure known as Syme's amputation.

COMPARTMENT SYNDROME

EXTREMITY

A compartment syndrome that develops following a thrombectomy requires a fasciotomy. Loss of sensation is an early sign of compartment syndrome. The presence of calf pain and loss of sensation in the distal extremity following a vascular procedure requires a fasciotomy. Compartment pressures should be checked in any patient who was in stirrups during an extended OR case and then presents with numbness or weakness. Casts should be removed in the setting of compartment syndrome. The anterior compartment is the most susceptible. This contains the deep peroneal nerve and may present as foot drop and numbness in the first toe interspace. Pain is the first presenting sign, especially with passive extension of the extremity. Compartment syndrome is diagnosed when intracompartment pressures are over 30mmHg.

ABDOMEN

A trauma patient with significant fluid resuscitation and rising airway pressures should be ruled out for abdominal compartment syndrome.

SYSTEMIC DISEASES

OSTEOPOROSIS

EPIDEMIOLOGY

Osteoporosis is the development of bone resorption leading to decreased integrity of the bony skeleton. Bones susceptible to fracture and damage are the result, leading to a significant amount of related morbidity and mortality. Osteoporosis affects some 10 million Americans; osteopenia affects nearly twice as many people. Internationally, osteoporosis can be found in 1 in 3 women and 1 in 8 men. Over a million fractures occur every year that are directly due to osteoporosis, leading to over 37,000 deaths annually from related complications. Few patients return to their baseline function after experiencing a fracture. Osteoporosis is most common in elderly patients, but a variant of osteoporosis can occur in any individual.

ETIOLOGY

Osteoporosis is the result of numerous distinct pathologies. More than one can be found in a patient with summative effects. While estrogen is protective in women prior to menopause, a paucity afterwards can accelerate osteoporosis. Hypogonadism

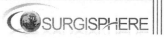

with low testosterone is a risk factor. Osteoblast defects, long term use of heparin, various antiseizure medications (such as phenytoin and carbamazepine), corticosteroid inhibition of new bone deposition, cyclosporine A, and aluminum-containing antacids have all been implicated as causing osteoporosis. Endocrinologic defects such as Cushing syndrome increase bone resorption. Alcohol and smoking have direct toxic effects on the bone. Cancer and lymphomas have been implicated as increasing bone resorption. Malabsorptive disorders such as anorexia or GI ailments can prevent proper absorption of calcium and essential vitamins.

PATHOPHYSIOLOGY

The summation of these risk factors along with various idiopathic causes leads to osteoporosis through decreased bone formation and increased bone resorption. Unopposed action of osteoclasts leads to removal of calcium and decreased bone mass and strength. Type 1 osteoporosis occurs mostly in postmenopausal women and is thought to be due to a shortage of estrogen (it can also occur in men from a testosterone decrease). Increased sensitivity to PTH with increased calcium loss contributes to osteoporosis in this population. Senile osteoporosis, which is type 2 osteoporosis, occurs due to decreased production of 1,25(OH)2 D3 from the kidney. Decreased bone formation with increased loss is the result. Finally, type 3 osteoporosis can occur in any person and is commonly due to medication-induced bone loss.

PRESENTATION

Osteoporosis is an asymptomatic disease. Identifying risk factors and correcting any underlying etiology is the method of choice for preventing the onset of osteoporosis and minimizing its effects. The first symptom of osteoporosis is often fracture, which is most likely to occur spontaneously in the thoracic or lumbar spine, or after falls in the forearm, hip, and femur. Rib fractures are more common with chronic steroid use.

DIAGNOSIS

Diagnosis of osteoporosis begins with blood tests to measure the level of calcium, phosphate, and alkaline phosphatase – all of which are normal in primary osteoporosis. This test is done to rule out other more reversible etiologies. Thyroid function is tested. Imaging studies center on locating regions of potential fracture. Plain films of the vertebral column are mandatory. Bone mineral density (BMD) testing is more precise and is a better predictor of fracture risk. A BMD score between -1 and -2.5 indicates osteopenia. Scores less than -2.5 are diagnosed as osteoporosis. BMD can be measured with a dual-energy x-ray absorptiometry (DEXA) scan, which is preferred over CT.

TREATMENT

Osteoporosis is best treated by preventing the onset of the disease. Calcium supplements, regular exercise, hormone replacement as indicated, calcitonin, selective estrogen-receptor modulators (SERMs), bisphosphonates, low dose PTH, and vitamin D intake are all beneficial. The majority of treatment is effective in preventing additional bone resorption. Weight-bearing exercise is highly beneficial. Alendronate sodium has recently been shown to lead to increased bone strength over a long period of use.

Table 329 Osteoporosis

Osteoporosis	
Types	1--postmenopausal women and is thought to be due to a paucity of estrogen. **2 (senile)**--occurs due to decreased production of 1,25(OH)2 D3 from the kidney. 3-- can occur in any person and is commonly due to medication-induced bone loss.
Presentation	Asymptomatic, first symptom is often fracture, which is most likely to occur spontaneously in the thoracic or lumbar spine, or after falls in the forearm, hip, and femur. Rib fractures are more common with chronic steroid use.
Diagnosis	Measure the level of calcium, phosphate, and alkaline phosphatase. Thyroid function is tested. Imaging studies center on locating regions of potential fracture. Plain films of the vertebral column are mandatory. BMD testing is more precise and is a better predictor of fracture risk. BMD can be measured with a DEXA scan, which is preferred over CT.
Treatment	Calcium supplements, regular exercise, hormone replacement, calcitonin, SERMs, bisphosphonates, low dose PTH, and vitamin D. The majority of treatment is effective in preventing additional bone resorption, alendronate sodium.

OSTEOARTHRITIS

EPIDEMIOLOGY

Osteoarthritis is one of the most common arthritic conditions that afflict people, with over 20 million people affected in the US alone. Over half of the elderly population is affected by OA. OA is a progressive disorder that occurs over many decades and leads to gradual decreases in mobility.

ETIOLOGY AND PATHOPHYSIOLOGY

OA is the result of articular cartilage breakdown due to degeneration and inflammatory processes. Weight bearing joints are affected the most, in addition to the distal interphalangeal (DIP) and proximal interphalangeal (PIP) joints in the hands. Cartilage loss is striking, and bony osteophytes develop throughout the body. OA occurs due to increasing age-related stress, obesity, following trauma or serious systemic infections, in repetitive stress injuries (RSIs), following inflammatory arthritis, and in various metabolic disorders. OA begins with a breakdown in the cartilage due to inflammation and degeneration, followed by erosion of the surface of the collagen. Inflammation and synovitis occurs followed by changes to the joint, formation of excess bone in an attempt to remodel and stabilize the affected region, and additional inflammation and breakdown.

PRESENTATION AND DIAGNOSIS

OA presents with pain, decreasing mobility, morning stiffness and stiffness following extended periods of rest, and joint instability. The stiffness typically improves with exercise. Physical exam findings include joint effusions, bursal inflammation, muscular spasms, joint crepitus, PIP and DIP enlargement, and limited ROM. ESR and CRP are not changed, and there is little WBC infiltrate in the synovial fluid. Plain films indicate numerous osteophytes and bony spurs with joint space narrowing and cyst formation.

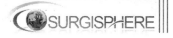

TREATMENT

Therapy for OA includes reducing stresses on the joints through weight reduction, exercise, physical therapy (PT) and occupational therapy (OT). Ice or heat application is sometimes beneficial. Pain control with NSAIDs and cyclooxygenase-2 (COX-2) inhibitors help alleviate symptoms. Narcotics may also be necessary in more severe OA. Osteotomy, removal of bony spurs, and arthroplasty are surgical options available in alleviating the sequelae of OA.

Table 330 Osteoarthritis (OA)

Osteoarthritis (OA)	
Etiology	Increasing age-related stress, obesity, following trauma or serious systemic infections, in RSIs, following inflammatory arthritis, and in various metabolic disorders.
Presentation	Pain, decreasing mobility, stiffness in the morning and following extended periods of rest, and joint instability. The stiffness typically improves with exercise.
Diagnosis	Joint effusions, bursal inflammation, muscular spasms, joint crepitus, PIP and DIP enlargement, and limited ROM. Plain films.
Treatment	Reducing stresses on the joints, exercise, PT and occupational therapy OT. Ice or heat application. Pain control with NSAIDs and COX-2 inhibitors. Narcotics may also be necessary in more severe OA. Osteotomy, removal of bony spurs, and arthroplasty.

ENTEROPATHIC ARTHROPATHY

ETIOLOGY AND PATHOPHYSIOLOGY

Arthritis due to various GI infections is referred to as enteropathic arthropathy. An immunologic predisposition towards antigens in various bacteria leading to an uncontrolled immune reaction and the development of an autoimmune disorder are blamed as the pathophysiology. This type of molecular mimicry is found with *Shigella, Salmonella, Campylobacter, Yersinia, Clostridium, Strongyloides stercoralis, Taenia saginata, Giardia lamblia, Ascaris lumbricoides,* and *Cryptosporidium* spp. Enteropathic arthropathy affects some 20% of patients with IBD.

PRESENTATION AND DIAGNOSIS

Enteropathic arthropathy presents like most other types of arthritis – an axial arthritis is present that is worse in the morning or with low activity. Peripheral arthritis may develop. Manifestations of IBD such as abdominal pain, hematochezia, aphthous ulcers, pyoderma gangrenosum or erythema nodosum, uveitis, and low grade fever are all prevalent. Symptoms similar to reactive arthritis may develop. Water diarrhea and abdominal pain are common in some patients.

TREATMENT

Treatment of enteropathic arthropathy involves modifying the underlying IBD, whether it is Crohn disease or ulcerative colitis. NSAIDs are sometimes used with caution, but sulfasalazine is more popular. Antagonists to TNF are used by some care providers.

Table 331 Enteropathic Arthropathy

Enteropathic Arthropathy	
Etiology	An immunologic predisposition towards antigens in various bacteria leading to an uncontrolled immune reaction and the development of an autoimmune disorder are blamed as the pathophysiology.
Presentation And Diagnosis	Axial arthritis is present that is worse in the morning or with low activity. Peripheral arthritis may develop. Manifestations of IBD such as abdominal pain, hematochezia, aphthous ulcers, pyoderma gangrenosum or erythema nodosum, uveitis, and low grade fever are all prevalent. Symptoms similar to reactive arthritis may develop. Water diarrhea and abdominal pain is common in some patients.
Treatment	Modify the underlying IBD. NSAIDs are sometimes used with caution, but sulfasalazine is more popular. Antagonists to TNF are used by some care providers.

GOUT

ETIOLOGY AND PATHOPHYSIOLOGY

Gout is the result of abnormalities with uric acid metabolism leading to arthritis and joint destruction. Excess stores of uric acid lead to tissue accumulation with subsequent urate crystal formation. Consumption of uncoated uric acid crystals by mediators of the immune system leads to an inflammatory reaction, which can subsequently cause joint damage through oxidative injury and direct toxic injury. Gout affects about 1 in 100 persons, and is highly amenable to medical intervention. Untreated gout can lead to tophaceous gout with joint destruction. Diseases associated with hyperuricemia include hypertriglyceridemia and HTN. African Americans are somewhat more affected than others, and males more than women. Cyclosporin A administration has also been tied to the onset of gout. Gout may be exacerbated by alcohol abuse, starvation, trauma, bleeding, diuretics, allopurinol, Lesch-Nyhan syndrome with hypoxanthine-guanine phosphoribosyl transferase (HGPRT) deficiency, von Gierke disease with glucose-6-phosphatase dehydrogenase (G6PD) deficiency, and fructose-1-phosphate (F1P) deficiency. Overproduction of uric acid can occur in tumor lysis syndrome, psoriasis, obesity, hemolytic anemia, and lymphoproliferative disorders. Hypothyroidism, hyperparathyroidism, and renal insufficiency are other causes of gout.

PRESENTATION AND DIAGNOSIS

Gout presents as monoarticular arthritis, especially affecting the lower extremities. The hallux is typically inflamed in a condition known as podagra, but this can be present in pseudogout and other arthritic conditions. Inflammation in gout reaches a maximum after about half a day with redness, swelling, and pain. Resolution of the initial attacks occurs within a couple of weeks, with recurrence over time. Polyarticular arthritis ensues over time with involvement of numerous other joints. Polyarticular arthritis develops over time and becomes chronic in course. Aspiration of synovial fluid and the demonstration of negatively birefringent crystals with sharp ends is diagnostic of gout. An elevated serum uric acid test is not diagnostic of gout, and asymptomatic hyperuricemia does not necessarily warrant treatment other than observation of renal function tests. Uric acid excess in a 24 hour urine sample is diagnostic of overproduction.

TREATMENT

Acute manifestations of gout are treated with NSAIDs, colchicine, and steroids. NSAIDs are the drug of choice, especially indomethacin. Colchicine is rarely used in the treatment of acute gout today due to its side effects and numerous contraindications. The chief complication of colchicine is granulocytopenia and so therefore requires WBC monitoring during administration. Gout prophylaxis involves the use of allopurinol or probenecid (absolutely contraindicated in acute attacks as

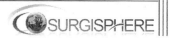

they can precipitate gout). Colchicine is used as prophylaxis along with NSAIDs. With a second attack of gout, lowering uric acid is undertaken, starting with probenecid, then sulfinpyrazone, then allopurinol. Dietary changes include avoiding alcohol and having a low-fat, low-cholesterol diet to avoid the ancillary disorders associated with gout.

Table 332 Gout

Gout	
Etiology	Abnormalities with uric acid metabolism leading to arthritis and joint destruction
Presentation	Monoarticular arthritis, especially affecting the lower extremities. The hallux is typically inflamed, but this can be present in pseudogout and other arthritic conditions. Inflammation in gout reaches a maximum after about half a day with redness, swelling, and pain. Resolution of the initial attacks occurs within a couple of weeks, with recurrence over time. Polyarticular arthritis ensues over time with involvement of numerous other joints. Polyarticular arthritis develops over time and becomes chronic in course.
Treatment	Gout prophylaxis involves the use of allopurinol or probenecid (absolutely contraindicated in acute attacks as they can precipitate gout). Colchicine is used as prophylaxis along with NSAIDs. With a second attack of gout, lowering uric acid is undertaken, starting with probenecid, then sulfinpyrazone, then allopurinol. Dietary changes include avoiding alcohol and having a low-fat, low-cholesterol diet to avoid the ancillary disorders associated with gout.

Table 333 Hyperuricemia Agents

DRUG	INDICATIONS	MECHANISM OF ACTION	COMPLICATIONS	NOTES
Colchicine	Gout Amyloidosis Scleroderma Mediterranean fever	Binds to tubulin to prevent cytoskeleton development and reduces inflammation by preventing neutrophil chemotaxis	GI Sx Neutropenia BMS Similar to arsenic poisoning	Alkaloid
Probenecid	Gout	Uricosuric agent	Can acutely worsen hyperuricemia symptoms	
Allopurinol	Gout	Inhibits xanthine oxidase to decrease formation of uric acid	Rash Hepatitis Eosinophilia	Also used for tumor lysis syndrome and nephrolithiasis

INFECTIOUS

PUNCTURE WOUND

A puncture wound through the finger tip requires an incision and drainage through the volar aspect across the IP joint.

OSTEOMYELITIS

ETIOLOGY AND PATHOPHYSIOLOGY

Osteomyelitis is the progressive destruction of the bone due to infection by GBS, *S. aureus, E. coli, S. pyogenes*, HIB, gram-negative bacilli, *Pseudomonas, Serratia*, and various anaerobes. Inflammation of the bone and subsequent damage is followed by new bone formation. The tibia and femur are the most commonly affected bones, but the vertebrae are also commonly affected in adults.

PRESENTATION AND DIAGNOSIS

Onset of osteomyelitis includes sudden development of fever, various constitutional symptoms, reduction in limb usage, and signs of inflammation and infection. A superimposed cellulitis or ulcer may be present in certain types of patients, especially diabetics. Blood culture is typically collected along with plain films and CT, but a bone biopsy is the gold standard for identifying the offending agent.

TREATMENT

Osteomyelitis is treated by identifying the offending organism and tailoring therapy against it.

Table 334 Osteomyelitis

Osteomyelitis	
Etiology	Osteomyelitis is the progressive destruction of the bone due to infection by GBS, *S. aureus, E. coli, S. pyogenes*, HIB, gram-negative bacilli, *Pseudomonas, Serratia*, and various anaerobes.
Presentation	Sudden development of fever, various constitutional symptoms, reduction in limb usage, and signs of inflammation and infection. A superimposed cellulitis or ulcer may be present in certain types of patients, especially diabetics.
Diagnosis	Blood culture is typically collected along with plain films and CT, but a bone biopsy is the gold standard for identifying the offending agent.
Treatment	Identify the offending organism and tailoring therapy against it.

EPIDURAL ABSCESS

ASSESSMENT

Abscess development can occur as a consequence of immunosuppression, IVDA in the elderly, or following epidural anesthesia for labor in pregnancy. Abscess formation can lead to circulation occlusion, nerve impingement, and spread to adjacent structures. It is commonly the result of infection by *Staphylococcus aureus*, gram-negative rods, and TB. An epidural abscess presents with fever, pain, progressive weakness, paresthesia, and a rise in WBCs.

MANAGEMENT

Epidural abscesses are treated with antibiotics after localizing the extent of the injury with MRI.

Table 335 Epidural Abscess

Epidural Abscess	
Etiology	Commonly the result of infection by *Staphylococcus aureus*, gram-negative rods, and TB.
Presentation	Fever, pain, progressive weakness, paresthesia, and a rise in WBCs.
Diagnosis	Circulation occlusion, nerve impingement, and spread to adjacent structures.
Treatment	Antibiotics after localizing the extent of the injury with MRI.

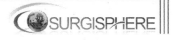

SEPTIC ARTHRITIS

ASSESSMENT

Septic arthritis not due to infection by *N. gonorrhea* is typically present in patients with a prior history of trauma to the affected joint. This monoarticular infective arthritis is due to a bacteremia that colonizes a region that sustained previous damage. Common bacteria include *S. aureus*, GBS, and gram-negative rods in young adults. Patients with sickle cell anemia are more likely to be infected with and *S. aureus*. IC patients and IV drug abusers (IVDA) are likely to be infected by *E. coli* and *Pseudomonas aeruginosa*. There is an increased risk of contracting nongonococcal septic arthritis with increasing age, patients with RA, presence of prosthetic joints, and in those with an immunodeficiency. Septic arthritis presents with the cardinal signs of infection, including redness, heat, pain, and swelling. Fever is also present. The affected joint is typically painful to move, so a limited range of motion is present on physical exam. Diagnosis is made by clinical history, an elevated ESR, and positive blood cultures on joint aspiration.

MANAGEMENT

Arthrocentesis is a diagnostic and therapeutic maneuver that can identify the over one million WBCs that may be present in the region, the low glucose level indicative of a bacterial infection, and the presence of numerous PMNs. Arthrocentesis may also decrease the joint pressure and permit increased ROM. In conjunction with antibiotics tailored to the infective organism, resolution is possible with resumption of near normal joint function.

Table 336 Nongonococcal Septic Arthritis

Nongonococcal Septic Arthritis	
Etiology	Due to a bacteremia that colonizes a region that sustained previous damage.
Presentation	Redness, heat, pain, and swelling. Fever is also present. The affected joint is typically painful to move, so a ROM is present on physical exam.
Diagnosis	Clinical history, an elevated ESR, and positive BCx on joint aspiration.
Treatment	Arthrocentesis and antibiotics tailored to the pathogen.

NECROTIZING FASCIITIS

ETIOLOGY AND PATHOPHYSIOLOGY

Gas gangrene refers to myonecrosis and soft tissue destruction through the production of toxins and gas by *Clostridium perfringens*, but other *Clostridium spp.* may also lead to infection. Low oxygen content and direct inoculation into the muscle make up the ideal conditions for infection. Numerous exotoxins are produced leading to destruction of collagen, hyaline membranes, fibrin crosslinks, lecithin, and overall hemolysis. The immune reaction is impeded through direct toxic injury to leukocytes and other mediators of inflammation. Vascular injury also impedes the ability of WBCs to enter the region of infection. Mortality can be very high, especially in spontaneous cases.

PRESENTATION AND DIAGNOSIS

Gas gangrene presents with sudden pain out of proportion to clinical findings. A history of trauma is often elicited, along with risk factors such as alcoholism, IVDA, or DM. Edema, erythema, tenderness, crepitus, discharge, and mental status changes are prevalent. Diagnosis is made by elevation of aldolase, potassium, LDH, CPK, and evidence of myoglobinuria. Anemia and metabolic acidosis may also be present. A positive sialidase test is also diagnostic.

TREATMENT

Treatment for gas gangrene involves hyperbaric oxygen exposure, debridement, IVF, and possible amputation to avoid death. Antibiotics are also used with penicillin, clindamycin, or chloramphenicol. The antibiotic for choice in a patient with clostridium infection and a penicillin allergy is clindamycin.

Table 337 Gas Gangrene

Gas Gangrene	
Etiology	Myonecrosis and soft tissue destruction through the production of toxins and gas by *Clostridium perfringens*, but other *Clostridium spp.* may also lead to infections.
Presentation	Sudden pain out of proportion to clinical findings. A history of trauma is often elicited, along with risk factors such as alcoholism, IVDA, or DM. Edema, erythema, tenderness, crepitus, discharge, and mental status changes are prevalent.
Diagnosis	Elevation of aldolase, potassium, LDH, CPK, and evidence of myoglobinuria. Anemia and metabolic acidosis may also be present. A positive sialidase test is also diagnostic.
Treatment	Hyperbaric oxygen exposure, debridement, IVF, and possible amputation to avoid death. Antibiotics are also used with penicillin, clindamycin, or chloramphenicol.

PRACTICE QUESTIONS

 A 52 year old female involved in a highway overpass collapse following an earthquake is trapped in her vehicle for 2 hours. She is finally extricated, but significant RLE entrapment is evident on transfer to the hospital. There is no popliteal pulse present, and the right leg is cold and mottled. The muscles are firm and the leg is insensate. What is the first step in management?

A. Above knee amputation
B. Below knee amputation
C. Femoral-popliteal bypass graft
D. Multiple compartment fasciotomy
E. Thrombolytic therapy

 The best answer is <u>Multiple compartment fasciotomy</u>. The first step in treatment is to proceed to the OR to decompress the edema and swelling that has occurred in the leg following prolonged entrapment. Although she has significant vascular compromise, she has a chance at limb salvage if fasciotomy is done in all compartments of her leg to relieve the pressures.

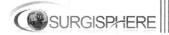

A 36 year old male who is four hours s/p hernia repair develops high fevers, altered mental status, and palpable air near his site of incision. What is the next best step in management?

A. Acetaminophen and observation
B. Intubation, pressors, and ICU care
C. Return to OR and wide local excision
D. Return to OR for small bowel resection
E. Vancomycin and piperacillin/tazobactam

 The best answer is <u>Return to OR and wide local excision</u>. This patient has necrotizing fasciitis due to clostridial infection. He requires immediate return to the OR for wide local excision of the affected area. Repeat excisions may be required. IV antibiotic therapy will also be required, but the first immediate step is surgery. Clostridial infections are composed of gram positive rods, and penicillin G is sufficient therapy.

 Which of the following requires an immediate trip to the OR for open drainage?

A. 1cm fluid collection near the LAR anastomosis
B. Enterocutaneous fistula
C. Infected skin boil
D. Localized pocket of pus on the skin
E. Tenosynovitis

 The best answer is <u>Tenosynovitis</u>. Tenosynovitis, pancreatic abscess, and perirectal abscess are all indications for immediate open drainage. Tenosynovitis can lead to permanent defects in function; pancreatic abscess can lead to death; perirectal abscess can lead to necrotizing fasciitis. The other options can be treated more conservatively.

 A 72 year old female involved in a motor vehicle collision presents to the ER with significant hypotension. A trauma series CT scan indicates pelvic bleeding. What is the next best step in management?

A. Angiogram
B. External fixation of the pelvis
C. Internal fixation of the pelvis
D. MAST
E. Surgical exploration

 The best answer is <u>External fixation of the pelvis</u>. Stabilization of the pelvis is the first step in management, followed by an angiogram to stop the bleeding via interventional means. Shock trousers are rarely used, and internal fixations are not done emergently. Surgical exploration is the very last option, due to the significant challenges of operating within the pelvic cavity.

A 32 year old male involved in a high speed motor vehicle accident is found to have a posterior dislocation of his femur. Prompt reduction and traction is completed. However, in this process, a femur fracture is discovered. What is the next best step in management?

A. Angiography
B. External fixation
C. Immobilization of the femur
D. Open reduction and internal fixation
E. Total hip replacement

The best answer is Immobilization of the femur. Due to the risk of bleeding, prompt immobilization of the femur is necessary following any femur fracture. Fixation is completed after the patient is stable but in the same hospitalization. Total hip replacement is an option in the elderly and with sufficient trauma. In the event of a posterior femur dislocation, traction should be maintained for one week, followed by the use of crutches.

 A 29 year old male involved in a fall from a high distance is found to have an anterior dislocation of his humerus. Which of the following nerves is likely to be damaged or compressed?

A. Axillary nerve
B. Median nerve
C. Musculocutaneous nerve
D. Radial nerve
E. Ulnar nerve

 The best answer is Axillary nerve. This patient most likely has compression or injury to his axillary nerve, which presents as loss of external rotation and abduction of the shoulder. Reduction is necessary. Another related fracture is a mid shaft humeral fracture – in this situation, wrist drop may occur, which should be treated with reduction and observation. Supracondylar fractures of the humerus may lead to median nerve injury and brachial artery injury. Distal radius fractures can lead to median nerve injury. Fractures of the scaphoid can lead to avascular necrosis, and occurs after falling on an extended hand. The development of a compartment syndrome in the forearm can lead to Volkmann's contracture due to degeneration of the flexor compartment with subsequent flexion of the distal extremity. Dupuytren's contracture is due to myofibroblast proliferation and is treated with fasciotomy; it can occur especially in alcoholism.

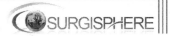

PEDIATRIC SURGERY

CHAPTER CONTENTS

GENERAL CONCEPTS

VITAL SIGNS

Table 338 Pediatric Vital Signs

Pediatric Vital Signs		
Age Group	**Blood Pressure**	**Heart Rate**
Neonate	70/40	120-160
3-12 months	90/50	90-140
1-6 years	100/60	80-110
6-12 years	110/70	70-100
12+ years	120/70	60-90

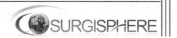

CANCER

Table 339 Pediatric Cancers

Pediatric Cancers
1) Leukemia
2) Brain tumors
3) Neuroblastoma (most common solid tumor under 2 years of age) / Nephroblastoma (most common > 2 years) Neuroblastoma is the most common posterior mediastinal mass

TRAUMA

Always consider abuse with pediatric trauma. The size of the little finger may be used to approximate the size of the trachea prior to intubation.

HEAD AND NECK

CONGENITAL AND STRUCTURAL

SPINA BIFIDA OCCULTA

Spina bifida occulta is failure of outer portion of vertebral column to close. There is no protrusion of spinal cord. A small tuft of hair may be present at the site. Spina bifida occulta presents with incontinence, slight ataxia, and minor loss of sensation to lower extremities.

MENINGOCELE

Meningocele is the result of damaged meninges protruding through a vertebral column defect. There is little loss of function. Meningomyelocele is the protrusion of meninges and CNS matter through vertebral column defect with visible cyst formation, and typically contains nerves and membranes. Meningomyelocele leads to paralysis and loss of sensation distal to site of damage with hydrocephalus. There is increased risk of occurrence in pregnant women taking medications for epilepsy and poor folic acid intake.

ARNOLD-CHIARI MALFORMATION

Arnold-Chiari malformation occurs in the small posterior fossa and leads to malformation of the cerebellum, herniation of the vermis, and hydrocephalus. It presents with stridor, lack of a gag reflex, dysphagia, spastic quadriparesis, nystagmus, syncope, progressive loss of function, and is associated with pneumonia and GERD.

DANDY-WALKER MALFORMATION

Dandy-Walker malformation occurs in the large posterior fossa and is associated with CSF foramen atresia with lack of a vermis. It presents with ataxia, syringomyelia, microcephaly, spina bifida, and cardiac abnormalities.

FETAL ALCOHOL SYNDROME

Fetal alcohol syndrome is due to significant alcohol exposure during pregnancy leading to severe mental retardation and a characteristic facies. It presents with stunted development, impulsive behavior, and mental illness.

LI-FRAUMENI SYNDROME

Li-Fraumeni syndrome presents with a defect in p53, a tumor suppressor gene. This defect occurs on chromosome 17p13. It presents with a dysfunction in cell cycle regulation leading to abnormal apoptosis with subsequent brain tumors, sarcomas, leukemia, and breast cancer development.

FAMILIAL RETINOBLASTOMA

Familial retinoblastoma is due to a defect in the RB1 tumor suppressor gene on chromosome 13q14. A defect in cell cycle regulation occurs leading to the development of retinoblastomas and osteogenic sarcomas.

NEUROFIBROMATOSIS

Neurofibromatosis I (NF1) is due to a defect in the NF1 tumor suppressor gene on chromosome 17q11. The defect lies with an RAS inactivation promoter, leading to neurofibromas, sarcomas, and gliomas. NFII is due to a defect in the NF2 tumor suppressor gene on chromosome 22q12. It leads to a defect in a cell membrane to cytoskeleton linking protein with subsequent vestibulocochlear schwannoma, meningioma, astrocytoma, and ependymoma formation.

CYSTIC HYGROMA

A cystic hygroma tends to present as a fluctuant neck mass. Complete excision is required, but even with a good operation, this tumor has a high recurrence rate.

CARDIOTHORACIC

EMBRYOLOGY

- Four stages of development
  - Stage 1: Tube-like heart similar to that of a fish
  - Stage 2: Double-chambered heart like that of a frog
  - Stage 3: Three-chambered heart like that of a snake
  - Stage 4: Four-chambered heart

Fetal Circulation

Waste from Fetus

Placenta

Food and Oxygen from Mother

Umbilical Cord

Ductus Arteriosus

Aorta

Foramen Ovale

Lung

Pulmonary Artery

Ductus Venosus

Liver

Lung

Left Kidney

Umbilical Vein

Umbilical Arteries

- Oxygen-rich Blood
- Oxygen-poor Blood
- Mixed Blood

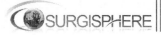

- Umbilical vein – ligamentum teres hepatis (round ligament of the liver)
- Umbilical artery – medial umbilical ligaments
- Ductus venosus – ligamentum venosum
- Ductus arteriosus – ligamentum arteriosum
- Foramen ovale – fossa ovale
- The median umbilical ligament is the allantois / urachus.
- The lateral umbilical ligaments are the inferior epigastric vessels.
- A right to left shunt presents as cyanosis, as in truncus arteriosus, tetralogy of Fallot, and transposition of the great arteries. A left to right shunt leads to CHF, as in ASD, VSD, and PDA. Eisenmenger syndrome occurs when a left to right shunt changes into a right to left shunt due to increased pulmonary vascular resistance. A heart-lung transplantation is required as definitive therapy.

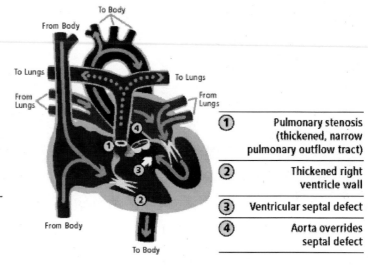

①	Pulmonary stenosis (thickened, narrow pulmonary outflow tract)
②	Thickened right ventricle wall
③	Ventricular septal defect
④	Aorta overrides septal defect

TETRALOGY OF FALLOT

- Etiology
  - Abnormal neural crest migration leading to displacement of anterosuperior infundibular septal development
- Pathophysiology: Pulmonary stenosis, RVH, overriding aorta, and VSD leads to R→L shunt and mixing of blood.
- Presentation
  - R→L shunt w/ cyanosis, clubbing, boot-shaped heart, syncope
  - Tet spells in ToF
- Significant endocardial cushion defect lead to a left to right shunt.
- Ostium primum defects are associated with significant ventricular septal defects and conduction abnormalities.

Tetralogy of Fallot (TOF or "Tet")

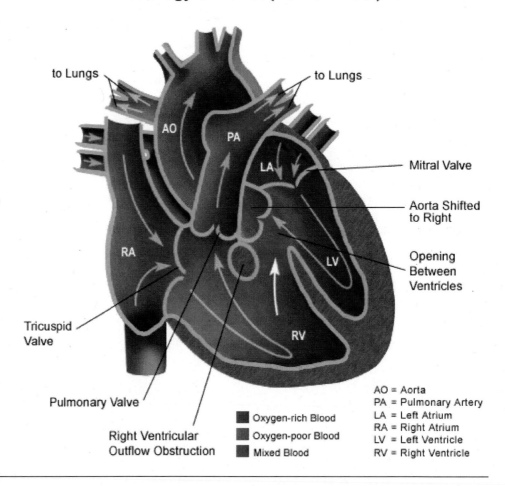

AO = Aorta
PA = Pulmonary Artery
LA = Left Atrium
RA = Right Atrium
LV = Left Ventricle
RV = Right Ventricle

Oxygen-rich Blood
Oxygen-poor Blood
Mixed Blood

AORTIC COARCTATION

- Type I

  - o Infantile: Aortic stenosis proximal to end of aortic arch

  - o Infantile occurs in Turner.

- Type II

  - o Adult: Aortic stenosis distal to end of aortic arch.

  - o Presents with notching of ribs, UE HTN, cerebral hemorrhage, infective endocarditis.

Coarctation of the Aorta

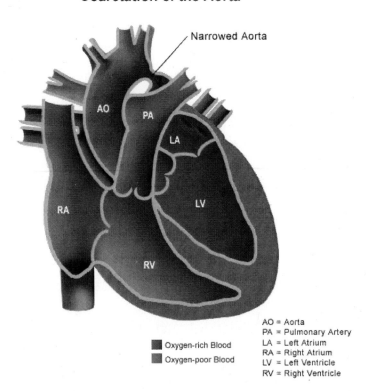

AO = Aorta
PA = Pulmonary Artery
LA = Left Atrium
RA = Right Atrium
LV = Left Ventricle
RV = Right Ventricle

Oxygen-rich Blood
Oxygen-poor Blood

TRANSPOSITION OF GREAT VESSELS

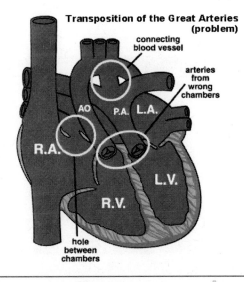

- The most likely cause of cyanosis in newborns is transposition of the great arteries.

- Transposition of the great vessels presents as arterial desaturation.

- Other causes of right to left shunts, which leads to cyanosis, include truncus arteriosus, tetralogy of Fallot, and transposition of great vessels.

- Causes of left to right shunts, which lead to CHF, include ASD, VSD, and PDA.

VENTRICULAR SEPTAL DEFECT

- VSD is the most common cardiac defect. About half close on their own. Failure to close spontaneously requires surgical intervention, especially if there is failure to thrive.

CONGENITAL DIAPHRAGMATIC HERNIA

A congenital diaphragmatic hernia presents with respiratory distress and a scaphoid abdomen. Diagnosis is made by CXR and ultrasound. Treatment begins with intubation, nasogastric decompression, reduction via a transabdominal approach, and repair. It is most commonly located on the posterior lateral left side.

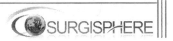

GASTROINTESTINAL

GASTROINTESTINAL DISORDERS

Table 340 Pediatric Cancers

Pediatric Cancers	
Duodenal atresia	Neonate
Meconium ileus	Neonate
Malrotation and volvulus	Neonate
Necrotizing enterocolitis	Neonate
Pyloric stenosis	1-2 months
Intussusception	Within the first year

ESOPHAGEAL ATRESIA

Esophageal atresia typically presents with a tracheoesophageal fistula leading to feeding intolerance. Esophageal atresia is diagnosed by the inability to pass an NG tube. A tracheoesophageal fistula is diagnosed by the presence of air in the GI tract. Up to half of all patients have associated abnormalities as part of the VATER syndrome: vertebral defects, imperforate anus, tracheoesophageal fistula, esophageal atresia, and renal abnormalities.

Table 341 Esophageal Atresia

Esophageal Atresia and Tracheoesophageal Fistula	
Type A	Esophageal atresia without tracheoesophageal fistula
Type B	Esophageal atresia with tracheoesophageal fistula at proximal esophagus
Type C	Esophageal atresia with tracheoesophageal fistula at distal esophagus (90% common)
Type D	Esophageal atresia with proximal and distal tracheoesophageal fistula
Type E	Tracheoesophageal fistula without esophageal atresia

GASTRIC OUTLET OBSTRUCTION

Gastric outlet obstruction is the result of pyloric obstruction, leading to projectile but non-bilious vomiting. Nausea and abdominal pain are also typically present. Diagnosis is made by X-ray, showing an absent air bubble in the stomach. Causes include PUD, tumors such as adenocarcinoma, lymphoma, stromal tumors, infections such as tuberculosis, and amyloidosis. Gallstones can also obstruct the stomach, leading to Boeveret's syndrome. Congenital pyloric stenosis is also a cause. Treatment depends on the cause, but the presentation can be ameliorated with proton pump inhibitors until surgery can be performed.

PYLORIC STENOSIS

Pyloric stenosis presents with nonbilious projectile vomiting at 1-2 months of age. It presents as a firm olive-like mass on physical exam and ultrasound that indicates a hypertrophic pylorus. Treatment is by way of a pyloromyotomy.

MALROTATION

Malrotation is due to incomplete midgut rotation during ontogeny leading to volvulus and possible ischemia. It typically presents with bilious emesis and is diagnosed by an upper GI series with small bowel follow through (SBFT). The presence of duodenum crossing the midline rules out the diagnosis of malrotation. Treatment of malrotation is surgical counterclockwise detorsion with appendectomy and colon placement in the left lower quadrant.

INTUSSUSCEPTION

Intussusception of the terminal ileum into the colon may lead to colicky abdominal pain with bilious emesis and currant jelly stools. Diagnosis is made by air contrast enema and treatment involves an attempt for pneumatic reduction. Failure to reduce or recurrent disease requires surgery.

Pyloric stenosis: Olive, nonbilious emesis
Malrotation: Duodenum does not cross midline
Intussusception: Currant jelly stools; Rx w/ air contrast enema

DUODENAL ATRESIA

Duodenal atresia presents as bilious emesis and presents as a double-bubble sign on KUB. An upper GI series with SBFT indicates a duodenum crossing the midline. Treatment is duodenojejunostomy. A multisystem examination must be completed prior to surgical intervention.

JEJUNAL AND ILEAL ATRESIA

Atresia of the intestines distal to the duodenum is likely due to a vascular accident occurring *in utero*. It presents with polyhydramnios, biliary emesis, and abdominal distention. Treatment involves excision but may lead to short bowel syndrome thereafter. Intestinal atresia is classified into four divisions.

Table 342 Intestinal Atresia

Intestinal Atresia	
Type I	Intraluminal diaphragm
Type II	Mesentery intact, fibrous cords between ends of intestine
Type III	Discontinuous bowel; either V-shaped or apple-core deformity.
Type IV	Multiple instances of atresia

MECKEL DIVERTICULUM

Meckel diverticulum is a derivative of the vitelline duct on the antimesenteric side of the small intestine. It may lead to painless rectal bleeding with ulceration, and may also lead to appendicitis-type complaints later in life. Atrophic gastric tissue is often present that may become ulcerated. Most are found incidentally and this is this is the most common gastrointestinal anomaly. About 2% of people are affected, with the diverticulum located within 2 feet of the ileocecal valve. 2% become

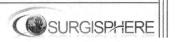

symptomatic, and one of two types of tissue are found within the diverticulum: gastric or pancreatic. Treatment is excision when symptomatic.

MECONIUM ILEUS

Meconium ileus is the development of a distal ileal obstruction due to the presence of meconium. It leads to abdominal distention with bilious emesis. A soap-bubble sign may be present and treatment involves enema-based decompression. Failure to decompress requires surgery. About 10% of patients will have concomitant cystic fibrosis.

HIRSCHSPRUNG DISEASE

Hirschsprung disease is also known as congenital agangliosis coli. It typically presents with bilious emesis and constipation. Diagnosis is by barium enema and rectal biopsy to search for ganglion cells. Treatment involves a colostomy with diverting loop ileostomy, followed by colostomy takedown and reanastomosis.

NECROTIZING ENTEROCOLITIS

Necrotizing enterocolitis leads to significant mucosal ischemia. It presents once feeding is started in a newborn and is accompanied with hematemesis and hematochezia. The main risk factor is premature birth. Air within the intestines is a telltale sign, and treatment involves nasogastric decompression, TPN, and bowel resection. Any bloody bowel movement in a child requires a barium enema.

C. DIFFICILE

The presence of C. difficile in a neonate is considered to be part of the normal flora, but it is not normal flora in an adult. Symptomatic disease may occur in neonates with Hirschsprung disease.

IMPERFORATE ANUS

Imperforate anus may present as either a high lesion or a low lesion. A high lesion is located above the puborectalis and may form a fistula with the urethra or vagina. A low lesion may lead to a fistula with the perineum. A high fistula requires a diverting colostomy, while a low fistula needs a sagittal anorectoplasty.

GASTROSCHISIS

Gastroschisis is an abdominal wall defect to the right of the umbilicus without overlying peritoneal sac. It requires primary abdominal wall closure and possible silastic silo if the bowel cannot be reduced. Free rupture of the umbilical artery may occur.

OMPHALOCELE

Omphalocele is an abdominal wall defect with a hernia coming out with peritoneal sac. It is commonly associated with other abnormalities, unlike gastroschisis. Silastic silo is used to close the wall if the defect cannot be reduced.

UMBILICAL HERNIA

Umbilical hernia tends to close spontaneously. A defect larger than 2cm or persistence into the second year of life are indications for surgery.

HYDROCELE

Hydrocele is a fluid collection within the scrotum. A communicating hydrocele is patent with the processus vaginalis. A non-communicating hydrocele will close spontaneously. Repair of the tunica vaginalis is necessary for communicating hydrocele.

HEPATOPANCREATOBILIARY

BILIARY ATRESIA

Biliary atresia leads to worsening jaundice in the neonate, and is diagnosed with a liver biopsy and HIDA scan. Treatment is to complete a hepaticojejunostomy, but may require a liver transplant. Extrahepatic disease occurs in 10% of cases. Surgery before 2 months of age is the most successful.

CHOLEDOCHAL CYST

The presence of a choledochal cyst requires surgical excision due to the risk of cancer. There are five types of cysts. Diagnosis is made by ultrasound and ERCP.

Table 343 Choledochal Cyst

Choledochal Cyst		
Type I	Extrahepatic cyst (most common type)	Hepaticojejunostomy
Type II	Cyst of common bile duct	Diverticulectomy
Type III	Choledochocele	Excision and sphincteroplasty
Type IV	Multiple cysts within and outside of the liver	Liver transplant
Type V	Diffuse intrahepatic cysts	Liver transplant

PRACTICE QUESTIONS

 Which of the following genetic defects can lead to the formation of a gastrointestinal stromal tumor?

A. Bcl-2
B. C-erb
C. C-Kit
D. p53
E. RBB

The best answer is C-Kit. Mutations in C-kit lead to the development of GIST tumors.

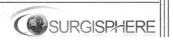

A two day old infant is born with a 7 cm fluctuant, multiloculated mass on her lower neck and upper thorax. What is the most likely diagnosis?

A.   Angiosarcoma
B.   Branchial cleft cyst
C.   Cutaneous lymphoma
D.   Cystic hygroma
E.   Thyroglossal duct cyst

The best answer is <u>Cystic hygroma</u>. Cystic hygroma is a hamartoma or vascular developmental anomaly arising from lymphatic vessels, manifesting as a raised, soft, shaggy, bubbly, pinkish-white lesion; cosmetic considerations may warrant attempted removal of lymphangiomas. They are fluid filled sacs that result from blockage of the lymphatic system. Most (90%) are either evident at birth or become evident before age 2 years. Most lymphangiomas occur in the posterior cervical triangle.

A 13 year old male with hereditary spherocytosis requires an elective splenectomy. When is the most appropriate time to immunize this patient?

A.   2 weeks prior to the procedure
B.   24 hours after the procedure
C.   24 hours prior to the procedure
D.   During the procedure
E.   Within 1 week after the procedure

The best answer is <u>2 weeks prior to the procedure</u>. All patients who are receiving an elective splenectomy should be immunized against H. influenza, meningococcus, and S. pneumoniae two weeks prior the procedure. Failing this, immunization within one week following the procedure is acceptable. The rate of overwhelming postsplenectomy sepsis is greater in the young than adults; it is also greater in elective splenectomy compared to trauma situations. The presence of an accessory spleen can be diagnosed with a technetium 99 scan; they tend to be located near the hilum of the existing spleen. Splenectomy is also done as a late treatment for ITP, an immune disease that forms IgG antibodies against platelets. The initial treatment of ITP is steroids, followed by IVIG if bleeding complications are present. Only if the ITP is refractory to maximum medical management is splenectomy completed. Platelets can be transfused in this situation after the splenic artery is ligated. The sole treatment for hereditary spherocytosis is splenectomy. A prophylactic cholecystectomy is also commonly done in the same setting. Splenectomy is also completed in the event of splenic vein thrombosis secondary to pancreatitis. Every attempt is made to preserve the spleen if it is damaged in a trauma situation.

CHAPTER CONTENTS

GENERAL CONCEPTS

PROMOTORS OF WOUND HEALING

Vitamin A has no effect on promoting wound healing. Complete epithelialization typically occurs in less than 5 days. However, vitamin A is indicated in reversing the effects of steroids. A daily dose of 25,000 units is used. Vitamin C augments proline crosslinks.

REPAIR AND REGENERATION

INFLAMMATORY PHASE

 Platelets → Neutrophils → Macrophages → Fibroblasts → Myofibroblasts

Wound healing starts with platelets coming to the site of injury and leading to hemostasis. Neutrophils migrate to the area within 24 hours, followed by macrophages within 3 days. Fibroblasts dominate the wound approximately 1 week following injury. These cells make up three phases of wound healing. The first phase is the inflammatory phase, which involves the neutrophils and macrophages. It is also during macrophage recruitment that the tensile strength of the wound is the least. As a result, the potential for a traumatic rupture, such as ventricular wall rupture following myocardial infarction, is the greatest approximately 3-5 days following injury. Fibronectin is also produced in high amounts by fibroblasts during this time to recruit fibroblasts to the area and assist in their binding to the ECM latticework that is being built.

PROLIFERATIVE PHASE

Once the wound is closed by the inflammatory phase, the proliferative phase begins and the tensile strength of the wound begins to increase. Collagen production increases significantly by recruitment of fibroblasts. Hydroxylation of hydroxyproline and hydroxylysine forms fibrils. This phase continues for about two months, with the greatest production occurring approximately three weeks following injury.

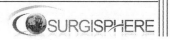

MATURATION PHASE

Thereafter, scar maturation occurs as part of the maturation phase. Tensile strength increases significantly via crosslinking and scar contraction begins to take place with the action of myofibroblasts. Remodeling of the scar also occurs during this time. Collagen breakdown is mediated by matrix metalloproteases. Tensile strength of the wound reaches 80% of its former strength by 6 weeks, and 90% by 6 months, which is the maximum.

IMPAIRED WOUND HEALING

Radiation during the proliferation phase leads to inhibition of collagen crosslinks, leading to significant weakening of the wound. As a result, radiation therapy following surgery typically occurs two or more months following operation to avoid breakdown of the wound. Defects in macrophages also impair wound healing, as macrophages are essential for breakdown of damaged tissue and recruitment of fibroblasts. Should the wound require reopening, it should be done at five days as all of the necessary cells to promote healing are already present and can lead to more rapid healing of the wound.

A number of other factors also impair satisfactory wound healing. Hypoxia leads to failure to hydroxylate the proline and lysine residues on collagen, preventing stabilization of the collagen and decreased tensile strength. Infection with bacterial counts over 100,000/g of tissue, foreign bodies, systemic diseases, poor hemostasis, malnutrition, steroid therapy, radiation, and cancer. Steroids lead to inhibition of wound healing by shutting down the inflammatory stage and preventing macrophage migration to the wound. This can be reversed with the administration of 25,000 units of vitamin A. Malnutrition impedes wound healing by the lack of availability of essential nutrients such as cystine, vitamin C, and zinc.

Overzealous healing of the wound may occur with keloid formation, which extends beyond the borders of the wound, and hypertrophic scar formation, which remains within the borders of the wound.

Table 344 Wound Strength

Wound Strength	
Two weeks	10%
Three weeks	20%
Four weeks	50%
Six weeks	80%
Six months	90% (maximum)

Table 345 Collagen Types

Collagen Types	
Type I	Bone, skin, tendon, scar. Most common type.
Type II	Cartilage
Type III	Embryonic tissue, vasculature, uterus, gastrointestinal tract. Abnormal in Ehlers-Danlos syndrome. Initial collagen type in wound. Replaced by type I collagen at 3 weeks.
Type IV	Basement membrane

HEALING BY SECONDARY INTENTION

Delayed wound healing is used in lieu of primary apposition of the wound to permit closure of a potentially contaminated surface. Serial debridements are possible with this method. Healing by secondary intention permits the use of a wound V.A.C. device to continue to keep the surface of the wound clean while granulation tissue forms.

SKIN GRAFTING

Table 346 Skin Grafting

Skin Grafting	
Full thickness	Limited contraction. Lower yield.
Split thickness	Increased contraction and higher yield. Donor site heals from appendages and hair follicles. Blood supply: diffusion from serum, followed by angiogenesis

CANCER

SQUAMOUS CELL CANCER

Squamous cell carcinoma of the tongue tends to be lateral in location and presents with an ulcerated appearance. Squamous cell carcinoma of the lip requires primary resection of 1/3 of the lip and a search for nodal disease. Squamous cell carcinoma of the nasopharynx may metastasize to secondary locations and can present several years later. Squamous cell cancer with one lymph node is considered stage I disease. Stage 2 disease has two lymph nodes on the same size of the diaphragm. Stage 3 disease has lymph nodes on both sides of the diaphragm. Stage 4 disease has positive lymph nodes in organ systems.

Squamous cell cancer of the skin is the most common cancer that occurs in humans, and the majority are due to exposure to ultraviolet radiation and chemical carcinogens. There are two stages for carcinogenesis. Initiation occurs following exposure to a specific stimulus and leads to a permanent change in the genome. In order for these cells to become tumors, promotion is required which leads to repeated exposure to adverse events leading to additional mutations. Hyperplasia results first, followed by metaplastic changes, then dysplasia, then frank carcinogenesis.

BASAL CELL CANCER

Basal cell cancer may be excised with **margins of 0.5mm**. It typically presents with a **pearly appearance** and is commonly located on the **face**.

MELANOMA

The presence of melanoma **less than 1 mm in size** requires a wide local excision with **1 cm margins**. No exploration for lymph nodes is necessary. The presence of melanoma **greater than or equal to 1 mm in size** requires 2 cm margins and a **sentinel lymph node** biopsy. If this sentinel lymph node biopsy is negative, no lymph node dissection is required. Melanoma is most likely to

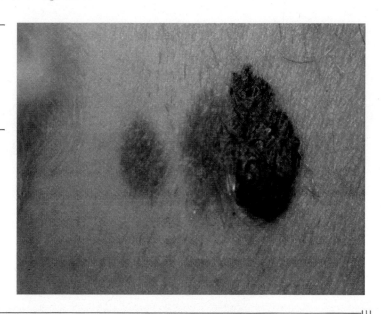

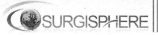

metastasize to the small bowel. If the primary source is unknown, an **exploratory axillary resection** has been shown to have a survival benefit. A full workup should be done beforehand, and the initial management is a CT of the abdomen and pelvis to ensure that there is not metastatic disease. Positive lymph nodes requires lymphadenectomy with interferon-alpha therapy. Any melanoma that has recently changed likely needs surgical excision; signs include an irregular border, change in color, and ulceration. Melanoma tends to metastasize to the small bowel.

Table 347 Types of Melanoma

Types of Melanoma
Superficial spreading (most common)
Lentigo maligna (best prognosis)
Acral lentiginous
Nodular (vertical growth phase, worst prognosis)

Table 348 Surgical Management of Melanoma

Surgical Management of Melanoma	
<1mm	WLE with 1 cm margin
1-2mm	WLE with 2cm margin and SLNB
>2mm	WLE with 2cm margin and SLNB

MARJOLIN'S SKIN

Marjolin's skin cancer typically occurs in patients with significant **burn** injuries. A five year course for development is typical.

TRAUMA

BURNS

FIRST, SECOND, AND THIRD DEGREE BURNS

A first degree burn extends only into the epidermis and typically leads to only redness, a small white plaque, and eventual resolution without scar formation. A second degree burn typically causes clear blistering with fluid and involves the dermis. Pain is variable depending on location and extent. Third degree burns are full thickness and typically lead to charring of the skin. Hard eschars are formed with a purple fluid. There is no pain with third degree burns. Cortisol may be elevated in burn patients several days following injury as part of the adrenal response to stress.

Table 349 Percentages of Total Body Surface Area

Percentages of Total Body Surface Area		
Body Part	**Adults**	**Infants**
Head	9%	18%
Anterior Torso	18%	18%
Posterior Torso	18%	18%
Perineum	1%	1%
Each Arm	9%	9%
Each Leg	18%	14%

FLUID RESUSCITATION

PARKLAND FORMULA

The fluid requirements in burn patients are significantly higher and depends on the total body surface area that is burned.

$$Parkland\ Formula = \frac{4\frac{ml}{kg}}{\%TBSA}\ burned\ \rightarrow \frac{1}{2}\ volume\ over\ 8\ hours, remaining\ \frac{1}{2}\ over\ 16\ hours$$

The fluid infusion timing should be started from when the burn occurred. Boluses should be avoided due to the net increase in fluid edema, thereby exacerbating total body fluid requirements. The amount of fluid that is necessary should be dictated by the patient's urine output; the Parkland formula serves as a guide for initial therapy only. Normal urine output for a young child is 1 cc/kg/hr. Children also are normotensive at lower blood pressures compared to adults. Trauma in children should be given 20 cc/kg of LR initially if they are hypotensive. Adults should make about 0.5 mL/kg. Lactated ringers is the initial fluid of choice.

SPECIAL CONSIDERATIONS

Electrical burns require a higher fluid output due to the presence of myoglobinuria. A target urine output of 100-150ml/hr and addition of sodium bicarbonate to alkalinize the urine should be done. Mannitol also has some benefit. D5W and colloid at a rate of 0.5ml/kg/%TSBA should be started.

BURN MANAGEMENT

Burn wounds require satisfactory management of the airway and adequate resuscitation. Initial debridement should be done in a burn operating room to minimize loss of heat. Bullae are debrided and gentle scrubbing is done to remove necrotic tissue. This is followed by a chlorhexidine bath. Silver sulfadiazine or another burn ointment is then used to cover the burned surfaces. Serial debridements and covering with ointment is done several times a day with monitoring for infection. The risk of infection is highest in patients with over 30% burns, children, and patients with multisystem failure. Biopsy should be done for any nonhealing wound due to the risk of infection. Excision of the burned tissue can start at 5 days and is limited to about 20% of the total burned area per occasion. Skin grafting should be done to heal the affected tissues. Early skin grafting is important as part of the treatment for burns to the face, hands, and circumferential neck burns.

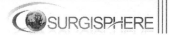

COMPLICATIONS OF THERAPY

A burn patient who has circumferential burns around an extremity requires an escharotomy to prevent compartment syndrome. The same is the case for full-thickness burns to the chest. Mafenide acetate, nitrofurazone, and sulfamylon are agents given topically to burn victims that can cause metabolic acidosis. Silver sulfadiazine (silvadene) is a topical burn remedy that can lead to leukopenia. Silver nitrate can lead to hyponatremia and hypochloremia. The most common infection in a burn patient is pneumonia. Burn patients should not be paralyzed with succinylcholine due to the hyperkalemia, which may lead to cardiac arrest.

PRACTICE QUESTIONS

 A 42 year old homeless man is seen by surgery in the ER for frostbite. What is the best initial therapy?

A. Amputation
B. Antibiotics
C. Moist heat
D. Splinting
E. Topical nitroglycerin

 The best answer is <u>Moist heat</u>. The best early treatment to minimize damage caused by frostbite is to apply moist heat to the affected appendage. Amputation may be required if substantial necrosis has occurred.

 A 13 year old boy falls and skids his knee while skateboarding. He is treated and released by you in the surgery clinic. During which period does maximum collagen production occur in the wound?

A. 24 hours
B. 5 days
C. 15 days
D. 30 days
E. 60 days

 The best answer is <u>15 days</u>. Maximum collagen production occurs by day 21, with significant increases in production occurring between 3 and 21 days. Following this period, significant crosslinking and strengthening occurs in the collagen lattice. Vitamin A given to patients on steroids can reverse the negative effects of steroids.

 Which of the following is an advantage of a split thickness skin graft compared to a full thickness graft?

A. Decreased contraction
B. Improved grafting with STSG
C. Increased vascularity
D. Less pain
E. Less scarring

 The best answer is <u>Improved grafting with STSG</u>. A STSG is favored over a FTSG due to improved graft outcome, increased contraction, and improved graft viability.

Which of the following agents used to treat topical burns can lead to a metabolic acidosis?

A.   Acetoacetate
B.   Bacitracin ointment
C.   Silvadene
D.   Silver nitrate
E.   Sulfamylon

 The best answer is <u>Sulfamylon</u>. Sulfamylon and mafenide acetate are associated with metabolic acidosis when used liberally as part of the treatment of burns. Sulfamylon inhibits the function of carbonic anhydrase, leading to acidosis. Mafenide acetate is also a carbonic anhydrase inhibitor that leads to hyperchloremic metabolic acidosis. Respiratory compensation leads to hyperventilation with low $PaCO_2$.

 A 76 year old man is treated for his myocardial infarction with tPA and recovers well. The penumbra surrounding his myocardial injury grows somewhat during this recovery phase due to reperfusion injury, which is mediated by which of the following immune cells?

A.   Eosinophils
B.   Fibroblasts
C.   Macrophages
D.   Natural killer cells
E.   Neutrophils

 The best answer is <u>Neutrophils</u>. Neutrophils mediate reperfusion injury with release of toxic byproducts that damages already fragile cells. They are also one of the first cells recruited to the area due to the surrounding inflammation.

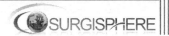

Which of the following cells is responsible for the release of elastase and collagenase as part of the initial steps in wound healing?

A. Eosinophils
B. Fibroblasts
C. Macrophages
D. Neutrophils
E. Platelets

The best answer is <u>Macrophages</u>. The first step in wound healing is formation of a platelet plug with production of fibrin and coagulum to provide early closure. Leukocytes then enter the area to remove any inflammatory debris and remove dead cells. Macrophages follow to breakdown the remaining membrane via the production of elastase and collagenase. Fibroblasts arrive within 24 hours to begin production of collagen and form a new basal epithelial layer. Hydroxylation of proline and lysine residues starts to occur at one week, with maximum collagen production occurring between 1-3 weeks. Vitamin C, iron, zinc, and oxygen all aid in wound management. Myofibroblasts in the region begin contraction of the scar at two weeks with subsequent remodeling occurring over the next month. The wound reaches 80-90% of its original strength over this period of time. The first type of collagen to be laid down is collagen III, followed by collagen I. Recall that vitamin A can be given to reverse the effects of steroids. There is no treatment for radiation damage that occurs during this time, leading to the production of abnormal fibroblasts. Fibronectin in the wound assists in the anchoring of fibroblasts. Degradation of collagen occurs with MMPs. Myofibroblasts are involved in closure of the wound through secondary intention.

SURGICAL ONCOLOGY

CHAPTER CONTENTS

HEMATOLOGY

GENERAL CONCEPTS

THROMBOXANE A2

Thromboxane A2 is a **vasoconstrictor** and **inhibitor of platelet aggregation**. It is released by activated **platelets**. The formation of TxA2 is **inhibited by aspirin**. Plavix leads to inhibition of platelet aggregation by inhibiting ADP. Plavix should be stopped five days prior to surgery.

TxA2 = vasoconstrictor, platelet aggregation inhibitor.
Prostacyclin = platelet aggregation inhibitor
NO = L-arg $\rightarrow$ cGMP $\rightarrow$ vasodilation, platelet aggregation inhibition

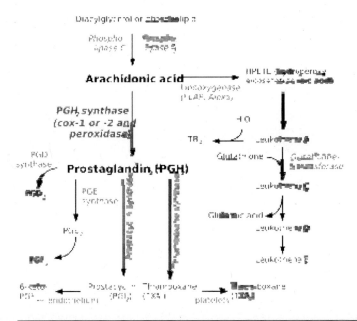

PROSTACYCLIN

Inhibitor of platelet aggregation. It is released from the endothelium and also promotes vasodilation, thereby antagonizing the effects of TxA2.

ANTITHROMBIN III

Antithrombin III is an inhibitor of thrombin, and factors IX, X, and XI. It is bound by heparin. Thrombin converts fibrinogen to fibrin and leads to the activation of platelets, and factors V and VIII. Fibrin forms fibrin split products which works with platelets to form a hemostatic plug. Fibrin crosslinking relies on factor XIII. Plasmin plays a role in anticoagulation and is activated by tissue plasminogen activator released by the endothelium. It leads to the destruction of the platelet

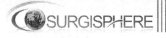

plug through degradation of factors V and VIII and fibrin. Plasmin is inhibited by alpha-2 antiplasmin. Antithrombin III deficiency is treated FFP.

BLOOD PRODUCTS

Cryoprecipitate is used as a therapy for von Willebrand disease due to the high concentration of vWF and fibrinogen. FFP contains all factors, proteins C and S, and antithrombin III. Factors VIII and vWF can be released by the endothelium through the administration of DDAVP.

BLOOD TRANSFUSION

A negative crossmatch is required between donor blood cells and recipient serum, in addition to satisfactory ABO compatibility. Postoperative transfusion criteria include a symptomatic low hematocrit, a symptomatic low central venous

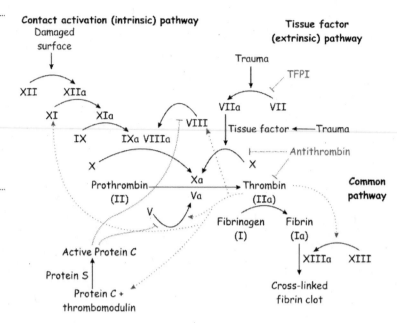

pressure, and a symptomatic low pulmonary capillary wedge pressure. The earliest intraoperative sign of blood mismatch is hypotension. The most likely risk of infection due to a transfusion is from CMV, followed by hepatitis C (1/500,000), then HIV (>1/2,000,000). The goal of a blood transfusion is to maintain oxygen carrying capacity when an increase in oxygen saturation alone would not be sufficient. Most practitioners will wait for a hemoglobin of 7 or hematocrit of 21 before transfusing a healthy person. However, there are studies that show that transfusing at a lower hematocrit would also be permissible. Blood transfusions for a hematocrit above 22 in most patients, or transfusing to a goal (i.e. 30) has been shown to be fraught with increased morbidity. Massive blood transfusions, such as following severe trauma, can lead to hypothermia, hypocalcemia, hyperkalemia, loss of platelets and clotting factors leading to additional coagulopathy, and metabolic alkalosis.

TRANSFUSION REACTIONS

ETIOLOGY AND PATHOPHYSIOLOGY

Transfusion reactions occur due to immune reactions against donated blood that does not match that of the recipient. Serious reactions can lead to death, and rapid identification and reversal are necessary. Acute reactions may be due to immune-mediated reactions with various antibodies; those antibodies against the major blood groups (AB) can lead to death through notable intravascular hemolysis. Non-ABO antibodies result in extravascular reactions and are milder. Nonimmune reactions occur with damage to the donated RBCs leading to hemoglobinuria and hemoglobinemia. The presence of various cytokines in the donated blood can precipitate additional APRs and lead to constitutional symptoms. Immune reactions can present as severe anaphylaxis and lead to shock and death. Fatal reactions affect 4 persons in a million; nonfatal immune reactions affect 1 in 10,000 persons. Allergic reactions occur in 1 in 300 persons, and anaphylaxis may occur in 1 in 50,000 persons. Multiparous women are more likely to have symptoms than other groups. The most common cause is clerical error.

PRESENTATION AND DIAGNOSIS

Transfusion reactions present with the aforementioned symptoms. Early signs include fever, dropping BP, flushing, anxiety, and wheezing. Later signs include DIC. In nonhemolytic reactions, only fever is present along with mild constitutional symptoms and hypotension. Allergic reactions may present with a maculopapular rash and pruritus. Anaphylactic reactions may present with dyspnea, wheezing, anxiety, bronchospasm, and hypotension. In transfusion-related acute lung injury (TRALI), SOB, hypoxia, and orthopnea with cardiac decompensation may be present due to clotting within the pulmonary capillaries. Diagnosis is made by workups for anemia and a direct Coombs test. Dilutional thrombocytopenia may also occur after massive transfusion.

TREATMENT

Transfusion reactions are treated by stopping the transfusion and careful observation. Prophylaxis against renal failure and DIC are necessary. Diuresis may be necessary. Acetaminophen is used for fever, diphenhydramine for mild allergic reactions, and epinephrine for anaphylactic reactions. Severe symptoms may require admission to ICU and supportive therapy. A workup for sepsis may be necessary. Transfusion of over 1 – 1.5L of hetastarch (hextend) can lead to an increased risk of bleeding.

Table 350 Transfusion Reaction

Transfusion Reaction	
Etiology	Immune reactions against donated blood
Presentation	Allergic reactions, anaphylaxis, shock. Early signs include fever, dropping BP, flushing, anxiety, and wheezing. Later signs include DIC. In nonhemolytic reactions, only fever is present along with mild constitutional symptoms and hypotension. Allergic reactions may present with a maculopapular rash and pruritus. Anaphylactic reactions may present with dyspnea, wheezing, anxiety, bronchospasm, and hypotension. In TRALI, SOB, hypoxia, and orthopnea with cardiac decompensation may be present.
Diagnosis	Diagnosis is made by workups for anemia and a direct Coombs test.
Treatment	Stopping the transfusion and careful observation. Prophylaxis against renal failure and DIC. Diuresis may be necessary. Acetaminophen is used for fever, diphenhydramine for mild allergic reactions, and epinephrine for anaphylactic reactions. A workup for sepsis may be necessary.

ANTICOAGULANTS AND THROMBOLYTICS

Table 351 Anticoagulants and Thrombolytics

DRUG	INDICATIONS	MECHANISM OF ACTION	COMPLICATIONS	CONTRAINDICATIONS	NOTES
Heparin	Anticoagulation Atrial fibrillation	Antithrombin III potentiation (similar to heparin sulfate proteoglycans on endothelial cells) leading to prevention of clot formation Inhibits factors II, IXa, Xa	HIT (early is benign; late is IgG mediated); treat with danaparoid sodium or lepriludin due to risk of thrombosis Can lead to white clot syndrome	Existing bleeding disorder Safe in pregnancy	Follow aPTT time Give protamine sulfate as antidote (beware of hypotension) Half-life: 90 mins Test factor VIII function if intrinsic elevation in PTT
LMWH		Factor Xa inhibition		Cleared renally	PTT is not followed

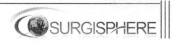

Warfarin		Inhibits epoxide reductase in liver to prevent formation of factors II, VII, IX, X, protein C, and protein S	Interacts with numerous medications (P-450) GI bleed Limb necrosis	Existing bleeding disorder Avoid in pregnancy Can lead to skin necrosis from lack of protein C – treat with heparin	Must monitor therapeutic index via PT/INR Half-life: 40 hours
Abciximab	Anticoagulation in PTCA	Prevents platelet aggregation and thrombus formation	TCP	Existing bleeding disorder	GPIIb/IIIa Ig inhibitor; similar to ticlodipine
Streptokinase	Fibrinolytic	Cleaves plasminogen to produce plasmin and breakdown clots	Allergic reaction on subsequent doses Bleeding	Hemorrhagic disorder	Usually given only once following MI Intrinsic elevation = malignancy
tPA	Fibrinolytic	Serine protease forms plasmin to breakdown clots	Bleeding	Hemorrhagic disorder	Used in MI and stroke within the first six hours of symptom onset
Clopidogrel	Hypercoagulability	Prevents platelet aggregation through ADP receptor blockade on platelets	Neutropenia TTP Hemorrhage	Safe in pregnancy	Plavix, ? MI and stroke risk Similar to ticlodipine
Aspirin	Hypercoagulability Fever	Increased bleeding time by impaired platelet release, inhibition of COX, and decreased thrombus formation Irreversible effects			Stop 7-10 days before surgery Prostacyclin inhibits platelet aggregation

Topical thrombin activates the fibrin glue used in surgery. Absolute contraindications to the use of fibrinolytics include a CVA within 2 months or active internal bleeding. Recent surgery, peptic ulcer disease, or trauma are major relative contraindications.

RED BLOOD CELL DISORDERS

MICROCYTIC ANEMIA

IRON-DEFICIENCY ANEMIA

ETIOLOGY AND PATHOPHYSIOLOGY

Iron-deficiency anemia is due to decreased iron stores following poor intake, excess loss, or poor absorption. Iron-deficiency anemia is the most commonly encountered anemia in general practice. It is most common in the reproductive years of women and in pregnant women. The most common cause in men is the result of an occult GI bleed. Other causes include alveolar hemorrhage, nosocomial loss, CRF treated with hemodialysis, following surgery, and various types of hemolysis.

PRESENTATION AND DIAGNOSIS

Iron-deficiency anemia presents with constitutional symptoms, exertional dyspnea, anorexia, melena, hematochezia, and / or hemoptysis, depending on the particular cause of blood loss. Objective signs include glossitis, angular stomatitis, koilonychias, pallor; iron-deficiency anemia can also be entirely subclinical. Anisocytosis and increased RDW are early signs of this disorder, and MCV indicates a hypochromic microcytic anemia. These results, combined with low ferritin, are diagnostic for iron-deficiency anemia.

TREATMENT

Treatment involves replacing iron stores and correcting any underlying etiology. Ferrous sulfate is the agent of choice to replenish iron stores in the body.

Table 352 Iron Deficiency Anemia

Iron Deficiency Anemia	
Etiology	Poor intake, excess loss, or poor absorption.
Presentation	Constitutional symptoms, exertional dyspnea, anorexia, melena, hematochezia, and / or hemoptysis
Diagnosis	Glossitis, angular stomatitis, koilonychias, pallor; iron-deficiency anemia. Anisocytosis and increased RDW are early signs of this disorder, and MCV indicates a hypochromic microcytic anemia, low ferritin.
Treatment	Replacing iron stores and correcting any underlying etiology.

SICKLE CELL ANEMIA

ETIOLOGY AND PATHOPHYSIOLOGY

Sickle cell anemia (SCA) is a commonly inherited disease that is associated with significant morbidity and decreased lifespan. An autosomal recessive defect in the beta chain of the adult hemoglobin (HbA) leads to the sickle cell hemoglobin (HbS). Due to defects in RBC deformability, obstruction of blood vessels leads to sickle cell pain crises and organ damage, in addition to anemia.

PRESENTATION AND DIAGNOSIS

SCA presents with constitutional symptoms and anemia. Painful crises occur intermittently due to vessel blockade (and possibly hand-foot syndrome) cause swelling and pain in the distal upper and lower extremities. Stroke is common, along with TIAs and RIND. Priapism may also occur with SCA. Acute presentations can include acute chest syndrome (ACS), which may present with severe chest pain due to blockade within the pulmonary vasculature. Chronic SCA can present with growth retardation, hepatomegaly, splenomegaly, pallor, jaundice, cardiomegaly with an SEM, skin ulceration, and cholelithiasis. A proliferative retinopathy is often present as well. Serious complications may also occur similar to an infection. Diagnosis of SCA is made by hemoglobin studies.

TREATMENT

SCA is definitively cured only by bone marrow transplantation. In most individuals, treatment centers on avoiding pain crises, giving prophylaxis for infection, and reducing the symptoms and damage from SCA. Fluid repletion is commonly the first step

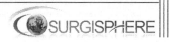

in any acute presentation. NSAIDs are the first line of treatment for pain management followed by hydroxyurea (by some clinicians). Penicillin is often given to avoid pneumonia, which is common in SCA, and folic acid supplements.

Table 353 Sickle Cell Anemia (SCA)

Sickle Cell Anemia (SCA)	
Etiology	Autosomal recessive defect in the beta chain of the HbA.
Presentation	Constitutional symptoms and anemia. Painful crises occur intermittently. Hand-foot syndrome may occur. Stroke is common, along with TIAs and RIND. Acute presentations can include ACS. Chronic SCA can present with growth retardation, hepatomegaly, splenomegaly, pallor, jaundice, cardiomegaly with an SEM, skin ulceration, and cholelithiasis. A proliferative retinopathy is often present as well.
Diagnosis	Made by hemoglobin studies.
Treatment	Definitively cured only by bone marrow transplantation. In most individuals, treatment centers on avoiding pain crises, giving prophylaxis for infection, and reducing the symptoms and damage. Fluid repletion is commonly the first step in any acute presentation. NSAIDs are the first line of treatment for pain. Penicillin, folic acid, hydroxyurea.

MACROCYTIC ANEMIA

MEGALOBLASTIC ANEMIA

ETIOLOGY

Megaloblastic anemia is the presence of immature erythroblasts with an increase in MCV. Megaloblastic anemia is commonly found in vitamin B12 deficiency or folate deficiency. The former may be due to an autoimmune defect leading to pernicious anemia, poor intake, or malabsorption due to ileal disease. The latter may be due to alcoholism, poor intake, chronic hemolytic anemia, or various malabsorption syndromes. Various chemotherapy drugs may also lead to megaloblastic anemia. Megaloblastic anemia is more common with increasing age. African American women and the elderly are most at risk.

PATHOPHYSIOLOGY

FOLATE DEFICIENCY

Folate deficiency may be the result of poor dietary intake, increased demand, as in pregnancy, or increased demand, as in chronic hemolytic anemias. Any number of hemolytic anemias may lead to an increased requirement in folate levels. Malabsorption syndromes such as Crohn disease or other enteropathies can lead to failure to properly absorb folate. Antagonists to folate such as methotrexate, or those agents that affect metabolism such as alcohol, sulfasalazine, triamterene, TMP-SMX, barbiturates, and nitric oxide can impede the use of folate by RBCs. Exposure to heavy metals or toxins such as arsenic or chlordane can also lead to retardation of folate utilization.

VITAMIN B12 DEFICIENCY

Vitamin B12 deficiency may be a result of many of the causes that lead to folate deficiency. In addition, pernicious anemia due to antibodies against parietal cells may lead to diminished amounts of intrinsic factor required for binding and absorption of vitamin B12. Lack of animal protein in strict vegetarian diets can also lead to deficiencies in vitamin B12. Diverticulosis and bacterial overgrowth, or infection by *D. latum* also lead to decreased vitamin B12 available for absorption.

PRESENTATION

FOLATE DEFICIENCY

Folate-deficiency megaloblastic anemia presents with pallor and glossitis. There are no neurologic deficits.

VITAMIN B12 DEFICIENCY

Vitamin B12-deficiency megaloblastic anemia presents with pallor, glossitis, and a peripheral sensory neuropathy that advances to a loss of deep tendon reflexes (DTR). Confusion and memory loss may be present. Delirium and dementia may occur in later stages.

DIAGNOSIS

Diagnosis of megaloblastic anemia is made by increases in MCV, identified decrease in folate and / or vitamin B12, and the presence of an anemia. Hypersegmented neutrophils may be present in pernicious anemia. A Schilling test may be done to test the ability to absorb vitamin B12. Methylmalonic acid is normal in folate-deficiency megaloblastic anemia but positive in vitamin B12-deficiency megaloblastic anemia. Antibodies to intrinsic factor can be demonstrated for pernicious anemia.

TREATMENT

Treatment for megaloblastic anemia is to replace the vitamin deficiency. Care should be taken in reversing a vitamin B12 deficiency by folate. Folate, however, will not prevent further progression of the neurologic symptoms from a vitamin B12 deficiency. Transfusion is occasionally undertaken in severe anemia, but pulmonary edema may develop. Vitamin replacement is the standard of care.

Table 354 Megaloblastic Anemia

Megaloblastic Anemia	
Etiology	**Vitamin B12 deficiency** due to an autoimmune defect leading to pernicious anemia, poor intake, or malabsorption due to ileal disease. **Folate deficiency** due to alcoholism, poor intake, chronic hemolytic anemia, or various malabsorption syndromes.
Presentation	**B12**-- pallor, glossitis, and a peripheral sensory neuropathy that advances to loss of DTR. Confusion and memory loss may be present. Delirium and dementia may occur in later stages. **Folate**-- pallor and glossitis, no neurologic deficiencies.
Diagnosis	Increase in MCV, identified decrease in folate and / or vitamin B12, and the presence of an anemia. Hypersegmented neutrophils, Schilling test, antibodies to intrinsic factor.
Treatment	Replace the vitamin deficiency, possibly transfusion.

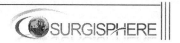

NORMOCYTIC ANEMIA

ANEMIA OF CHRONIC DISEASE

ETIOLOGY AND PATHOPHYSIOLOGY

The most common cause of a normocytic anemia is anemia of chronic disease (ACD); ACD is also the second most common type of anemia. While ACD tends to be a normocytic normochromic anemia, some presentations may have a microcytic anemia. ACD is due to decreased bone marrow production of erythrocytes after longstanding chronic disease, itself the result of a combination of erythropoietin resistance, decreased production, and decreased RBC half-life. ACD may also be due to chronic inflammation, cancer, and systemic diseases.

PRESENTATION AND DIAGNOSIS

ACD tends to develop with a moderate- or low-grade anemia and is typically subclinical in presentation. More severe cases may present with symptoms of anemia.

TREATMENT

Treatment of the primary disease is the only way to resolve ACD. Blood transfusions are rarely required.

Table 355 Anemia of Chronic Disease (ACD)

Anemia of Chronic Disease (ACD)	
Etiology	Decreased bone marrow production of erythrocytes after longstanding chronic disease. It may also be the result of chronic inflammation, cancer, and systemic diseases.
Presentation/Diagnosis	Moderate- or low-grade anemia, which is typically subclinical. More severe cases may present with symptoms of anemia.
Treatment	Treatment of the primary disease.

SPECIFIC ANEMIAS

HEMOLYTIC ANEMIA

ETIOLOGY AND PATHOPHYSIOLOGY

Hemolytic anemia leads to early destruction of RBCs and presents with anemia when the bone marrow cannot compensate for the loss of RBCs. Numerous causes exist, but major ones include G6PD deficiency, hereditary spherocytosis, sickle cell anemia, DIC, HUS, TTP, prosthetic valves, and PNH. It is present in about 1 in 20 anemias and leads to symptoms only with severe anemia.

PRESENTATION AND DIAGNOSIS

Hemolytic anemia presents with symptoms of anemia. Tachycardia, dyspnea, and weakness are typically present in severe cases. Bilirubin pigmented stones may lead to cholelithiasis. Repeated transfusions may lead to hemochromatosis. A history of use of certain medications, such as penicillin, quinine, or L-dopa may be responsible for an immune reaction leading to hemolytic anemia. Favism is especially common in the Mediterranean type of G6PD. Pallor, jaundice, splenomegaly, leg ulcers, and other symptoms of anemia may be present on physical exam. Diagnosis is made by peripheral blood smear and standard tests for anemia.

TREATMENT

Treatment for hemolytic anemia is similar to that for any other type of anemia – transfusions with symptomatic, severe anemia, avoiding triggers that worsen the anemia, and treating reversible causes.

Table 356 Hemolytic Anemia

Hemolytic Anemia	
Etiology	G6PD deficiency, hereditary spherocytosis, sickle cell anemia, DIC, HUS, TTP, prosthetic valves, and PNH.
Presentation	Symptoms of anemia. Tachycardia, dyspnea, and weakness, cholelithiasis. A history of use of certain medications, favism. Pallor, jaundice, splenomegaly, leg ulcers may be present on physical exam.
Diagnosis	Diagnosis is made by peripheral blood smear and standard tests for anemia.
Treatment	Transfusions with symptomatic, severe anemia, avoiding triggers that worsen the anemia, and treating reversible causes.

GLUCOSE-6-PHOSPHATASE DEHYDROGENASE DEFICIENCY

ETIOLOGY AND PATHOPHYSIOLOGY

Glucose-6-phosphatase dehydrogenase (G6PD) deficiency is an X-linked disorder that affects nearly half a billion people around the world. Its protection against malaria is the likely reason G6PD deficiency is so prevalent. Defects in the ability to oxidize certain reactions lead to excess glutathione, which in turn leads to free radical formation and premature damage to RBCs.

PRESENTATION AND DIAGNOSIS

G6PD presents with neonatal jaundice and acute hemolytic anemia. Drug-induced hemolysis or consumption of fava beans leading to hemolytic anemia is common. Jaundice and splenomegaly is found on physical exam. Most patients are entirely asymptomatic. Diagnosis is confirmed by measuring the activity of G6PD enzyme.

TREATMENT

Alleviating symptoms by discontinuing the offending agent is the only treatment necessary, in addition to avoiding fava beans and giving supportive therapy in acute exacerbations.

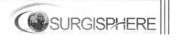

Table 357 Glucose-6-Phosphatase Dehydrogenase Deficiency (G6PD)

Glucose-6-Phosphatase Dehydrogenase Deficiency (G6PD)	
Etiology	X-linked disorder.
Presentation	Neonatal jaundice and acute hemolytic anemia. Drug-induced hemolysis or consumption of fava beans leading to hemolytic anemia is common. Jaundice and splenomegaly.
Diagnosis	Measure the activity of G6PD enzyme.
Treatment	Discontinue the offending agent, in addition to avoiding fava beans and giving supportive therapy in acute exacerbations.

PLATELETS AND COAGULATION DISORDERS

IMMUNE THROMBOCYTOPENIC PURPURA

ETIOLOGY AND PATHOPHYSIOLOGY

Also known as idiopathic thrombocytopenic purpura (ITP), this bleeding diathesis presents with thrombocytopenia, purpura, and petechiae along with a predisposition towards hemorrhage. The presence of autoantibodies against platelets leads to decreased platelet longevity due to macrophage phagocytosis in the spleen. The antibody appears to be against a GPI anchor. ITP is a relatively rare disorder due to its subclinical nature in most patients. Concurrent SLE, AML, CML, or MDS may be present; the disorder may also follow infection by EBV, VZV, CMV, rubella virus, HAV, HBV, HCV, HIV, or a generic URI. Medications that can lead to sensitization include quinine, cephalothins, rifampicin, gold salts, NSAIDs, HTN medications, diuretics, and abciximab. Heparin-induced thrombocytopenia (HIT) may also lead to ITP.

PRESENTATION AND DIAGNOSIS

ITP may lead to morbidity through intracranial hemorrhage or bleeding in other parts of the body. Petechiae and ecchymoses are typically present. Neurologic exam may be positive for findings, and a hemopericardium may be identified in some individuals. Diagnosis is confirmed by CBC and large platelets found in peripheral blood smears. Antiplatelet antibodies may also be present. A positive Coombs test is common. Marrow biopsy is normal.

TREATMENT

ITP is treated with corticosteroids, IVIG or Rho immune globulin (RhIG), and platelet transfusions, if severe bleeding is present. Splenectomy results in remission in 70% of cases. Platelets should be given only after the spleen has been removed or the splenic artery is clamped. IVIG should be given prior to splenectomy to permit a transient rise in platelets. Either two weeks prior or prior to discharge, immunizations for *H. influenzae*, *S. pneumoniae*, and *N. meningitidis* are necessary.

Table 358 Immune Thrombocytopenic Purpura (ITP)

Immune Thrombocytopenic Purpura (ITP)	
Etiology	Idiopathic
Presentation	Intracranial hemorrhage or bleeding in other parts of the body. Petechiae and ecchymoses. Neurologic exam may be positive for findings, and a hemopericardium may be identified.
Diagnosis	CBC and large platelets found on peripheral blood smear. Antiplatelet antibodies may also be present. A positive Coombs test is common.
Treatment	Corticosteroids, IVIG or RhIG, and platelet transfusions if severe bleeding is present. Splenectomy results in remission.

HEMOPHILIAS

HEMOPHILIA A

ETIOLOGY AND PATHOPHYSIOLOGY

Hemophilia A is an X-linked recessive disorder with factor VIII leading to a bleeding diathesis through disruption of the normal coagulation cascade. Spontaneous bleeding can occur, and significant bleeding with trauma is possible. Incidence is 1 in 5,000 persons but the lifespan is normal if no blood-borne illnesses are transmitted through transfusion. Males are significantly more affected; females tend to be carriers.

PRESENTATION AND DIAGNOSIS

Hemorrhage occurs frequently with hemarthrosis, CNS complaints, GI bleeds, genitourinary bleeds such as hematuria, epistaxis, hemoptysis, compartment syndromes from hematomas, and contusions. Physical exam elicits signs of hemorrhage including tachycardia, tachypnea, hypotension, and orthostatic hypotension. Lab studies indicate a normal PT, elevated aPTT, normal platelet count, and deficits in factor VIII levels. Severity of disease is related to the extent of factor VIII deficit.

TREATMENT

Hemophilia A is treated with factor VIII infusions (recombinant factor VIII is preferred). Oral hemorrhage may be treated with a combination of factor VIII and epsilon aminocaproic acid to reduce fibrinolysis. DDAVP may increase levels of factor VIII. Cryoprecipitate is also used successfully.

Table 359 Hemophilia A

Hemophilia A	
Etiology	X-linked recessive disorder in factor VIII.
Presentation	Hemorrhage occurs frequently with hemarthrosis, CNS complaints, GI bleeds, genitourinary bleeds, epistaxis, hemoptysis, compartment syndromes from hematomas, and contusions.
Diagnosis	Tachycardia, tachypnea, hypotension, and orthostatic hypotension. Lab studies indicate a normal PT, elevated PTT, normal platelet count, and deficits in factor VIII.
Treatment	Factor VIII infusions. Oral hemorrhage may be treated with a combination of factor VIII and epsilon aminocaproic acid. DDAVP may increase levels of factor VIII.

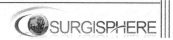

HEMOPHILIA B

ETIOLOGY AND PATHOPHYSIOLOGY

Hemophilia B is an X-linked recessive disorder that leads to defects in factor IX and subsequent hemorrhage. 1 in 5,000 persons are affected and lifespan is normal in the absence of blood-borne illness from transfusion. It is less common than hemophilia A.

PRESENTATION AND DIAGNOSIS

Hemophilia B presents like hemophilia A. Hemoglobin, PT, and platelets are normal. aPTT is increased. Factor IX is decreased significantly.

TREATMENT

Hemophilia B is treated with recombinant factor IX infusion; epsilon aminocaproic acid is used with oral bleeds to prevent fibrinolysis. FFP can also be used successfully, and is preferred.

Table 360 Hemophilia B

Hemophilia B	
Etiology	X-linked recessive disorder in factor IX.
Presentation	Like hemophilia A.
Diagnosis	Hemoglobin, PT, and platelets are normal. aPTT is increased. Factor IX is decreased significantly.
Treatment	Recombinant factor IX infusion; epsilon aminocaproic acid is used with oral bleeds.

VON WILLEBRAND DISEASE

ETIOLOGY AND PATHOPHYSIOLOGY

Von Willebrand disease (vWD) is a bleeding diathesis that prevents hemostasis in response to vascular damage. Adhesion to platelets is impaired and stabilization of various coagulation factors never occurs. vWD is rather rare (1:10000) and morbidity varies. vWD is an inherited autosomal condition with onset at a young age; females especially present at onset of menarche. vWF is secreted by endothelial cells. vWF assists with platelet adherence to collagen.

PRESENTATION AND DIAGNOSIS

vWD presents with bleeding diatheses leading to epistaxis, easy bruising, and hematoma formation. Significant menstrual bleeding is possible. GI bleeds do not occur as frequently. A deficiency in von Willebrand factor (vWF) is diagnostic. This activity of vWF can be measured using a ristocetin activity test, while the presence of vWF can be determined with an antigen test. A PTT is increased in vWD, while PT is normal. The most severe vWF disease occurs in type III disease.

TREATMENT

Treatment of type I vWD involves DDAVP which leads to a rise in vWF due to release from storage vesicles. Type II vWD is treated with DDAVP as well, but concentrates with factor VIII and vWF may be necessary prior to surgery. Treatment of type III vWD involves vWF-containing factor VIII concentrates. Platelet transfusions are also therapeutic. Prolonged bleeding times in patients on dialysis should be treated with 20 mcg of DDAVP. Cryoprecipitate contains vWF.

Table 361 Von Willebrand Disease (vWD)

Von Willebrand Disease (vWD)	
Etiology	Autosomal disorder.
Presentation	Bleeding diatheses leading to epistaxis, easy bruising, and hematoma formation
Diagnosis	Ristocetin activity test, while the presence of vWF can be determined with an antigen test. PTT is increased, while PT is normal.
Treatment	**Type I vWD** involves DDAVP, low vWF level. **Type II vWD** is treated with DDAVP as well, but concentrates with factor VIII and vWF may be necessary prior to surgery. Poorly functioning vWF. **Type III vWD**-- vWF-containing factor VIII concentrates. Platelet transfusions. Low vWF level.

ANTITHROMBIN III DEFICIENCY

A defect in antithrombin III leads to a disinhibition of coagulation and leads to permissive activation of factor IX, X, and thrombin. The result is an increase in incidence of thrombosis, both arterial and venous. This autosomal dominant disorder occurs in up to 1 in 2000 patients. Initial therapy is heparinization, followed by lifelong anticoagulation.

FACTOR XI DEFICIENCY

Factor XI deficiency is an uncommon disorder that has few clinical effects. This autosomal dominant disorder can be corrected with FFP on a PRN basis.

DISSEMINATED INTRAVASCULAR COAGULATION

Disseminated intravascular coagulation (DIC) is the result of a prothrombotic state such as following a major obstetric procedure, the development of shock, TTP, burn, massive transfusion, major operation, infection, or cancer. It leads to consumption of clotting factors and platelets leading to diffuse bleeding and spontaneous coagulation in the periphery. Treatment is to give FFP and cryoprecipitate together with platelets as needed.

PROTEIN C RESISTANCE

Protein C resistance is an autosomal dominant disorder that is associated with factor V Leiden mutations. It is treated with heparin prior to surgery. The incidence of DVT is elevated in this patient group.

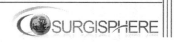

PRACTICE QUESTIONS

A 61 year old male with von Willebrand disease presents with signs and symptoms of acute appendicitis. Which of the following is recommended to minimize the risk of bleeding in this patient?

A. Cryoprecipitate
B. Fresh frozen plasma
C. Packed red blood cells
D. Platelet transfusion
E. Vasopressin
F. Whole blood transfusion

The best answer is <u>Cryoprecipitate</u>. Von Willebrand disease leads to a functional deficiency in platelet adherence to collagen. A prolonged bleeding time is the effect, and may be disastrous in surgery. Either cryoprecipitate or DDAVP can be given to help reverse this defect.

A 44 year old male diagnosed with hemophilia A is a candidate for a liver transplantation due to longstanding cryptogenic cirrhosis. Prior to undergoing this procedure, which of the following is the best infusion to minimize intraoperative bleeding?

A. Factor IX
B. Factor VIII
C. Fresh frozen plasma
D. Packed red blood cells
E. Platelet infusion

The best answer is <u>Factor VIII</u>. Recombinant factor VIII is the best treatment for patient with hemophilia A who require an operative intervention in order to minimize intraoperative bleeding. Factor VIII deficiency is manifest as an increase in PTT.

What is the half-life of albumin?

A. 12 hours
B. 2 days
C. 2 months
D. 3 weeks
E. 4 hours

The best answer is <u>3 weeks</u>. Albumin has a half-life of 21 days. Pre-albumin should be used as a measure of nutritional repletion as it has a half-life of 2 days.

Which of the following is a major contributor to blood oxygen content leading to perfusion of peripheral tissues?

A. Heart rate
B. Hemoglobin concentration and %SO2
C. Hemoglobin concentration and PaO2
D. PaO2
E. PAO2

The best answer is <u>Hemoglobin concentration and %SO2</u>. The greatest contributor to oxygenation is hemoglobin concentration and percent of oxygen saturation within the blood. The initial treatment to improve peripheral oxygenation is to increase oxygen saturation to 100%. Further increases lead to an increase in dissolved oxygen within the blood, but this has a negligible effect at low oxygen flow levels. The next step is to give blood transfusions as clinically indicated in order to improve oxygenation. The relevant equation is 1.37 x oxygen saturation x hemoglobin concentration + 0.003 x PaO2.

 Which of the following leads to a decrease in the affinity of hemoglobin to oxygen?

A. Decrease in hemoglobin concentration
B. Decreased 2,3 DPG levels
C. Decreased CO2 levels
D. Increased acidity
E. Platelet transfusion

The best answer is <u>Increased acidity</u>. The affinity of hemoglobin to oxygen is decreased by a drop in pH, increase in 2,3 DPG levels, and an increase in CO2.

 Which of the following has the greatest chance of being transmitted from one person to another in the course of a blood transfusion?

A. CMV
B. HBV
C. HCV
D. HIV
E. HTLV

The best answer is <u>CMV</u>. Cytomegalovirus is the most common infection transmitted from one person to another in the course of a blood transfusion, and routine screening is not done due to the high rates of endemic infection. Over 20% of patients are positive by age 20, and 70% are positive by age 70. White blood cells are the carrier for infection, and for this reason, washing blood when giving it to immunocompromised patients is recommended. The risk of contracting hepatitis A, B, or C is up to 1 in 30,000. The risk of HTLV is up to 1 in 250,000. The risk of HIV is over 1 in a million.

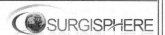

A 32 year old patient is found to have von Willebrand disease as part of a coagulation workup after experiencing excess bleeding following removal of his appendix. Which of the following best describes the source of vWF?

A.   Endothelium
B.   Fibroblasts
C.   Macrophages
D.   Platelets
E.   White blood cells

The best answer is <u>Endothelium</u>. vWF is released by the endothelium. vWF serves as a carrier for factor 8 and assists in the binding of glycoprotein Ib on inactivated platelets and GP IIb/IIa on activated platelets. There are three times of deficits: type 1 is the most common and is the mildest – treatment involves DDAVP only; type 2 is somewhat worse, and type 3 is the most severe as it is a homozygous defect – type II and type III are treated with cryoprecipitate and factor IIX. Diagnosis is made by increased bleeding time and PTT; PT is normal. Of note, DDAVP is also used as an adjunct to reversing a coagulopathy in patients with ESRD and CRF.

A 22 year old female who receives coumadin due to atrial fibrillation develops peripheral skin necrosis. Which of the following factor deficits can this be attributed to?

A.   Factor II
B.   Factor IX
C.   Factor X
D.   Protein C
E.   Protein S

The best answer is <u>Protein C</u>. This patient has a deficiency in protein C, leading to warfarin-induced skin necrosis. A heparin to coumadin bridge is essential in preventing the onset of this hypercoagulable state. Protein C deficiency can occur in up to 5% of the population. Factor V Leiden deficiency is a related defect that prevents protein C from binding to factor V, leading to hypercoagulability. In the formation and breakdown of clots, there are several important mediators. One of them is urokinase, which is responsible for the breakdown of fibrin through activation of plasminogen. In the event of an overdose of this clot-breaking medication, amino-caproic acid and cryoprecipitate can be given. Heparin can lead to thrombocytopenia, which presents as white clots and is due to antibodies against the heparin. Platelet aggregation is the end result, leading to vascular thrombosis. Reversal of heparin with protamine may lead to hypotension.

Which of the following is one of the changes that occurs to packed red blood cells after prolonged storage?

A. Breakdown of 2,3 DPG
B. Decrease in osmotic fragility
C. Decrease in potassium
D. Increase in calcium
E. More basic pH

The best answer is <u>Breakdown of 2,3 DPG</u>. Stored blood tends to have very little 2,3 DPG, an increase in osmotic fragility, a decrease in calcium due to binding with citrate, an increase in potassium, and a more acidic pH. On a different note, platelet aggregation and vasoconstriction can be induced by thromboxane A2; production of TxA2 is inhibited via downregulation of prostaglandin conversion by aspirin. Other mediators that can cause platelet aggregation include serotonin and ADP. Release of platelet granules can occur via platelet factor 4. The administration of mismatched blood during an operation will present as bleeding.

A patient receiving coumadin has monitoring of his INR until it becomes therapeutic. Which of the following factors is NOT affected by coumadin?

A. Factor II
B. Factor IX
C. Factor V
D. Factor VII
E. Factor X

The best answer is <u>Factor IX</u>. Warfarin leads to a prolongation in PT / INR, which affects factors II, V, VII, and X. Fibrinogen is also affected. Liver disease also leads to similar effects. Warfarin administration can be reversed with the administration of vitamin K, which leads to gamma-carboxylation and increased concentrations of factors produced by the liver. Warfarin may be more active with the concomitant administration of alcohol, metronidazole, amiodarone, and cimetidine. Warfarin may be inhibited with rifampin, phenytoin, and barbiturates.

A 36 year old female suffers significant blood loss during a lysis of adhesions when the surgeon inadvertently transects a major vessel. Once the patient is stabilized, which of the following changes is the body making to compensate for isovolemic anemia?

A. Decrease in cardiac output
B. Increase in 2,3 DPG
C. Increase in blood viscosity
D. Increase in dissolved oxygen
E. Increase in peripheral resistance

The best answer is <u>Increase in 2,3 DPG</u>. The body will seek to increase 2,3 DPG to promote greater unloading of oxygen along the oxygen-hemoglobin dissociation curve. Other effects will be a decrease in pH, increase in temperature, an increase in cardiac output to improve peripheral oxygen delivery, decreased blood viscosity to decrease resistance to flow, and decrease peripheral resistance to improve flow.

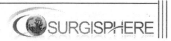

HIGH-YIELD TOPICS

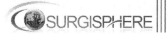

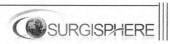

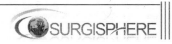

INDEX

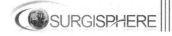

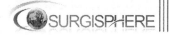

C

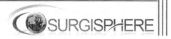

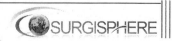

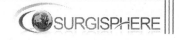

I

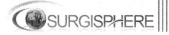

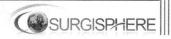

P

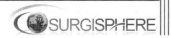

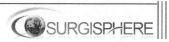

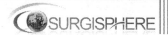

W

X

Z

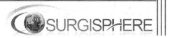

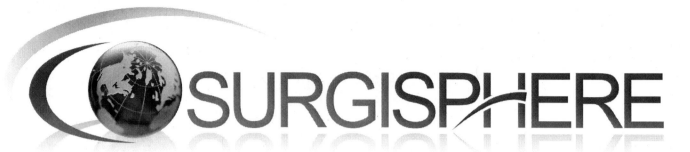

Visit us on the web at www.ClinicalReview.com

Welcome!

CONGRATULATIONS ON YOUR PURCHASE! With your membership, you have a unique opportunity to access the most comprehensive and high-yield resource for surgery. This multidisciplinary review course follows the content outline developed by the American Board of Surgery and covers concepts essential to the modern practice of surgery.

Your purchase may include a textbook, the Online Review Course, or the Comprehensive Review Course. By purchasing the Comprehensive Review Course, you have taken a major step to increasing your fund of knowledge and improving your practice of surgery.

If you purchased either the textbook or online review course, use the coupon code below to upgrade your purchase to the Comprehensive Review Course. By purchasing the component you are missing, your online account will automatically be upgraded so you can enjoy all of the benefits of the Comprehensive Review Course.

CONTENTS

COUPON CODE: ClinicalReview

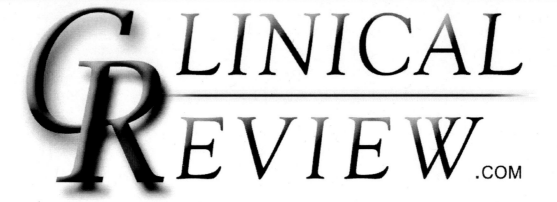

Visit us on the web at **www.ClinicalReview.com**

Comprehensive Review Course

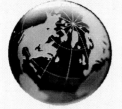

The Comprehensive Review Course is our multidisciplinary high-yield review for surgery that now includes a weekly reading course. It rigorously follows the content outline produced by the American Board of Surgery and is the ideal review for the ABSITE and surgery written examinations. This review course consists of high-yield textbooks, thousands of practice questions with detailed explanations, comprehensive PowerPoint presentations, audio and video lectures, a system to keep track of your progress and performance, and weekly quizzes and reading assignments that reference major surgery textbooks and the literature.

All of our textbooks are included online and a published copy of the Clinical Review of Surgery, ABSITE Edition is mailed to you. Also available on Amazon, this detailed textbook has hundreds of tables, images, equations, and high-yield notes to highlight essential concepts in surgery.

Diagram: Comprehensive Review Course (center), surrounded by: Published Textbooks, Interactive Practice Questions, PowerPoint Slide Presentations, Audio/Video Lectures, Real-time Feedback.

The online course uses the latest technologies to bring you over a thousand practice questions with detailed explanations. Practice questions are separated according to their relevance to the junior and senior ABSITE examinations and by body system. Several practice examinations are also available. You can go through these practice questions as many times as you desire.

PowerPoint presentations cover high-yield concepts in surgery. A lecture series breaks down difficult topics into easy-to-remember parts. Special emphasis is placed on topics essential to the modern practice of surgery. This lecture series can be downloaded to your iPod or other portable music player.

According to a recent study, residents who complete our Comprehensive Review Course have scored up to 20% higher on the ABSITE. Our multidisciplinary approach leads to increased exposure to essential concepts in surgery, ample opportunity for practice with over a thousand questions, and retention through reinforcement with multiple textbooks, slide presentations, and didactic lectures. This is test preparation for the 21st century.

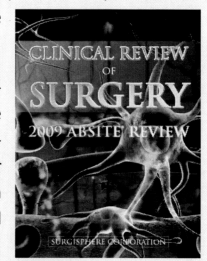

Online Review Course

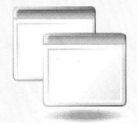

The Online Review Course is the only surgery review program to offer over a thousand carefully vetted questions and detailed explanations in a format that faithfully follows the content outline developed by the American Board of Surgery. All of the questions come with detailed explanations.

Choose questions by subject area. Questions and their choices are randomized, so no two exams are alike. Our sophisticated exam interface gives you instant feedback, permits you to keep track of your performance, and compare it to that of your peers. Several practice examinations are also available to help you gauge your readiness for the ABSITE.

The Online Review Program comes with a PowerPoint slide review that goes through all of the high-yield concepts that are essential for the modern practice of surgery. A comprehensive lecture course also comes with the online program. View streaming video covering all of the high-yield topics and take it with you on your iPod. There is no other review course like this in the world.

Review a research article that describes how our students score up to 20% higher on the ABSITE at Preview.ClinicalReview.com.

Original Article

Improvement in ABSITE Performance Using a Multidisciplinary Surgery Education Program

Mark Kent
Surgisphere Corporation, 3604 Witherspoon Blvd, Suite 111, Durham, NC 27707
Correspondence to Mark Kent, Support@ClinicalReview.com

Background	Over 50,000 surgery residents complete the American Board of Surgery In-Training Examination yearly. Numerous review materials exist to assist residents with test preparation, but no decisive studies have proven the efficacy of any particular method.
Methods	250 surgery residents from programs across the United States were randomly selected from the pool of first-time subscribers to the multidisciplinary Comprehensive Review Course produced by the Surgisphere Corporation. 160 residents completed the entire review course, submitted both their 2007 and 2008 ABSITE scores, and completed a brief survey.
Results	Average scores on the 2007 ABSITE for the entire pool of residents was 56 ± 1.4 (mean $\pm$ SEM). Residents that completed the entire review course scored an average of 18 points higher, with a mean of 74 ± 1. 25 PGY 1 residents had a mean score of 74 ± 3, 43 PGY 2 residents had a mean score of 79 ± 2 with a 24 point improvement compared to their 2007 score ($p<0.001$), 42 PGY 3 residents had a mean score of 75 ± 3 with a 17 point increase ($p<0.001$), 28 PGY 4 residents had a mean score of 70 ± 3 with a 13 point increase ($p<0.01$), and 22 PGY 5 residents had a mean score of 71 ± 2 with an 11 point increase ($p<0.001$).
Conclusion	Residents that completed the entire multidisciplinary Comprehensive Review Course produced by the Surgisphere Corporation scored up to 32% higher on the 2008 ABSITE compared to their 2007 ABSITE performance.

Introduction

The American Board of Surgery In-Training Examination (ABSITE) is taken yearly by surgery residents in the United States. The purpose of this examination is to measure resident progress and serve as an evaluation tool to objectively quantify resident familiarity with essential concepts in surgery.[1]

Numerous studies have examined the role of various educational resources on improving resident performance on the ABSITE.[2][3][4][5][6] One successful approach has been to use a problem based learning module to stimulate resident education in surgery.[2] Weekly reading assignments and didactic sessions have also had a positive outcome in resident education.[4][6]

The role of web-based competency assessments has also been proven to play a beneficial role in ABSITE preparation.[5] Until now, no single educational resource combines a weekly reading program with problem-based learning, a didactic series, and real-time competency assessments easily accessible to surgery residents.[7]

The Comprehensive Review Course for the American Board of Surgery In-Training Examination is a multidisciplinary review program consisting of published textbooks, interactive practice questions with explanations, slide presentations, audio/video lectures, and real-time feedback.[7] This is the only available review course that tracks resident progress and performance and provides this feedback automatically to program directors.[7]

Textbooks

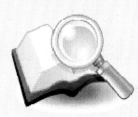

Multiple textbooks are available to help you review for your next surgery examination. Our textbooks cover essential topics you are required to master by the American Board of Surgery. We faithfully follow the content outline created by the ABS to ensure that we are doing everything we can to help you prepare.

The <u>Clinical Review of Surgery</u>, ABSITE Edition is our flagship review textbook for the American Board of Surgery examinations. This is a vital resource for any surgery resident, covering important topics in surgery that you are required to master. This comprehensive review guide includes extensive tables, high-yield facts, photographs, drawings, and a highly organized structure to maximize your learning. This textbook is available on Amazon.com, and is part of the bestselling Comprehensive Review Course.

Other textbooks are also available, including a Pocket Edition that fits in your white coat pocket and can use as a reference guide during busy rotations, a High-Yield edition that serves as a rapid review just before the examination, a Q&A book that includes hundreds of practice questions with detailed explanations, a flash card book that quizzes you on important topics, and a PowerPoint review book that includes all of our online slides.

Frequently Asked Questions

Contact us anytime for help! A more detailed list of commonly asked questions can be found at Support.ClinicalReview.com.

Important Links

- **Customer Support** Support.ClinicalReview.com
- **Product Preview** Preview.ClinicalReview.com
- **Review Course** ABSITE.ClinicalReview.com
- **Online Store** Store.ClinicalReview.com

Important Information

Comprehensive ABSITE Review Course

 *The most comprehensive review course for the American Board of Surgery In-Training Examination*

- 470 page HIGH-YIELD REVIEW TEXTBOOK that follows the content outline created by the American Board of Surgery for the ABSITE and surgery qualifying examination.
- Over 1,000 peer-reviewed QUESTIONS AND DETAILED EXPLANATIONS covering concepts covered on previous examinations.
- Special High-Yield Edition covers the most frequently tested topics and permits a rapid review prior to the examination.
- PowerPoint presentations can be used in resident conferences to permit group reviews.
- Didactic lecture series that you can take with you on your iPod.
- **Weekly surgery reading course that follows Cameron's and Sabiston's**

This review course has been VALIDATED BY PROGRAM DIRECTORS and PEER-REVIEWED. Residents who used our product last year rated it as the #1 REVIEW SOURCE FOR THE ABSITE. Residency programs around the country sign up their residents to use our review course. **We are the definitive review resource for surgery.**

In a survey we completed in 2006, residents that used our review course reported a 10-20% improvement in their ABSITE scores. They found it to be a key resource in continuing surgical education and organizing their study efforts. Join our new weekly reading course today!

FIVE STAR RATING BY OVER A THOUSAND RESIDENTS

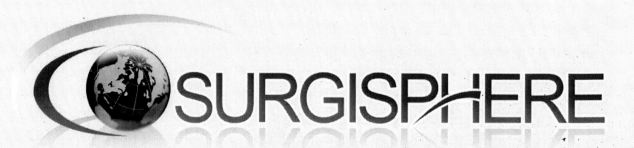

The Surgisphere Corporation pushes the boundaries of innovation and creativity to improve the quality of healthcare. As a market leader in medical education, consulting, and professional services, we strive to deliver more effective solutions using the latest technology.